A Cop Doc's Guide to Public-Safety Complex Trauma Syndrome: Using Five Police Personality Styles

Daniel Rudofossi, Psy.D., Ph.D.
New York University

Death, Value, and Meaning Series
Series Editor: Dale Lund

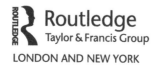

Routledge
Taylor & Francis Group

LONDON AND NEW YORK

First published 2009 by Baywood Publishing Company, Inc.

2 Park Square, Milton Park, Abingdon, Oxon OX14 4RN
711 Third Avenue, New York, NY 10017, USA

Routledge is an imprint of the Taylor & Francis Group, an informa business

First issued in paperback 2017

Library of Congress Catalog Number: 2009002105
ISBN 13: 978-0-89503-348-2 (hbk)

Library of Congress Cataloging-in-Publication Data

Rudofossi, Daniel, 1961-
   A cop doc's guide to public-safety complex trauma syndrome : using five police personality styles / Daniel Rudofossi.
      p. ; cm. -- (Death, value, and meaning series)
   Includes bibliographical references and index.
   ISBN 978-0-89503-348-2 (cloth : alk. paper)   1. Police--Mental health. 2. Police--Job stress. 3. Post-traumatic stress disorder. I. Title. II. Series: Death, value, and meaning series.
   [DNLM: 1. Stress Disorders, Post-Traumatic. 2. Grief. 3. Personality Assessment. 4. Police. WM 170 R917c 2009]

   RC451.4.P54R83 2009
   616.89002'43632--dc22

                                                                    2009002105

ISBN 978-0-89503-348-2 (hbk)
ISBN 978-0-415-77207-5 (pbk)

Table of Contents

PART III
Eco-Ethological Existential Analytic Therapy on the Front Line

Foreword

Dr. Daniel Rudofossi's *A Cop Doc's Guide to Public-Safety Complex Trauma Syndrome: Using Five Police Personality Styles* is an original sequel to his seminal and groundbreaking work *Working with Traumatized Police Officer-Patients: A Clinician's Guide to Complex PTSD*. With Dr. Rudofossi's expansive framework and fresh, relevant, and diverse case examples, clinicians have a new roadmap of treatment as his theory and novel interventions effect and alter the impact of complex trauma and losses in a collaborative journey. His theory and treatment of trauma and losses are anchored in his eco-ethological existential analyses, which effectively illustrate "when, why and how to intervene with real clinical illustrations leading to conceptually fleshed out public-safety personality styles." Daniel Rudofossi developed these techniques as the first uniformed psychologist of the New York Police Department (NYPD). He did research involving 2% of NYPD's 40,000 officers and folds those findings into his knowledge gained from his therapy experiences with hundreds of police and other emergency responders.

    A Cop Doc's Guide to Public-Safety Complex Trauma Syndrome: Using Five Police Personality Styles is a unique and holistic approach about and treatment of police and public-safety personnel. The genesis of this work may lie in the urban intensity of the NYPD, yet it is relevant to emergency responders and public-safety personnel anywhere. With his original theory of Complex PTSD in public-safety populations, he offers evidence and clinically significant case examples to illustrate the coordinates that shape the five public-safety profiles. He takes the why of Complex PTSD and how it impacts and develops in the context of personality differences hidden in complex losses. This guide will help bridge further work with other populations that have experienced Complex PTSD. A new theoretical and practical approach to the treatment of Complex PTSD in the context of five police personality styles is delivered. While the focus is on complex posttraumatic stress disorder, application of the protocols can be generalized to understanding, treating, and intervening in less severe conditions before they become more malignant. Along with his first book, the sequel should be a required text for mental health professionals seeking competency to work with this police and public-safety population.

For me, another important aspect of Dan Rudofossi's writing is that he unravels the Gordian knot of how police and public-safety officers come to be. He became a police officer before he became a psychologist. As he says, "he became a participant before he became a participant observer." As such, he was able to experience the paradoxical morphology involved in transforming from civilian to cop. As a rigorous professional psychologist, Dr. Rudofossi is able to describe the forces that shaped and molded him. He does this in both psychological and pragmatic terms. I cannot overstate the importance of this accomplishment.

I believe that all of public-safety is an underserved population in terms of available and acceptably competent psychological services. This is due, in large measure, to the misapprehensions public-safety personnel have about psychologists. In larger measure, psychologists contribute to this dilemma through ignorance about and ambivalence toward treating this population. Another complication is that the majority of psychologists and the majority of public-safety personnel are characterologically different.

Dr. Michael Roberts, a renowned police psychologist, is the civilian director of police psychological services for the San Jose California Police Department and has conducted psychological testing of emergency responders for over 30 years. I asked him to address the issue of differences between police officers and psychologists in reference to my review of Dr. Rudofossi's book.

> When I think about the various reasons it is difficult for the typical psychologist to work effectively with police officers I usually start with how and why these two occupational groups differ. Perhaps the most important difference between psychologists and police officers, and the reason that the two don't usually mix well, is that they have a much different view of the world and the people in it. The California Psychological Inventory (CPI) includes two scales that describe an individual's basic approach to the world and the people in it. When these two scales are combined they produce four different "Types" or ways of approaching the world. The gulf between most psychologists and most police officers is apparent in that over 75% of police can be described as Alpha or Beta Type, that is, rule enforcing and abiding. [Note, the eco-ethological conceptualization of Dr. Dan Rudofossi's presentation of the five public-safety personality styles.] Sixty percent of officers are Alphas who are outgoing, dominant and rule enforcing, and an additional 20% are also rule enforcing and abiding, but they are described by others as much more self-contained or rigid and "by the book." By contrast, 75% of psychology graduate students are either Gammas or Deltas, sharing a disposition to challenge the norm, be somewhat rebellious, and rule-resistant. (Dr. Mike Roberts, Director of San Jose Police Psychological Services, 6/18/03)

This understanding is conceptualized and presented in terms of Dr. Rudofossi's eco-ethological theory of Complex PTSD. This gives a frame of reference for use by clinicians and researchers. Although his emphasis is on assessment and treatment, the far-reaching implication is key to public-safety psychology and expands and complements our findings for treatment of Complex PTSD in police personality styles. To the extent that these differences exist, there is a danger that each group will construct and hold derogatory stereotypes of the other. When they do, there exists an inverse ratio of compatibility, not to mention interference with the establishment of a therapeutic alliance. Police officers and, to a varying degree, all public-safety personnel lose the most in this circumstance. They are the ones who need the support and professional insights to deal with the trauma, loss, and isolation that, too often, come with their occupation. They need education and coaching to make sense of the conflicting demands placed upon them. *A Cop Doc's Guide to Public-Safety Complex Trauma Syndrome: Using Five Police Personality Styles* encourages and educates mental health professionals to work with emergency responders, even in the worst of circumstances. It seeks to illuminate a complex culture and simplify it through knowledge. In the process, resistances and misapprehensions will diminish on both sides. Differences, even characterological ones, will be reduced to the level that they "do no harm." You are commended for embarking upon this intellectual and spiritual quest.

Dr. Rudofossi illustrates that public-safety personnel must embrace what are generally considered maladaptive coping techniques to be effective emergency responders. An example I use is the utilization of dissociation in the service of functioning during crisis. Another would be the constant suppression/denial of normal emotions in order to retain control and objectivity. Inevitably, these techniques generalize to all aspects of the emergency responders' life and, over time, accumulate and can become emotionally toxic: our strengths become the other side of our weaknesses. I was a San Francisco Police Officer for 35 years, mostly in all aspects of uniformed patrol. I entered police psychology in the late '70s. An ongoing challenge has been to attempt to explain law enforcement to clinicians and psychology to cops, particularly the effects on police officers' personality styles. I feel I never fully succeeded in this effort. Now, Dan Rudofossi has given us a comprehensive description, cause and effect, and the psychological interacting elements involved. We owe him a debt of gratitude for his thoroughness and his personal candor.

In *A Cop Doc's Guide to Public-Safety Complex Trauma Syndrome: Using Five Police Personality Styles,* Dr. Rudofossi points out the forces, both pervasive and subtle, that are at work. He describes his own metamorphosis. He starts by pointing out the ecological factors in play during the police academy and the various cultural imperatives along the road to efficacy and acceptance. Throughout the book there are brilliant examples of officers' survival adaptations gone awry. The reader will come to appreciate the humanity of the emergency responders and how they came to their debilitating conditions. With this appreciation comes an understanding of how and why Dan Rudofossi's eco-ethological existential analysis of the five police personality styles works.

The glue that cements *A Cop Doc's Guide to Public-Safety Complex Trauma Syndrome: Using Five Police Personality Styles* together is the love that Dr. Rudofossi has for his work. Time and again you will be struck by his integrity, his depth of understanding, and his deep caring for the emergency responders who are both his patients and his colleagues. This book will spark a great deal of wholesome debate. This, in turn, will cause further modifications, extensions, and theory building in the treatment of what can now be recognized as Complex PTSD in the police and public-safety population. I intend to make it required reading for my graduate students. Dr. Rudofossi is retired from active police work. He teaches at New York University as an Adjunct Professor, he writes, consults, and continues to see emergency responders in his private practice as a licensed psychologist in New York. He is an active consultant for the Saybrook Graduate School's Police and Public Safety Psychology Program. He is certified in Rational Emotive Behavior Therapy (REBT) and Psychoanalytic Psychotherapy, and as a Clinician Diplomate, Existential Analyst/Logo therapist. Many sought him out to work through the horror of the terrorist attack and collapse of the twin towers. We seek him out for consultations on the West Coast. We will hear a lot more from him in the years to come. Psychology in general, police and public-safety psychology in particular, will greatly benefit from his continued professional contributions. Finally, as a Cop Doc with over 2 decades of experience and thousands of officer–patients in tow, I have witnessed my personal friend and colleague work as a Cop Doc: Dr. Daniel Rudofossi's novel theory and treatment approach, "eco-ethological existential analysis," captures the reality of hidden losses and trauma, transforming them into healing intervention that works with real police officers. This is the only book of it's kind. Get it, read it, and start using it!

Allan W. Benner, PhD

Preface

Dan Rudofossi occupies a rare vantage point. Once a police officer, he now is a therapist. Dr. Rudofossi thus is uniquely suited to address the grief and trauma that shadows the careers of public-safety officers. In his first book, *Working with Traumatized Police Officer-Patients: A Clinician's Guide to Complex PTSD Syndromes in Public Safety Professionals,* Rudofossi sensitized clinicians to the unique elements of police culture that both can facilitate and complicate a police officer's response to critical traumatic incidences, grief, and PTSD. This work, *A Cop Doc's Guide to Public-Safety Complex Trauma Syndrome: Using Five Police Personality Styles,* follows on that earlier success. Here Rudofossi offers sage counsel on ways to approach different types of police officers as they struggle with loss and trauma.

Three themes dominate in this exceptional work. The first is individuality. While the concept of personality types is a model one may or may not resonate with, it ultimately emphasizes the very different ways that persons, in this case police officers, respond to traumatic incidents. The work emphasizes, therefore, that therapeutic interventions have to be tailored to individual clients. No one size fits all—a critical insight in a field where models of debriefing fight for the right to be the new orthodoxy. Rudofossi's work stresses that interventions need to take into account the very personal characteristics and needs of the officers involved. Even partners may benefit from diverse interventive strategies.

A second theme accentuates the need for validation. In the closed culture of police, it is critical for officers to have their sense of loss, as well as their trauma, acknowledged. Failing to do so disenfranchises their grief, further isolating them from the civilian society they are sworn to protect.

A final theme is resilience. While police officers may witness the worst that society has to offer and face traumatic incidences that most of the public is spared, Rudofossi reminds us and reaffirms that police officers are resilient. Most return to work even after the most horrendous experiences. This notion of post-traumatic growth is a significant theme in contemporary studies of grief. It reminds us of the strengths that all of us draw upon. Even in grief and loss, trauma and violence, humans still retain the power of growth. This central fact offers a bond, putting on a badge and a blue uniform makes one no different.

After a particularly difficult, even scary caving trip, my young godson once remarked that this was one of the events that his dad said made one either grow up or grow down. Grief and trauma are such events. They either diminish us or force us to grow—to gain new insights or skills, more confidence, and perhaps even a deeper spirituality. Rudofossi offers a road map—a way, even in loss, to assist police to grow up rather than down.

Kenneth J. Doka, PhD

Acknowledgments

First, and in profound appreciation for my ability to have survived and grown in my faith in the highest being—the highest spiritual force, God! I often reflect, as many greater folk than I have said, "There go I but for the grace of God." It has been my good fortune to have so many blessings that follow:

My wife CSRR, Sarah Rudofossi of whom we have shared the best of my heart and soul in our marriage and whom I love dearly. In our love we experience the power of love, forgiveness and commitment to transcend even the darkest corners and seek the light by the grace of G-d. There is nothing in this world like the power of love it is Divine Inspiration: In the face of love G-d's Intuition emerges as the magnet that draws two to become as one: When it is real nothing—can draw either apart . . .

with gratitude and appreciation,

Daniel

Thank you Dr. Dale Lund for seeing in my book a valuable addition to the literature on trauma and loss—that is a privilege and honor. I thank the excellent staff at Baywood Publishing Company, especially Bobbi Olszewski, Astrid Loveless, Julie Krempa, Lorna Roher, and Anthony Green, the copy editor, for their high level of commitment, professionalism, and amiable approach to a complex process with equanimity.

My close friend and mentor of the highest caliber, Cop Dr. Al Benner, inspired me by his apolitical honesty, integrity, and fellowship during rough times. *Indisputably, Doc Benner is the Cop Doc's Cop Doc.* His service is legendary. His courage is indefatigable! A true pioneer who blazed unexplored paths in police psychology by his incredible ingenuity, humility, fraternity, and profes-sionalism. Dr. Professor R. R. Ellis—a superb clinical psychologist who did his best by his humanity—being the exemplary educator, clinical supervisor, and gentleman he is. A decade-and-a-half of our lives have evolved together into a personal friendship and collegiate relationship. Dr. Ellis gave countless hours in editing with a wonderful openness, sense of humor, and love; his sagacious and acute critiques are magnificent. What he planted in his students is harvested in the here and now. Dr. Stuart Young, physician, novelist, co-author, exra-ordinary scholar, colleague, and friend for life—a true breakfast club pal. Dr. Al Ellis, your inimitable style and clinical supervision of how to put your therapy into practice remains invaluable. Dr. K. Doyle, colleague and friend of extraordinary integrity, who gave of her energy, support of my ideas, and editorial suggestions and my 3-year journey at the Institute for Rational Emotive Behavior Therapy. Dr. N. Pelusi, an excellent leader in REBT/CBT and for a good dose of humor, PRN. Dr. R. Balter, PhD, JD, a rare friend, as judicious as she is keen in her wisdom as an attorney and psychologist. Dr. Terry Jordan, whose research brilliance helped me in my passage from doctoral candidate, through my disser-tation, to my own as a researcher and clinician in counseling psychology; and a decade-and-a-half as a colleague working in tandem through different clinical and research populations—our ongoing friendship for many years is a rich treasure I cherish. Thank you Dr. Bill Schiff for your brilliant teaching as an ecological physicist and support toward my own ecological–ethological approach in understanding complex trauma with police at NYU in 1993-1994. Dr. Bill Worden's superb advice and poignant insights into trauma and grief are also appreciated.

I have been enlightened by the genius and erudite supervision of Dr. Charles Brenner, the father of the science of conflict as a Psychodynamic Psychotherapist. It is not only his cognitive genius, but his emotional as well that surfeits over his fecund mind: if one grabs Diogenes' torch in darkness, in search of an honest man with humanity and humility, he will find him in Dr. Brenner. I am grateful for the privilege afforded by his generous sharing of perspective, extending way beyond "the hours" of clinical supervision—my eco-ethological approach toward PPS-CPTSD has benefited from his prolific perspicuity. I have been greatly enriched by Dr. Bob Scharf's and Dr. R. Weiss' inimitable psychoanalytic ability, skill, ingenuity, and humanity, with cherished gratitude to the New York Psychoanalytic Institute and Society.

Thank you Dr. Bob Barnes, president of the Viktor Frankl Institute and Hardings Simmons University for your incredible courage, fraternity, wisdom, kindness, and finest of humane excellence and education. Without doubt the achievement of the Diplomate Clinician as an Existential Analyst was sown in the long hours of supervision through the generosity and clinical skill of Dr. Ann Graber. Professor Jo Anne Thorp, most astute of forensic observers—a great friend with genuine brilliance and generosity from which I have learned firsthand.

Dear friends, thank you for your support and intellectual stimulation: S. Southwick, MD; R. Montgomery, DDS, MPH; S. Luke, MA; Professor Jo Ann Thorpe; Catrine Giery, MA; Det. M. Hennessy; Mary Henessy, MSW; J. Kreiger, MA; Bert Breiner, PhD; Michael Perlin, JD; N. Pelusi, PhD; B. Schayes, MD;

S. Young, MD; M. O'Keefe, PhD; M. Bellsheren; P. Stevens, PhD; H. Schwartz; L. Ellis, PhD; E. Albert, MPH, JD; D. Valentine, MD; K. Doka, PhD; M. Yusaf, PhD; R. Balter, JD, PhD; W. Schiff, PhD; E. Nalplant, PhD; R. Hirsch, EdD; R. Katz, PhD; D. Cohen, PhD, B. Hutzell, PhD; V. Hutzell, PhD; O. Cruz, MA; D. Panitz, MA; Luigi Valenti! The best photographer I know, Det. Sal Vitale, thanks. Being a Cop Doc was strongly supported by the vision of the *finest of the finest bosses on the job and off:* Retired Chief Mansfield, MA and Inspector V. Werbkay, MA, selfless leaders who gave much of their time, support, and commitment to ensuring I could deliver to police members the best of care. Thanks to Mr. Genet, MBA, and of course, the SBA President Sgt. Ed Mullin, PBA, Pat Lynch, LBA and CBA, and of course, *thanks to each peer-support officer to a person who always exemplified what I considered as outstanding in commitment and skills: the heart and soul of the NYPD.*

Det. Jimmie Giery, a cops cop, fourth-generation crime-scene investigator, the best of the best, a true buddy! Lt. J. LaTorre, another true buddy, who covered my back and sprung for Macanudo cigars on the PA Deck and cappucino to boot! Sgt. Louis Vilenti, MA, dapper, true blue pal. To my other crime-stopping street colleagues: the midnight crew, PSA 1, 3, 3A, and 4; my partner, Captains D. Sosnowik, MA, and J. Dillon; G. Suarez, JD; V. Sheehan; B. Sans Castett. Lts J. LaTorre, BA; B. Chlan; P. Kelly, MA, JD; S. Jones, A, Sgts B. McNally; A. Medina; M. Miselewisch; Jerry Wong; and, of course, Louis Vilenti, MA, Det's M. Hennessy; R. Otting, MA; S. Mohammed; J. and K. Geary; E. F. Matis; and Phil Gibutosi—you all remain the finest! I salute you all: now and always! To a truly great film producer, visionary, and friend Emanuel Defeliciantonio, cheers!

Inside the beat of the NYPD Cop Docs, I have the following salutation to offer: Chief Surgeons Thomas and Dr. M. Symond, who served as my personal supervisors in the NYPD (both deceased and served till their deaths), I salute you! To the Brave Agents of the DEA and Dr. Mike Pons, DEA-EAP; Dr. E. Sharpe, DEA-EAP; Dr. Hector Torres, DER-EAP; and Dr. M. Neuhaus; FBI Special Agent J. Reese; Dr. H. Schlossberg, Det. NYPD (a psychologist with a gun); Det. Dr. G. Mack, NYPD; and fellow Sgt. Dr. Henry: An honor to be in your company! My gratitude for PC, NYPD Dr. R. Kelly, JD, LLM, who appointed me as the first uniform psychologist with Chief Mansfield and Inspector Werbkay, the ingenuity and courage of Commissioner John Walsh, HRA PD, appointing me the honor of being the police surgeon on call.

I thank my family: Mom, an inspiration to me in her abundance of lifelong love—through thick and thin—whose compassion lightened my darkest moments of trauma. In beloved memory of two of the most courageous men: my father, Harry, a combat veteran with four ribbons in WWII, USN; my grandfather, Morris, an infantryman in WWI, U.S. Army. To WWII decorated Veteran Pop,

Mr. I. Friedman, I salute your courage, humanity, and friendship! To my son, Jonathan, USMC, my hero, who keeps me laughing with his humor and love. Their war stories will never be forgotten nor will their courage. My grandmothers, who loved wholeheartedly. To my sisters, who are lifelong friends: Vicky and Mara. Spiritually—Rabbis Kalman Packouz, M. Rubenstein; and J. Kolokowski: thank you for your timeless noetic wisdom and for combating the complacency in anti-Semitism/racism hidden and disenfranchised. In partnership with the finest officer–patients, I owe my education and wisdom still learning from you all. Each journery hopefully enlightened your path as it did mine! To Cop Doc peers, paving new roads without forgetting our own beaten paths! To my students at NYU, the brightest and finest—the best with love!

Engaging Public Safety Officers Suffering from Police Complex PTSD Syndromes: An Ecological-Ethological Existential Analysis of the Five Police Personality Styles

An esteemed colleague and expert on Terrorism and the Psychology of Combat and Killing Lt. Colonel Grossman (Retired U.S. Army) *New York Times* best-selling author, Professor West Point, and public speaker who educates FBI, DEA, Intelligence Officers, national and international; Executive Branch level Legislators, and countless public safety audiences and their families affirms his evaluation of my work in his own words,

> Wow. This is "Deep Wisdom" making a powerful and valuable contribution. Useful and applicable to therapists who care for law enforcement, fire fighters, **and (I would submit, based on my own personal experience) the military.** Dr. Rudofossi's "five public safety personality types" is of great value not just to the therapist, **it would also be useful to any supervisor (law enforcement, firefighter or military) who wants to gain a deep understanding of the lives and careers that have been entrusted to his care.**

> And Dr. Rudofossi's "Epilogue: Toward an Antidote to Terrorism" is worthy to stand alone as a booklet that would help us to grasp the nature of our battle against those who would wield terror as a weapon. He shows us that terrorism ranks with despotism and tyranny as "psychopathological" behavior, with "victimization results [that] are perniciously psycho-physiological." This is a powerful insight that he uses to illuminate a path toward defeating terrorism while still protecting our own national and individual psyches.

> As he so well states, we must "not glorify or romanticize what is on one hand human illness and on the other human depravity and evil. . . . In order to flesh out the antidote for dealing with terrorism, we must understand the poison that has been ingested. . . . Arguably even the perpetrators are victims of their own human illness and human depravity we have become afraid to characterize for what it genuinely is, 'evil'!" And "It is in healing [this evil, psychopathological behavior] that we heal as well."

"Dr. Dan" has served as both a cop and as a therapist. From this unique perspective he can well and truly state that: "To serve is a profile in courage! Therapists serve, too. The deeper the excavation the more resplendent the shine of darkness into the fulgent light of hope."

Well done, Dr. Dan. And many thanks for the bright light of hope that you shine forth, upon our brave men and women who go in harm's way, upon those who would wield terrorism against us, and upon ourselves.

And I take up the prayer with which Dr. Rudofossi chooses to conclude his book: "May G-d balance the scales we choose to embrace, justice and liberty to eternities grace!"

Lt. Col. Dave Grossman
U.S. Army (ret.) Author, *On Killing and On Combat*

With such a privileged introduction by a leader and esteemed colleague in the field of Counter-terrorism and the Psychology of Combat and Killing, I will now add in my own words why this book is as important as the first one I wrote in this series.

My book offers an insider perspective on what police and public safety officers experience on the job. It is designed to give the clinician-scientist an in-depth understanding of the complex and hidden trauma and loss experienced by public safety officers. This guide offers a viewpoint of public safety that uses the Scientific Practitioner Model. The content emerges from over a decade of intensive work with police officers.

As a participant observer, I was officially appointed as the first Uniform Psychologist, New York Police Department. *I am a licensed psychologist who has also been a street cop, a police sergeant, and commanding officer* of a police unit in one of the largest police departments in the world.

My street experience as a patrol officer included the city projects, subways and streets where I received line of duty injuries and commendations. During this time, I had been active as a police officer including patrolling "urban war zones" and effecting over 200 arrests without a complaint for abuse of authority or force. This experience and credibility has helped me numerous times in relating to officers and working through assessment, crisis, and therapy with hundreds of officers. I helped put the successful program of Member Assistance Program, known as PAPA today, on the MAP of peer support and ambulatory intervention in the world of policing and psychology. What I offer here is the result of more than a decade of ambulatory assessment, therapy, and research with the officers I was privileged to work with.

The problem with the few guides or books published on public safety stress is that they contend that the real stress is administrative. The problem itself lies in the types of questions and assumptions underlying most researcher bias in this field.

Administrative stress, common to every profession, has been **overemphasized** *rather than events associated with trauma and grief responses that police experience.* This misplaced emphasis on administrative stress is due, in part, to the understandable denial of officers (conscious and unconscious) to identify trauma and grief. This in turn, is also denied by many police administrators and the communities officers serve as well. What confounds research findings is the assumption that what is considered trauma and loss events for public safety officers is accurate; this is mainly based upon anecdotal interpretation.

This book is written in response to a need for an advanced specialized guide for clinicians to operationally define, understand and responsibly treat Complex Post Traumatic Stress and Grief Syndromes as it emerges in the unique varieties of police personality styles. This sequel book culls the depths where the first book on *Working with Traumatized Police Officer Patients: A Clinician's Guide to Complex PTSD Syndromes in Public Safety Professionals,* left off.

The term "police" is used synonymously with public safety and military professionals. Each chapter has a specific domain. Working with public safety personnel is at once stimulating, exciting and very serious in potential applications. Mapping out the spires of loss into a hub that coheres a perspective of complex trauma with individual differences in clear focus are proffered in this book: *Theory is wed to practice and practice to effective interventions with police-officer patients.*

This follow up book to my first book titled *Working with Traumatized Officer-Patients: A Clinician's Guide to Complex PTSD in Public Safety Professionals* holds the "psychological imagination" of a wide audience of professional clinicians of varied orientations. That varied audience includes police and public safety/military mental health practitioners, criminal justice practitioners, military practitioners, trained para-professional responders, peer-support officers, undergraduate and graduate students in criminal justice, criminology, psychology and psychiatry, counseling and social work. This is not another pop self-help book; it is not written after interviewing a few officers and coming up with a grand plan. It is not created from an ivory tower, nor is it a political or a journalist's book.

This is a passionate book with one agenda; that is, understanding and advocating professionally for better health and welfare for all public safety officers. To this end, my book offers a thorough assessment and intervention guide for the clinician and public safety professionals who would like to gain a deeper psychological understanding of the public service officer. There is no other book in the field of trauma that is based upon my original approach to do a comparative analysis with except my current book, *Working with Traumatized Officer-Patients: A Clinician's Guide to Complex PTSD Syndromes in Public Safety Professionals.*

Filling in the gaps between my current book and what is being proffered in my sequel is an expansion of my theory of Police and Public Safety Complex

Trauma (PPS-CPTSD). In this book the focus shifts the paradigm of PPS-CPTSD into the ground of a personological framework which helps differentiate "how" and "why" a clinician's approach is made highly effective by understanding the distinct personality style officer-patient's present with. My approach segues into difficult examples which bolster and highlight each officer-patient's eco-ethological field experience of loss in trauma with a focus on enhancing resilience and motivation to heal losses—otherwise left disenfranchised. It is complementary to my first book [aforementioned above]. The present expands the Ecological-Ethological Existential Analysis of Complex PTSD into the context of *personality styles* with an emphasis on resilience—without ignoring the pathological aspects of loss that often envelop officer-patient trauma syndromes.

This work provokes clinicians to use their *psychological imagination* with other populations as the reader is moved along the different spires that have remained disconnected: These disconnected spires are now encountered in the hub of loss that re-connect missing links that fill in a complex puzzle in-deed and with effect for clinician, researcher and criminal justice practitioners alike. My intervention extends into the areas of the returning veteran in which a significant number are also public safety officers. Regardless an Ecological-Ethological Existential Analysis may be applied to military branches in the field of operations. Military Clinicians as well as supervisors may assist soldiers (Commissioned or Non-Commissioned) who have experienced trauma and losses. This achievement is collaboratively accomplished with the clinician provoking inner resilience via an existential analysis which cannot be prescribed but re-experienced in the crossfire of the officer's life's traumas and losses one soldier at a time.

Delivering an expansion of my theory of Police and Public Safety Complex Trauma is achieved via my integration of other models of trauma and loss into an original both/and operationally defined intervention model. Practicing an existential-analysis as an effective clinical approach that deals with personality differences in public safety is sown from a field of loss and despair. The existential analyses are delivered through clinical case composite examples of personality differences selectively shaped by the impact of repetitive losses in multiple experiences of hidden trauma.

My book discusses why, where, how, and when the clinician can intervene effectively by understanding and discriminating one police personality style from the other. Understanding subtle differences in personality styles can make the difference in securing or losing the therapeutic alliance. Without this specialized knowledge the trained therapist may lose the alliance; the untrained counselor will almost certainly forfeit the alliance in a generalist approach.

What does exist is a series of fine books that capture trauma and grief in other populations (except public safety) in a way that validates the patient's experiences in depth, while gaining an understanding of the various aspects of the general culture as context. *My book goes far beyond that goal in validating trauma and loss in a developmental clinical context for the clinician desiring to work with individual differences that public safety officers bring to the table of trauma therapy.* The fact is, at the time of this book's publication an inaccurate singular uni-dimensional public safety officer exists subtly as a treatment prototype, as just another administratively stressed out professional. The hope is that this book will put that impoverished speculative myth to rest. This book has an applied approach that gives the reader a deep understanding of what it is like to deal with each officer as uniquely varying in his/her personality style of presentation within the context of their police experiences. Each profile is a composite of at least three patients from each cluster. In order to protect their identity, many distinguishing factors are changed. The clinical and meaningful material or words are not.

Excellent articles, monographs, guides and books exist for the diverse and varied community of mental health professionals who are actively involved in the treatment of patients who suffer from Post Traumatic Stress Disorder (PTSD), Grief, and the multitude of Mental and Behavioral Disorders. Yet, there is a dearth of material for the practitioner to identify and assess the specific problems that emerge in the context of what police and public safety/military officers encounter, and in light of the different personality differences officers present with. *Indeed, police and public safety/ [military commissioned and non-commissioned] officers are—one of the last hidden minorities who have endured significant extraordinary experiences in their daily lives as public safety personnel. This book answers that need by offering the psychotherapist, peer support and supervisor practical methods in treatment of public safety populations from a personality perspective.* The psycho-pharmacologist will find the assessment and intervention chapters useful in targeting symptoms through prescriptive medication in the context of personality traits. Nowadays that psycho-pharmacologist may include the licensed psychologist as well.

The complexity and diversity in styles of officers presented rests on a firm clinical and empirical foundation. I offer the clinician an original, operationally defined presentation of five differential police personality styles. Profiling is not new, nor is the effectiveness of defining, diagnosing and treating various personality styles. The wisdom of personology in highlighting the general styles of personality has informed clinical practice for decades. My work is expanding this application to police and public safety populations including the military. Moreover, my approach is not parochial. I offer the dynamic, cognitive, behavioral and existential therapists a different focus for intervention, integration, or a singular, more traditional approach to treatment. I also enjoin you to use my method in the context of your own clinical and personal skillfulness with this unique and worthy population.

It is in doing an Ecological-Ethological Existential Analysis that the wounded soldier officer patient who is always there for us, may in their hour of need be gently and assertively guided to "internally witness" their own hidden and inner strength with you. *May that in-deed inspire you to always find hope in tragic optimism that frames our paths as healers who remain healed!* As a sage much wiser then I said, there is no such thing as despair! There is nothing that has been broken that can not be repaired with hope, courage and optimism!

PART I

Foundations:
Theory of Police and
Public-Safety Complex PTSD

CHAPTER 1

Police and Public-Safety Complex PTSD (PPS-CPTSD): Toward an Integration of the Five Hubs of Loss

Complex trauma and grief symptoms are as disturbing, unexpressed, and denied in multiple ways as are the diverse populations experiencing them. Three different researchers examining different public-safety and military personnel groups have come up with similar findings:

> It is frequently remarked by nonmilitary psychiatrists that the military service or a state of war produces no new types of psychiatric reactions. However, there occur in *military service certain florid schizophrenic like states with sudden onset and rapid recovery which are seldom seen under other circumstances except perhaps in penal institutions.* (Solomon & Yakovlev, 1945, p. 535)

The quote above is a field observation during World War II. The clinicians observed schizophrenic-like symptoms in combat-stress conditions. Moving on, 40 years later, Tanay suggests another broad facet of this syndrome.

> We eliminate the victims we are guilty of creating on a symbolic level by denying the existence of the condition from which they suffer. The endless debates over whether there is shellshock, combat neurosis, or concentration camp survivor syndrome fulfill our manifestations of denial. (Emanuel Tanay, MD, Kelly, 1985, p. 38)

This description generalizes to what I observed time and again in public-service officers. In a publication specific to public safety, titled *The Dissonance of Trauma and Grief* is my reflection:

> Without the skills or support to reintegrate the *impact of events of trauma and loss many police officers endure, on a frequent and intense level, an almost schizophrenic disintegration of a sense of self likely* engendered through physiologic and psychic processes of oppositional conflict. (Rudofossi, 1997, p. 109)

9

Our first move toward identifying trauma as evidenced in public-safety and police officer-patients is our choice of an appropriate term. That term must underscore the complexity of trauma and loss. Fortunately, such a phrase as well as a concept exists and has support from a wide range of research and clinical experience: Complex Post Traumatic Stress Disorder (C-PTSD). In this chapter, the conceptual basis for understanding what I have termed, Police and Public-Safety Complex PTSD (PPSC-PTSD) is presented.

My conceptualization is achieved through clarifying four branches connected by loss, which are expressed in the presentation of PPSC-PTSD. My presentation of that hub is made comprehensible by connecting multiple losses as one of the major motive forces that drive traumatic-stress syndromes. The four branches are: complex trauma and dissociative identity disorders (Chu, 1998; Cohen, Berzoff, & Elin, 1995; Gottlieb, 1997; Herman, 1992; Marmer, 1980; Putnam, 1989; Terr, 1990); complicated and disenfranchised loss and grief (Bowlby, 1975; Doka, 1985, 1989, 2002; Doka & Martin, 2001; Ellis, 1992, 1994; Rudofossi & Ellis, 1999; Rando, 1984; Worden, 2001); the noogenic neurosis and the triad of existential despair and psyche ache (Barnes, 2007; Frankl, 1978, 1988, 2000; Graber, 2003; Schneidman, 1996; Southwick, 2007) and the stress and strain of attempts toward adaptation to losses within an ethological-ecological and neurological perspective (Giller, 1991; Gibson, 1966, 1986; Gibson & Gibson, 1955; Gould, 2002; Hartmann, H., 1958; Hartmann, E., 1984; Helson, 1964; Lorenz, 1971, 1972, 1973; Lorenz & Leyhausen, 1973; Morris, 1967, 1969a, 1969b, 1971, 1977; Morris & Morris, 1966; Myers, 1940; Pavlov, 1941; Rappaport, 1971; Rudofossi, 1994a, 1997, Rudofossi & Ellis, 1999; Schiff, 1979; Southwick, 2007; Tinbergen, 1948, 1969; Van Der Kolk, Greenberg, Boyd, & Krystal, 1985; Van Der Kolk & Saporta, 1991; Vaillant, 1977; Wolpe, 1952; Yehudi, Resnick, Kahana, & Giller, 1993). A complementary approach to loss binds all four branches into a dynamic view that capture's the patient's presentation. That complementary conceptual approach combines theory with its extension into treatment. It gives you an applied framework that furthers your effectiveness in working through the real loss you are likely to encounter with officer-patients. That insight provides explanatory power that ultimately will increase your effectiveness with officer-patients. The presentation of my eco-ethological approach to trauma projects from a structure that reflects a prism of insight from evidence as articulated in an earlier publication (Rudofossi, 1997, 2007).

We will go forward in this chapter with the strength of a comprehensive theoretical basis that offers an integration of police and public safety Complex PTSD, as my theory moves from the vantage point of a conceptual to an applied clinical method. That synergistic goal is achieved via a number of composite clinical examples that elucidate different areas of complex trauma and loss. My focus will bring us closer to a conceptualization that flows into an existential insight-oriented treatment approach. That orientation toward insight may offer an intervention model that addresses whatever "gestalt" is pressing in the officer-patient's presentation.

Gestalt used appropriately does not mean all encompassing, something my work hardly can accomplish. Rather, it means the problem the officer-patient freely associates about is attended to in "our work" session by session. That gestalt may help us develop an understanding of what the patient presents both on a conscious level and symbolically on an unconscious level from an ecologically relevant niche and within the drives that are ethologically motivated.

Your awareness of this understanding will likely help you develop your own sense of how to approach each officer-patient individually. The same applies to your development of cultural competence. Your insight may help you reach the difficult task of repeatedly unraveling the officer-patient's conflicts and maladaptive beliefs in a way that yields meaningful change. Unraveling is hard work, ripe with resistance on a conscious, unconscious, existential, ethological, and socially constructed level.

COMPLEX TRAUMA AND DISSOCIATIVE IDENTITY DISORDERS

Some clinicians present compelling evidence that specific groups of individuals are more at risk to develop Complex PTSD (Herman, 1992). To understand that vulnerability in its appropriate context is to realize it is not by personal defect. That vulnerability includes being subject to experiences we have defined as critical incidents. That is, these individuals form groups identified by shared experiences of trauma and loss. The groups may gain their cultural identity, defenses, and shared responses anthropologically, in addition to some endogenous vulnerability. I suggest to split "nature or nurture" in conversation is to speak ideologically, not logically, empirically, or scientifically. Therefore, I choose to present examples of vulnerable patients identified as anthropologically vulnerable groups such as children of incest, severely repeated physical abuse, victims of repeated sexual assaults and rape, combat veterans, and victims of political torture, assaults, and terrorism (Chu, 1998; Figley, 1985; Freud, Ferenczi, Abraham, Simmel, & Jones, 1921; Fromm, 1973; Herman, 1992; Kardiner & Spiegal, 1947; Kelly, 1985; Krystal, 1968; Krystal, Kosten, Perry, Southwick, Mason, & Giller, 1989; Meek, 1992; Myers, 1940; Terr, 1990; Solomon & Yakovlev, 1945). The rich foundation for Complex PTSD and the relationship to complicated grief are defined and confronted in the works of Terr, Herman, and Chu respectively.

In a far-reaching review of the literature, Judith Herman presents a new argument for looking at Borderline Personality Disorder (BPD) and Multiple Personality Disorder/Dissociative Identity Disorder (MPD/DID) on a continuum of disorders that are all related to the etiology and influences of repetitive trauma. Dr. Herman suggests that repetitive trauma needs to be viewed in the historical perspective of the participant. Hysteria and the histrionic personality have roots in the history of medicine that are associated with an exaggeration on the part of the victim or survivor. Hysteria may still carry some of the archaic remnants of that epoch.

Some colleagues present a different view, in which distinctions are clearly and diagnostically important. They focus on separating the borderline character and narcissistic disorders from trauma syndromes as extant, evident, and important (Kernberg, 1984, 1995; Masterson, 1976, 1988). Evidence suggests their points are well supported.

Others have argued against the dissociative disorders/syndromes, especially DID as not diagnostically correct (Mersky, 1992). These same authors also argue that acute stress disorder, somatic disorders, and PTSD all add to needless complex taxonomies, and at worst, iatrogenic classifications that support fictitious disorders and malingering (McNally, 2003; Merskey, 1992). We will not settle these disagreements here. However, regardless of differentiation of diagnosis between disorders, what may be more relevant is an extensive category that defines an approach. That category can handle the many variations or branches that have evolved in our combined searches for what constitutes trauma and loss. Again, that is searching for commonality as well as difference under one concept. What is clear is that despite theoretical differences among colleagues, the character disorders and clinical syndromes we have highlighted are arched by a syndrome that revolves around loss and trauma. Arguably, that arch brings us back to Complex-PTSD, which can hold its weight in research, clinical support, logic, and science.

Mardi Horowitz, a leading theorist and clinician in trauma, supports Herman's argument for the establishment of Complex PTSD as an umbrella diagnosis. Since the 1970s Dr. Horowitz has been at the leading edge of work in trauma and loss integration within a conceptual framework of a stress-response syndrome. He has presented an evolving framework of cognitive-psychodynamics (Horowitz, 1974, 1976, 1998, 1999, 2003), to his present configurational analysis and may be viewed as one of the leaders in complex-trauma formulations (Horowitz, 2003). Although Dr. Horowitz does not use the direct C-PTSD differentiation, that may be more of a lexicon emphasis, but etymologically not a real semantic differentiation.

LEONORE TERR, MD:
TOO SCARED TO CRY—COMPLEX TRAUMA

Of many contributions Terr makes, one that stands out is the one between what she labels Type I Trauma and Type II Trauma. The victim of a Type I Trauma endures a single traumatic experience, whereas in the latter the victim suffers a series of traumatic experiences.

One commonality among members of all these groups is that they disavow their experiences of trauma. The repetition of these events alters one's perception of trauma as "just routine" in culturally acceptable terms. Violence becomes part of the regular landscape of experience as "par for the course." However, nothing could be further away from the reality of the survivor's intrapsychological experience. Accompanying the survivor to the beginning of his therapy may be an intrapsychic trauma lying deeply buried. If that is so, then you may intelligently ask, "Why shouldn't these survivors protest and release a ceaseless flow of tears?"

Please notice that first I used the word "victim" and then "survivor." Why did I not use "survivor" or "thriver"? Allow me to clarify my conceptualization of all three terms. Although the words survivor, and thriver, enjoy prolific use, they may have evolved into almost meaningless terms. This meaninglessness may fail to distinguish victim from survivor, and certainly from thriver. Perhaps today too many people, including some clinicians, use these terms interchangeably, as if one can simply become a survivor and thriver when these terms are applied. That application may be a move toward minimizing the gains patients make during or outside therapy. I suggest stop and pause! I suggest we explicitly define and correspond each term to the different phases that an officer-patient moves through in the experience of trauma. That is, we can say that the patient is in the "victim-stage" when the shells of terror, numbness, denial, and the symptoms of withdrawal are replete. When the patient moves into therapy, trauma is brought into awareness. The officer-patient participates in the "participant-survivor stage" through gaining understanding and working through emotional, behavioral, mental, and existential strain from a prior level of impoverished insight. That is, the patient moves into the "survivor stage" by establishing self-care and having an interest in healing. Having reached this point, the officer-patient can reclaim the meaning of his world and pursue life within the perspective of repositioning the traumatic event in his personal history as a thriver-participant.

In her milestone classic opus, *Too Scared to Cry* (1990), Lenore Terr spelled out why silence around trauma is so prolific. In her promise of making us all more aware, she includes her description and insight into trauma syndromes.

She relates her rich clinical experience through the voices of children and adult victims in Chowchilla, California, who were buried alive, felt death, and escaped to breathe life again. Chowchilla is a quaint, unsuspecting town which was the site of one of the major kidnappings of the twentieth century. Terr interviewed the victims. Her experience and research into the evolution of victims into survivors and thrivers suggest that consequent scars of psychic trauma remain in adults, although altered. She provides insight into adults who have been subject to traumas similar to those her Chowchilla "heroes" had experienced. In her book, the depth of loss is ever-present. In the following section, we will start with why silence is so prolific, in spite of commonsense wishes for the contrary, that is, the wish to wail forth in pain and terror.

Massive Denial and Numbing

Massive denial helps keep away the pain for a while, but it returns, as do most repressed conflicts and wishes to make it go away. For example, consider the amazing success of the rescue efforts of the police officers of Madera County's Sheriff's Department to liberate the child survivors of Chowchilla's kidnapping. Dr. Terr describes the massive denial through the blind spot of emotional omission.

> No old pictures of law enforcement men bringing in the Chowchilla Victims graced the wall of booths (during Chowchilla's Frontier Days of street and historical days), nor was there a shot of the three kidnappers being escorted to their arraignment. One might have thought that the Madera county sheriff's department would have been proud of its most famous case. From the law enforcement point of view, the outcome was highly successful. But no. No one attending the frontier days on the day I attended would have known that a bus kidnapping had ever happened in Madera County, unless, that is, the person already knew. The Chowchilla kidnapping was to be denied. . . . The need to forget the disaster and to put it out of mind far outweighed any civic pride in its "successful" outcome. What was left was a blank spot, a blank spot in group memory and a blank spot in feeling. (Terr, 1990, p. 77)

Terr taps out more than one key note in her perceptive pick-up of what illustrates denial through omission. When it comes to loss, silence may indicate a special resistance through massive denial, which is not borne of ignorance; the spots where "civic pride" in one's wishes and actions are fulfilled are intentionally left blank. Those blank spots are often the missing acknowledgment of the law-enforcement officers expectation. That blank spot on an unconscious level may be the denial of what is meaningful in one's approach as a police officer. The officer-patient may be "shooting blanks into the space" of what he has invested so much into making meaningful—expectations, ideals, and real good work, all in the saddle of public service.

The silence of emptiness where meaning may be expected to fill the void is left alone. Time, the officer-patient and others suspect, ought to fill the void, which is even more surreal without the context of what is lost.

That emotional loss may be associated with unprocessed and unrealized trauma. At times the experience of trauma appears to be frozen under the surface of intellectual facades. While trauma is denied, the culture of silence does not forget. It may socialize officer-patients in ways similar to how other communities of victims become socialized to trauma: through pretending as if it does not and never has existed as a painful experience.

Traumatic Anxiety and Amnesia

Dr. Terr (1990) found that children who experienced Type II trauma had an amnesia for memories of the fear, pain, and violence after traumatic experiences. Amnesia is a forgetting, although the memory is intact. As she explains, the most disturbing traumatic material, in comparison with ordinary memory, may have a different pathway in processing and storing information. Keeping this in mind, traumatic amnesia may be related to states of dissociation.

I posit from an evolutionary point of view that this would make sense in conferring on the victim a way of not being overloaded by the direct content of the trauma. That direct content may be associated with guilt, rage, anxiety, and a changed perception of most of what preceded that event as a defense against the strain and stress of intense mourning. The freeing of energy is a biological tendency in all living beings. The energy needed may be cut off through a redirection of forgetting what is too traumatic to remember.

Yet clues exist: fantasy, dreams, and reenactment are all paths that may lead to assessing this dissociated amnesia (Gottlieb, 1997). There are four kinds of repeated dreams of trauma: exact repetitions, modified repetitions, deeply disguised, and terror that cannot be remembered upon awakening (Hartmann, 1984).

Dreams of terror (domestic or foreign terrorism) may leave the dreamer with only the vague and uncomfortable nervous feeling of a signal anxiety.

Terr suggests,

> Freud says what lies behind this tendency to repeated dreaming is a kind of anxiety unique to psychic trauma, "traumatic anxiety." But ordinary dreams are not equipped to dissipate traumatic anxiety, the anxiety of the external. The anxiety stirred up by trauma is far too massive, far too intense, to be handled by one or two ordinary nightmares. Dreams do not work after massive horror, terror, and disgrace. Dreams, simply are too weak a mental mechanism to handle this kind of intensity. Traumatic anxiety does not spontaneously dissipate during ones lifetime. Once this anxiety is set into motion, it may recur with new life stresses especially those that carry echoes of the old helplessness and loss. (Terr, 1990, p. 214)

It may be that separation anxiety is inextricably linked and reenacted through the traumatic stress and anxiety that emerges in losses never acknowledged, leaving the victim with a "narcissistic injury" and belief that he is helpless and alone. The possibility that this separation anxiety hearkens back to childhood takes away nothing from its viability in the here and now. It may be more than coincidence that when officers were fatally wounded, many called for their mothers. That evidence exists, despite being mature and healthy adults, prior to the tragic shooting. Regression serves a protective tendency that makes sense as adaptive functional dissociation and telescoping of trauma (Rudofossi, 1997).

Terr (1990) illustrates traumatic anxiety with a real example through William Manchester, the prolific writer and historian. Manchester, in his fiction and nonfiction, may have repeated his earlier experiences of war trauma. Terr explains Manchester's own history and struggles in dealing with the assassination of his friend, President John F. Kennedy.

It was after his profound loss of a beloved friend that traumatic dreams emerged. In those dreams, he was "tired, scared, angry and always climbing a hill." Put in historical perspective, Terr gives us the background of Manchester's earlier combat traumas. That background included Manchester's deception about his age, idealistic fervor, and his enlistment in the armed services. He fought "fierce battles with the enemy," during late adolescence and into early adulthood. That enemy never perished. That enemy reemerged in the symbols kept alive and reenacted on the dormant battlefield through repeated traumatic dreams. As Terr suggests, the assassination of Kennedy triggered the release, reenactment, and reexperiencing of Manchester's earlier combat trauma. John F. Kennedy was murdered 35 years after Manchester's experience of combat trauma. But it was the murder of the President that triggered the release of traumatic loss 35 years past being reexperienced in the traumatic nightmares he wrote about in *Good-bye darkness: A memoir of the Pacific war* (Manchester, 1979). This functioning of a telescope from a current trauma contracting to an original quantum psychic trauma (Rudofossi, 2007) is compelling and will be illustrated in a later chapter.

Terr's presentation of William Manchester as an example clarifies her admonition that unlike the common folklore and popular portrayal of trauma in which victims always freeze and are total immobilized, a striking difference occurs in reality. In reality, she points out, the victim usually tries to go on as if everything is okay. She presents Stephen King, Alfred Hitchcock, and Virginia Woolf as three highly gifted (geniuses) who presented their childhood traumas through the lens of their own struggles with repetitive traumas. Perhaps that is why the one who is afraid of Virginia Woolf is the Virginia Woolf afraid of letting down her veil of anger and alcoholism that deceives all, including herself, about the unmourned death of her son. From the open door to her own son's death does the moribund air clear and mourning may begin in earnest. On the other hand, we may also, as readers and consumers, be "amusing ourselves to death" as the late Neil Postman (1994) suggested, in the way we get bits of information that cheat us out of meaningful discourse on one level, and on another leading to silence through all the quick summaries of tragedy in an intellectual nutshell.

What further obfuscates clarity is that to block genuine expression is a societal demand and reinforcement for sound bites and not an individual mechanism of defense by intellectualizing. Intellectualization on a social level of media diffusion of trauma reinforces the tendency to whisk away the pain of loss in a "snap-out-of-it" mentality.

With that snap-out-of-it mentality on a social level, I suggest that Terr's (1990) work illustrates a critical point that may be lost: the time span between the experiencing of a trauma and the emergence of any expression of loss related to that prior trauma suggests a long pause. I suggest that pause extends to rethinking two troublesome areas. The first is time-limited protocols for trauma and grief work. If memories of trauma are repressed, distorted by intense anxiety, dissociated and compartmentalized in memory for decades, our humility and our realism demands a therapeutic attitude (to not shrink our hours into working "therapeutic magic").

The second troublesome area is usually inadequate to the task of describing delayed trauma processing. That delay in expressing trauma symptoms, I suggest, is almost always linked to loss, and not primarily to shock. Shock is always an aspect of loss; it is a disruption of what is expected to be there in the psychological space we create in the repetitive reliability of our own ecological niches. This time distortion in trauma where grief emerges in the context of "complicated" and "disenfranchised" grief is in the quantum nature of loss. An example of that is suggested by Manchester's (1979) 35 year delay of his expression of his loss. To iterate this will become relevant in my conceptualization of what I call "telescoping of trauma" in the eco-ethological approach. For now, I suggest we return to the unfinished business in the context of Terr's commentary on Manchester's rich work for building up our understanding of loss through trauma and the subtle economics of unmourned loss and objective fear.

That assessment of fear in trauma is that, while catastrophizing may occur and is amenable to therapy, especially via cognitive behavioral approaches, it has its roots in reality and objective fear. If we forget that reality, we may collude in an unprofessional judgment about the officer-patient's reactions to trauma in his misperception that we are judging rather than facilitating healing. A modified cognitive-behavioral approach may open up the maladaptive aspects of how to approach avoidant and withdrawing behaviors and cognitions that have evolved over time in the officer-patient's repertoire.

From a psychodynamic level, the maladaptive "why" may be opened up wide while using Terr's example of Mr. Manchester's creative writing about his own hidden trauma through characterization and plot. Some psychiatrists and psychologists conjecture that the writing and presentation of authors (which is no less than our patient's) dealing with trauma, may be viewed as a cathartic purging and even an abreaction on a creative level of expression (Gabbard & Gabbard, 1987; Gabbard & Western, 2003). I suggest while in many cases that outcome may be true, and without any therapy, it may occur as a self-initiated therapeutic intervention. In many more cases it may not. Why and in what way can this be contradicted by the evidence?

If we view a purpose of sharing one's trauma through creative writing, such as a book, poem, or song, that reaches many others, at least two purposes may be realized. One purpose may be a public confession, on one hand helping one purge (usually fantasized) guilt, and on another a wish fulfillment to get others to acknowledge what the survivor has lost. Both wishes of public confession, as well as acknowledgment and validation by others, may be unconsciously satisfied. That satisfaction can be achieved unconsciously by getting readers to mourn the author's losses. Mourning those losses may be achieved in a vicarious way, maintaining safety and distance for the author. That safety may be achieved through expressing the visual and nonverbal depiction of ecological aspects of trauma to the anonymous, yet intimate mass of readers. Nonverbal and visual means of ecological aspects of trauma are safer for the author than speaking about and expressing his real losses; this is met by knowing others are enticed to get involved on a nonverbal, nondirect level. The vicarious experience may be achieved by the audience, not by the entertainer. The entertainer is disenfranchised from the direct responsiveness of the audience as a dissociative experience. The written account may also be a transitional object of sorts, in which acknowledgment gets to be mourned in a public sense, accepted, and normalized through indirect means, without any resolution.

If my theory is correct, unfortunately and sometimes tragically, the author displaces the burden of his own grief work onto the anonymity and ever-present reading audience. The reader is burdened by the author displacing his own mourning and bereavement through others. That author, although poetic, artistic, and intellectually gifted, may elude his own conscious awareness of his real need to grieve his own losses.

That displacement may create a paradox that is counterintuitive: the more beautiful, touching, and evocative the artistic expression, the more displacement, intellectualization, and repression may be occurring, especially in a social and media context where trauma is dissociated and the grief work is put off onto others. Included in those others are you and me, the therapist. Included in those who may displace their work onto others are the officer-patients, who have striking similarity to authors and other artists who may project and displace onto us the symbolic representations of trauma and loss. Symbolic representations of trauma and loss are orchestrated best in "choir practice," a process where peers share war stories. The war stories are celebrated within the ethology that mimics the field of trauma: heightened release of sexual anonymity, altered states of consciousness with alcoholic relish, aggressive play and risk taking via passionate upstarts, with deft dispassionate retreat into withdrawal of depression and existential voids.

That displacement of symbols may become evident in the transference to us in our identity as his therapist. That transference, while unique in some ways within therapy, is different when we become aware and do not reenact what others do. This means we do not react judgmentally, and we do respond with empathy in timing our interventions (Benjamin, 1993; Brenner, 1974, 1976, 1982). We may also appreciate what is delivered to us in these expressive works as invitations to engage the officer-patient as we may do with an author's publication. I suggest our engagement may not preclude our appreciation of the expressive work as art in its own right; but we may make a real difference by being consciously aware of our responsibility to explore the loss being revealed to us. Like authors, public and police professionals can be intriguing and exciting in their presentations. In our approach as mental health professionals, we may be alert to the possibility of losing our attention to that exciting intrigue, which, while seductive in an all too human manner, in the long run may sabotage our ability to reach the officer-patient, who may never mourn his losses.

Maintaining our attention is a responsibility that extends to many of our interventions; for example, interpretations, cognitive reappraisals, supportive assurance, paradoxical intervention, and existential confrontations, to name a few. In your therapy with an author, no less than with an officer-patient, you may be presented with provocative details through war stories, diaries, and records of trauma. While we can accept and even cherish these as privileged gifts, our work is made meaningful by helping to redirect the meaning and loss for the officer-patient toward gradually expressing and mourning his losses. Expressing and mourning losses emotionally help reduce rage and the tedium of denial, which may abound around the corner of vengeance and consequently lead to acting out. That is to say, many a talented genius of letters and words spared least of all himself: Marlowe, Plath, Poe, Camus, Pope, are but just a few . . . (Gabbard & Gabbard, 1987; Styron, 1997).

Identification with the Aggressor—Vendettas

Anna Freud (1936) came up with the description of *identification with the aggressor,* later called the Stockholm Syndrome and made famous by Patti Hearst's abduction by the SLA. This condition is typified by a victim identifying with the power wielded by their aggressor. The victim begins to mimic her oppressor, perhaps as a compensatory wish to regain power and control now lost in the relationship. In the original psychoanalytic conceptualization, it is libido that is invested in this form of identification. Libido appropriately defined means aggressive and sexual energy that is in part a motive force and a drive derivative (Brenner, 1974; Richards & Willick, 1986).

While Terr's (1990) focus remained on childhood trauma, she made the suggestion that vengeance may underlie shocking events of aggression. From school violence to the Chowchilla's kidnappers, outrageous acts of violence may be passed off as legitimate ways of getting back at those who initiated the violence. Although that retribution may exist as fantasy or confabulation, it is too costly to ignore the impact of this distortion of thought process. Our conversation is limited to the victims who radically change in ways that may mimic the inflexible pattern of antagonism the aggressor exhibits. It is reasonable to speculate that the aggressor is aware on an unconscious level, if not a conscious level, that they may provoke such a response in the victim/survivor. A vendetta may be a partial motivation in the schemas of perpetrators, as Dr. Terr suggests. That vendetta is in response to what is perceived as a "slight" that triggers some fantasized disempowerment in the aggressor. The devaluation of the so-called oppressor becomes a conduit for all types of terrorism, domestic and foreign, as well as a convenient excuse.

However, our frame of reference in this book is understanding the officer-patient's identification with the aggressor. We may need to rethink our schema about officer-patients as being enforcers, and at times consider them as being victims/survivors of abuse and aggression. To that end, I suggest it is conceivable that disproportionate levels of violence toward victims in response to a trivial slight may be seen more clearly through the lens of earlier and multiple violations, where vendettas stew from initial losses that remain hidden. Those losses may remain silently hidden. Simultaneous with losses is resentment that may be translated into a vendetta, which accretes energy through some cultures that condone revenge or aggression rather than mourning. Communication through violence may be almost entirely nonverbal and primary, as in the ecological niche of police war zones, and aggression may get "acted out" in the most perverse of expressions: violence and death. That perversity may include pleasure at release of violence, adding energy to this destructive force.

I opine this may be relative to what public-safety officers experience in "war zones" as a "conspiracy of silence," suggested by Terr (1990). That silence to others outside the circle is an accounting of the abuses, humiliations, and terrorism endured. Some actual examples of brutality against officer-patients are: bottles thrown at them from roofs, shots fired at them from high caliber firearms, assaults and other injuries targeting them while rendering emergency health care, and nasty invectives (pigs and fascists) shouted at them during mass public rallies. The officer-patient may find fear, humiliation, and lack of support more tolerable while channeling negative emotions through destructive expression of aggression. That aggressive expression may be acceptable in the general culture of the war zones; grief and mourning may not be.

This physical and verbal barrage is a pattern of abuse. It may set a climate for anger and rage. In many officers, that anger may rarely be acted out in all of its ugly permutations. That extreme may happen from time to time when a victim of long-standing trauma acts against the aggressor in the same way the aggressor attacked her. Like the victims in the war zones, some officer-patients may learn to associate and identify with the behavior and communication of aggression exacerbated by the unacknowledged losses that accumulate and get acted out in spectacular and tragic ways as vendettas. This can take the form of a unit or platoon acting as if they were the criminals they have been pursuing. One example that stands out is the 77th Precinct in Brooklyn. There are many more officers in my experience who have exhibited any number of unacknowledged losses via aggressive fantasies of vendettas against the perpetrators who offend both the civilian population and the officer-patients. Perpetrators can focus the effects of their own hidden losses directly toward officers; they do this through direct and repetitive gestures of hostility and aggression. In expanding Terr's

(1990) conspiracy of silence, we move on to consider the fear of even thinking about trauma.

Traumatophobia—Terr (1990) suggests we not forget the novel concept that Sandor Rado, MD, former director of Columbia University's Psychoanalytic Institute coined, *phobia to trauma or traumatophobia*. This may be viewed as a predictive research and clinical hypothesis. Rado (1939, 1956) asserted that soldiers in World War II would "anticipate a fear response," and "remain fearful of fear being expressed." Traumatophobia is seen as "feeling terrified of expressing that an event is traumatic" in the first place (this is true of terror victims and may be true of police officers as well); that is, being too scared to cry and even to speak about the trauma as a way of keeping away the terror associated with the event. Herman offers the what of complex trauma in three phases as follows.

HERMAN'S THREE PHASES OF COMPLEX PTSD IN TRAUMA AND RECOVERY

Judith Herman, MD presents a case for complex trauma in a number of populations (1992). Particular emphasis is given to populations subject to dissociation. Attention focuses on incest survivors, political prisoners, and child sexual-abuse victims. In fact, the populations that Herman present includes combat trauma, complicated posttraumatic stress disorder, and multiple-personality disorder. All are helpful in understanding police and public-safety trauma. That relationship will emerge as we move forward. What she saves in parsimony of presented stages she does not neglect in elegance of theory and treatment (1992).

Herman states a qualification up front: "No single course of recovery follows these stages through a straightforward linear sequence. Oscillating and dialectical in nature, the traumatic syndromes defy any attempt to impose such simple-minded order" (1992, p. 155). The core of her approach is beauty in simplicity through three stages she describes as follows:

- *Safety*: In this stage, the trauma therapist facilitates the establishment of safety. This stage cannot be rushed, she insists, as is prevalent among other major complex trauma and grief therapists. Prior to exploratory work, safety has to be ensured within a consistent therapeutic alliance. The importance and necessity of investing time in ensuring safety in the relationship by gaining trust in the therapist is integral to any approach in treating trauma.
- *Remembrance and Mourning*: Establishing the contextual framework for the emergence of the meaning of traumatic loss is key. A number of goals include achieving a reconstruction of the survivor's own story and transforming the traumatic memory through the process of mourning the traumatic losses. Validation of what is important in the specific history of the individual is

achieved through an alliance with the therapist, which begins within the therapy and extends outside the therapeutic hours. Validation outside therapy is achieved through strong social support, ensured and enhanced in the "safety stage." What moves into memory is not reenacted; it is abreacted through remembering, validating, and mourning the loss.

• *Reconnection:* The patient achieves this stage by finding meaning and getting involved in day-to-day living. That is a quality-of-life choice without the level of prior shame, denial, guilt, and its manifestations of withdrawal, avoidance, and enduring patterns that perpetuate loss, trauma, and dissociation. It is not necessarily returning to a former state of living and relating to others, but usually is more of an emphasis on preparing for the struggle of genuine living, which includes being able to attend to the issues and involvement in everyday life with pleasure and engaging in relationships with others. The trauma is reconstructed as one's story—one's own history. In Herman's conceptualization, both the therapist and patient acknowledge and make explicit the trauma without attaching labels, such as histrionic or borderline. The new category, Complex PTSD, arguably may be a more elegant and appropriate diagnosis than the weighted implications of pejorative labels and their implications that accompany a diagnosis of histrionic and borderline character disorders. The responsible treatment of Complex PTSD is also a clear objective in the work of Dr. James Chu.

JAMES CHU, MD:
REBUILDING SHATTERED LIVES

Prior to exploratory work, Dr. Chu (1998) pointed out that the responsible treatment of Complex PTSD requires patients to achieve certain skills, which precede any attempt at abreaction. As Chu suggests, abreaction work done prematurely may result in the patient experiencing overwhelming and dysfunctional isolation, provoking regressive and self-destructive behavior. To preempt that destructive behavior, patient mastery of the earliest stage of treatment is presented in the acronym, SAFER.

Earlier Stage Treatment—SAFER
S— Self-care and Symptom Control
A—Acknowledgment of Traumatic Antecedents
F— Functioning
E— Expression of Affect (appropriate to stage of trauma work)
R— Relationships that are supportive—(therapeutic alliance as well).
(Chu, 1998, p. 162)

Chu's Caveat about groups is similar to Terr and Herman's.

Overly intensive self-help groups that focus on traumatic experiences may bring on intrusive thoughts feelings and recollections as well as autonomic arousal in the forms of heightened anxiety, irritability, and nightmares. Changes in the patient's external environment are frequent precipitants to de-compensations. . . . (Chu, 1998, p. 162)

One of many important problems patients with Complex PTSD bring to therapy is *chronic disempowerment.* Chu explains this as a sense of self as hateful and defective, with intense difficulties in relationships, dependency on others for soothing when dysfunctional, and rigid responses to the environment (Chu,1998).

One ingenious program offering promise as well as an innovative solution to an alternative means of achieving this early and very difficult stage of SAFER may exist. It has achieved initial success.

A Successful Experiment of Reempowerment— Post Trauma Retreat: Capt. Dr. Benner

The *Post Trauma Retreat* was developed and is continually being refined in the highly competent and creative hands of Dr. Albert Benner, Dr. Hayden Duggan, and Ms. Valerie Duggan, CSW. It was conceived by Dr. Duggan and Ms. Duggan in the northeast and by Dr. Benner on the west coast and Dr. Fay (Benner, 1991, 1998, 2001). It offers a retreat where clinicians facilitate the trauma and loss work in a structured and supportive group process. I believe the program's value lies in the ability of the clinicians as well as the motivation and trust established with the police and public-safety personnel. The reputations of Dr. Benner, Dr. and Ms. Duggan, and Dr. Fay in the community of police and public safety, precede them as genuine and perspicacious in the application of their expertise. This program is one of intensive exposure to actual work-related traumatic events.

Clinicians with the assistance of peer support provide a therapeutic and safe environment. While so much is accomplished in a week of intensive support, the program responsibly seeks to place officer-patients with appropriately trained, empathic, and responsible therapists for continuation of the important work underway.

Middle-Stage Treatment—Abreaction, in part, is the reconstruction of a comprehensive articulation and verbal narrative of traumatic events. Chu recommends that abreaction is best achieved from a position of strength in the patient's self-concept (1998). He explains that your awareness (as a clinician) of the following problems, addressed in this middle stage, may require and strain your motivation and tolerance as a member of the therapeutic dyad:

Rigid and Repetitive Reenactments of trauma occur in relationships; of course that includes the officer-patient's transference to you. Patients usually tend to be rigid. Often their negative thoughts revolve around self-blame for the trauma, shame, misery, and torment about self-despair and helplessness.

Anger and Enmeshment—In dealing with anger and projection of anger onto the therapist, clinicians need to be active and involved in a way that fosters trust and attachment. However, Chu warns the therapist about becoming overly identified with the patient and cautions against the trap of fostering dependence and enmeshment in the patient's developing relationship with the clinician. Deep mistrust arises initially in the patients and is difficult to deal with clinically. On the other side of that misattribution, you will likely encounter the patient holding onto "idealized hope" of your rescuing him.

Control and Manipulation—This odious pair may initially appear easily in public-safety and police populations due to the dysfunctional myths reviewed in an earlier work (Rudofossi, 2007). Instead of collaboration, you may encounter an "us versus them" mentality. This is a reminder of why, after stabilization and containment is ensured, abreaction may follow.

Fixation on the Trauma—For patient safety and welfare, dismantling defenses is appropriate only when the current environment is safe from both internal and external threat, including the trauma of self-perpetuated abuse. Premature abreaction, says Chu, "is not only overwhelming, but self perpetuating" (1998, p. 81).

Tendency to use self as a vehicle of tension relief and control—Destructive, addictive disorders, pseudorelief, and control mechanisms need to be identified and neutralized.

Some of the major defenses against the complex trauma and loss in Chu's presentation are massive denial, depersonalization, derealization, and dissociation (1998).

Effective abreaction takes place in an outpatient office setting with a trained therapist, as Chu illustrates very nicely in the following:

Common Phases of Abreaction

    A. *Increased Symptomatology*—This phase includes intrusive memories in which reexperiencing the trauma, including the visceral aspects, are likely to be recalled and emerge in many sessions.

    B. *Intense Internal Conflict*—Psychodynamically, this is on a structural level of conflict in terms of aggressive drive derivatives and their expression via relational modes of anger and agitation in competition with the desire to achieve healthier compromise formations (Brenner, 1976).

    C. *Acceptance and Mourning*—In this stage, the patient moves toward expressing what has been identified as the loss in the trauma. The process of mourning has begun.

    D. *Mobilization and Empowerment*—Acceptance of past aggressive behaviors, as opposed to rejection and disavowal, leads to the resolution of these internal conflicts.

    E. *Working Through Trauma*—This is a progressive process that is accomplished over time.

Late-Stage Treatment: Consolidation of Gains and Increasing Skills

In this stage, the patient presents an increased confidence in his investment in genuine relationships, including friendships, without overt patterns of manipulation and hostility. The patient moves forward on a continuum of becoming fully active in living and accepting pleasure. This stage also may include further abreaction and integration of self-concept, ego strength, and resilience. Chu suggests this is no easy task.

> When therapists assume that patients naturally understand empowerment and are inclined to move toward feeling more empowered an impasse often occurs based on therapist's empathic failure. Patient's react by becoming more resistant, distant, or angry, and therapists tend to become overwhelmed. Moreover, because patients understand only their own disempowered world, they may have difficulty articulating what is wrong; they simply feel confused, misunderstood, and unheard. . . . (Chu, 1998, p. 183)

Chu suggests that traumatic and dissociative disorders of a repetitive nature be described as umbrella disorders under Complex PTSD. He offers logic and evidence to validate comorbidity with complex trauma-based syndrome. The salient point is that complex traumatic syndromes and dissociative disorders belong together. In another acronym for dissociative disorders, BASK, Chu credits the four parameters to Bennett Braun, MD (1988). This acronym suggests the four domains of dissociation as follows: *B*ehavior; *A*ffect (Emotion); *S*omatic sensation; *K*nowledge; Chu adds *I*dentity (1998).

Braun (1988) and Chu (1998) suggest each experiential state of dissociation has its own unique set of BASK-I. Chu suggests identity is impacted by constant use of certain experiential reliance on dissociation, which has a healthy component as well as a normative aspect to that experience. Excessive reliance on dissociation as a defense against losses has a very different result, which may be the development of the Dissociative Identity Disorders (DID). Identity is a key factor in DID (or what was called Multiple Personality Disorder), one of the more controversial constructs of psychology and psychiatry.

Dissociative Identity Disorder (DID) and PPSC-PTSD

Moving forward, we can review the basis for how trauma syndromes are placed into a developmental perspective. Ellin presents such a perspective in his developmental model of trauma, which has a focus on trauma and violence as antecedents to DID and other related dissociative disorders (Cohen et al., 1995; Kluft, 1986, 1992; Putnam, 1989). In this conceptual model, trauma is no longer repressed or acted out in one's life; it becomes a defensive constellation through the process of dissociation.

While DID remains the most trying and controversial of diagnoses, that controversy is far from settled; it is one that cannot easily go away. Much evidence has balanced the controversy between false memories and genuine trauma. Although false memories cannot easily be denied, neither can the qualitative and empirical evidence that has accumulated from the days of Janet's work at Harvard on dissociation to date (1907). No one has done more reliable and valid research in this domain than Dr. Elizabeth Loftus (1979). She empirically illustrated how *suggestibility* can mold the expression of recovered memories, including false memories—evidence which cannot be ignored. Gottlieb (1997) suggests a similar hypothesis and uses a case example to illustrate how fantasies about dissociation may add another dimension similar to a heightened suggestibility in patient and therapist in the diagnostic process. He puts forward a compelling hypothesis to consider in our understanding of Multiple Personality Disorder (MPD): "Fantasies and enactments of multiplicity imply a prior set of fantasies, that allow for the possibility of multiplicity" (p. 930). That some patients present exaggerated memories is not remarkable in the history of any medical or psychological disorder, but it is a real problem. Whatever side you take, the evidence shows that multiple, intense, and repetitive traumatic experiences all contribute to dissociative disorders.

Evolutionary Perspective of DID

In the evolution of our understanding of dissociative disorders, the issue of loss of one's own identity may shade the realization that an integrated sense of self and identity may be nonexistent (Kohut, 1971, 1977). Ellin suggests that dissociation functions as a silent defense against overwhelming trauma but may contribute to a disintegration of identity development (Cohen, Berzoff, & Ellin, 1995). This disintegration of development may be reenacted through *projective identification* and *projections onto significant others* (Kernberg, 1984, 1995; Kohut, 1971), which invariably includes the transference onto the psychotherapist.

Labile emotions so common in borderline rage, anger, separation anxiety, and imagined abandonment is heightened in this disorder and are likely to emerge in the officer-patient's emotional reactions to trauma, abreaction, and projected onto you. That labile emotional valence may be a clue for you to hang in there and slowly let the material emerge.

I suggest the organization of these different alterations of identity and striking disparity in presentation may be influenced by attempts to respond to different contexts of evolutionary influences that mean survival or death in police and public-safety patients (Lorenz, 1971, 1973; Lorenz & Leyhausen, 1973; Morris, 1967, 1969a, 1969b; Morris & Morris, 1966; Rado, 1956; Tinbergen, 1948, 1969). The emotional valence that may have originally been adaptive may be transferred to other situations in which officers are not in danger. Officer-patients may continue to react in the same way that served a survival value initially and has now become maladaptive.

> Krystal and colleagues (1989) suggest, from the perspective of evolutionary biology the resistance of traumatic learning to modification probably reflects the fundamental importance of avoiding catastrophic situations at all costs. However, from the therapeutic standpoint, the inflexibility of traumatic responses makes it likely that long-term or periodic treatment might be necessary to maintain clinical improvement in some PTSD patients. (Krystal et al., p. 190; In his book; see also Giller, 1990, p. 10)

The support of a positive relationship between dissociation and traumatic events has been collaborated (by Janoff-Bulman (1989, 1992). Also, physiological studies have supported dependent differences on a number of parallel levels of development in the domain of memory, cognitions, language, and visual perception (Cannon, 1914; Cohen et al., 1995; Giller, 1990; Southwick, 2007). DID is postulated as being caused in part through information disregulation, which may be a product of different capacities for memories related to different states of consciousness, which may run parallel to memory and alterations in personality (Rappaport, 1971).

Memory Along Parallel Lines of Development and Altered Personality

Putnam suggests that multiple trauma influences the context of separate parallel processes of memory and development (1989). These alternate parallel branches may develop along different processes in which memory and perception are imprinted in different ways through the dominance of one alteration of personality in comparison with another. It is important to understand that the memory does not reproduce veridical memories, but does produce reconstructive memory. Both confabulation and fantasy may shape memory.

The therapist employs a key by using the transference to analyze conflicts associated with traumatic experience, while not acting in response to it as other people may. Through material gathered by free association, the patient and therapist work on understanding the dynamics between the structural conflicts (id, ego, and superego) that surround trauma outcome. This type of assessment, diagnosis, and therapy is not without controversy within, and certainly without, the circle of trained clinicians. However, it seems fair to say psychoanalytic psychotherapy has informed serious inroads toward identifying and treating multiple personality disorders (Marmer, 1980), including case studies (Smith, Buffington, & McCard, 1982) that support multiple alterations on a number of empirical levels.

Bessel Van Der Kolk and colleagues (1985) suggest *traumatic memory encoding* may be precognitive or prelinguistic and may lend itself at first to somatosensory expression (Goleman, 1992, 1994; Southwick, 2007; Van Der Kolk, 1987, 1989; Van Der Kolk, Greenberg, Boyd, & Krystal, 1985; Van Der Kolk & Saporta, 1991). Somatosensory overload in the survivor may be experienced along with hypervigilance, hyperemotional excitement, escalating anger, and anxiety that usually follows PTSD (Benner, 1991; Figley, 1985; Hendin, 1983; James, 1994; Peterson, Prout, & Schwartz, 1992; Reese, 1991; Southwick, 2007; Thorpe, 2007).

I suggest those somatosensory overload feelings may be experienced as painful, confusing, and without insight and can lead to the pains, aches, and suffering in silence that officer-patients exhibit. However, they may also lead to altered dissociative states as a defense against overwhelming anxiety associated with loss. That loss may have arterial roots in disenfranchised shame and guilt over fears of abandonment and loss of ethological security in the ecology of the units niche. Existential loss is primary in losing the bonds forged in the crucible of survival in life-and-death moments. Specifically, unexpressed shame and guilt related to the secondary formation of dissociative states that emerge in the ecology of trauma, and the need for ethological survival may exacerbate officer-patient confusion. Shame implies a loss of one's face, a belief one has not been up to par and deserves or receives humiliation as a result. Public shame has many levels of loss and may lead to avoidant behaviors. What the survivor hides at all costs may be a fear of losing his *belonging with* his fellow officers if he discloses the real terror and loss that comes with somatosensory overload. The need to survive in an ecological niche offers a selective advantage by allowing emotional investment in one's fellow officers while hiding emotional empathy and denying the meaning of losing one's unit members in the throes of terrorism and war occluding the heavy weight of these experiences trapped in disenfranchised losses.

My own clinical experience as well as others have validated that the officer who may be most in need of his peers may become separated from them if the true state of affairs is disclosed. Fellow officers may be the traumatized officer's major social support network (Benner, 1991; Lambert, 1986; McNamara, 1967; Mitchell, 1988; Silverstein, 1992; Southwick, 2007; Thorpe, 2007). Guilt may be conceived of as a loss of one's ideal self-image in his ecological niche, which may evoke a massive denial due to fear of disclosure as well as guilt about what he has failed to do from the officers ideal vantage point. Until the unconscious conflict around loss is made conscious, no abatement of guilt and its dissociative impact is likely as altered states of consciousness continue. That is critical on a psychodynamic as well as existential perspective.

We will look at an illustration by means of a composite case example, when we review Rando's complicated mourning in this chapter.

Switching to Altered States of Consciousness

Kluft sheds light on how repetitive severe trauma may act like a "switch" that triggers dissociative disorders (1986, 1992). That switch may be multi-directional. Putnam suggests that a switching occurs as multiple states of consciousness are altered in trauma survivors (1989). The multiple altered states he posits are psychobiologically rooted and may be thought of as related to self-schemas, which include symbolic representations: cognitive, affective, emotional, and nonverbal. A critical mass may be reached when the patient crosses a threshold, provoking triggers for dissociation. Kluft's four-factor model of dissociation is very useful:

1. The survivor's ability or tendency to experience dissociation is necessary.
2. The survivor is exposed to traumatic events that are intense and repetitive.
3. The survivor experiences factors that support this dissociation, including environmental factors and the lack of supportive adults who promote adequate expression of the loss and trauma (significant other, friends, and relatives.)
4. The survivor is not protected from traumatic experiences and does not have support to process the trauma. (Kluft, 1986)

I suggest that the four-factor model of Kluft reads as a check list for what we have seen as evident for the officer-patient's unusually high probability of developing dissociation (Rudofossi, 1997, 2007). To be a public-safety officer, one has to adapt to a number of conflicting roles, which may indicate a dissociative ability. The lack of support in expressing grief is not rare not only in the public-safety culture but in the family as well. Protection from further trauma is not realized in most public-safety departments. While combat veterans get a rotation from the battlefield, no such privilege exists in police and public-safety cultures in general. This is regardless of repetitive and intense trauma. It appears that the vast majority of officers are subject to the factors involved in dissociation disorders. The four treatment stages suggested for DID (Cohen et al., 1995) are as follows:

Initial Phase—Social support is enlisted, ongoing relationships that exacerbate trauma are confronted, and warning the patient about the lengthy work ahead is honestly approached. A firm foundation is laid out as soon as possible before beginning memory-processing work.

Middle Phase—The survivor's interpersonal communication skills and cooperation is enhanced, negotiating adaptive solutions to problems, correcting cognitive errors, processing traumatic memories, and devising nondissociative coping strategies. Notice that trauma-memory processing is a small component of this work.

Late preintegration phase of therapy—In this stage, the survivor consolidates treatment gains, thereby strengthening and practicing nondissociative defenses. Grief work and reprocessing of the impact of the trauma are moved along. Integration of alter personalities culminating in full integration and resolution is made into an active task.

Postintegration Phase of Therapy—Manage with life as an integrated individual—The survivor's ability to reach out to others is achieved before stress reaches a critical and overwhelming mass. The socialization skills gained here complement a higher frustration tolerance to be able to deal with the "thousand natural shocks that flesh is heir to" without reoccurring decompensation. That is a major achievement, whether accomplished in part or in whole.

A major point throughout all these stages is the fact that grief work addresses losses accumulated over a lifetime of splitting and dissociative processes. It took decades to create the defensive process of dissociation, as Braun (1988) put it. The goal of grief work is creating an internal strength from within the officer-patient, what R. R. Ellis calls a healing process in grieving (1994); that is, moving on in the grief work without resorting to comorbid addictions ranging from drugging, boozing, and random sexual flings to numb and deny losses. Relapse prevention as well as acceptance is a preparation for the joint venture between patient and therapist (Lazarus, 1972; Linehan, 1993).

The grief work can take a very long time. It is reasonable that it may take years of supportive trauma therapy to reach the stage of insight and cognitive-behavioral therapy to work through the grief and mourning process. Dr. Henry Schwartz reminds us, "Treatment of character and of trauma requires attention to competing subjectivities in the context of an empathic relationship" (Schwartz, 1994, p. 229). The alliance is the ongoing process in which both participants, the officer-patient and you, can achieve respective goals of healing via healing interventions, which include your relating empathy.

C-PTSD AND DID: RELEVANCE FROM A POLICE AND PUBLIC-SAFETY PERSPECTIVE

Police and public-safety populations experience a cultivation of complex factors that we have reviewed, which contribute to a harvest of dissociation and C-PTSD. The late teens to young adulthood are the years when the identities of the public-safety and police officer emerge. Repeated events of murder, violence, and meaningless hostility are thrust at the officer. In the identity formation of an officer, the introduction to trauma is often abrupt and shocking and develops in a dynamic ecology and culture. The repeated exposure to trauma is compounded by the difficult and often contradictory roles an officer may be thrust into during an event she experiences. What happens to that experience in relation to her self-concept, concept of peers, community of people she serves, and significant others? How can she express her loss when it is said to be a part of being an officer? And as the culture and ecology suggests, if he/she cannot accept the blood and guts of the job and toughen his/her skin, then give it up (Neiderhoffer, 1967; Spielberger, Grier, & Greenfield, 1982).

As therapists, we are keenly aware that the rote repetition of an event of trauma the officer-patient experiences is not grief work. That loss is vast; it embraces expectations, ideal self-concepts, ideal behaviors, unidentified wishes, actual behaviors, and activities not meeting the mettle of internal standards. The officer accords little if any acknowledgment of these losses, which may include the event itself, as in traumatophobia. Feelings, ideas and behaviors during the event, and fantasies about the event that have been dissociated may not be acceptable to the officer on a conscious level. What is unacceptable may not be admitted into conscious awareness.

What is not admitted into conscious awareness may be even more important for understanding the development of the individual officer-patient than what is admissible to consciousness. Complex trauma and dissociative disorders are what remain unidentified and disavowed as unacceptable. In officer-patients, the real trauma and loss may remain hidden for decades, as in the case of William Manchester. It is that disavowal of reality through the use of fantasies, defenses, and splits in identity that may remain far from conscious awareness. That distance does not preserve, but may drain the officer-patient by consuming energy. This is not unusual with sufferers of human anguish and depravity that push the boundaries of human endurance.

More to the point is that loss may be fundamental to the process of dissociation itself. Personality styles may be (in part) cumulative responses to survival and adaptation in which the survival value in an ecology of traumatic losses leads to denying trauma, which includes a loss of self-awareness, and autonomy. It is tragic in its cost and comic in that it renders the officer-participant impervious to self-awareness. The officer is a closed conduit for effecting the very developmental change required. That paradoxical development is perhaps a real approximation to what the Greeks meant by tragic-comedy. This is a far cry from losses being expressed and worked on. The multiple losses of all populations presented here are likely to be denied, and forced into censorship. In addition to this potent disadvantage, we need to include additional cultural and ethologic-ecological influences and the developed niches within police and public-safety populations. That brings us into our next investigation of the core of PPS-CPTSD: the domain of disenfranchised, complicated, and complex loss.

COMPLEX LOSS: DISENFRANCHISED
AND COMPLICATED LOSS

Disenfranchised Loss

The phrase disenfranchised loss and grief was coined by the world's leading expert in this area of loss, Dr. Ken Doka, a gerontologist and Lutheran minister who pioneered what I suggest may be conceptualized as a core of Complex PTSD, disenfranchised loss. The patient who experiences many major losses may not understand what is hidden and unacknowledged from her conscious awareness. When losses are not accepted, sanctioned, openly acknowledged, socially supported, easily recognized, or publicly mourned, they become disenfranchised grief (Doka, 1985, 1989, 2002). Doka and Martin (2001) offer examples such as disability, unemployment, addiction, chronic pain, separation, divorce, and serial losses.

If we compound the disenfranchised losses with the impact of trauma and the dissociative processes that follow developmentally, there is abundant complexity to the presenting problem the officer-patient may bring to the therapy hour. In making that complexity palatable, keep in mind that when loss is disenfranchised and not adequately identified, even less so grieved, one's sense of what is important and real may feel threatened.

The absence of a validation of reality is the trauma and loss officer-patients experience. A dissociative approach to life may gain a superior advantage in which depersonalization, derealization, and surrealism may develop. The cost for those who have a tendency to dissociate is that fantasy may overwhelm a realistic view of life. That denial may be intrapsychic and compounded by cultural and eco-ethological influences. Massive denial may have its consequence: massive decompensation. The ignited keg that may be implicated in both massive denial and massive decompensation is likely to be found in disenfranchised loss. The experience as a whole, or in part, may become disenfranchised from the participant. That has been persuasively shown in other populations as a potential trigger for development of disenfranchised grief (Doka, 2002; Ellis, Williams, & Zinner, 1999; Rudofossi, 1994b; Schneidman, 1996; Silverstein, 1992; Worden, 2001). I suggest this is significant in varying levels in C-PTSD and dissociative disorders. It need not be repeated in our review of the clinical and research literature supporting that inference as feasible and prominent.

The significance of this disenfranchised traumatic loss may disrupt the development of identity in a hierarchical-based culture, as almost all police departments are. This hierarchy reinforces the explicit roles of rank with power and privilege. The implicit power derived from labels given by peers is not easily shaken. For example, being a "cop's cop," a "hero," a "rogue," or "psycho cop" in the internal power struggles for dominance and subordination in the context of identity and security, may remain subtle yet potent. The loss of status by application of a negative label may be associated with shame, humiliation, degradation, self negation, and deprecation from others. An officer-patient with a positive label as a hero can receive the brunt of ridicule if expectations that are too high are not met consistently: an impossible situation with consequent loss and narcissistic injury.

Legitimacy of rites for expressing loss and the right to grieve may become delimited, in Doka's conceptualization of sociological influences and rules. He supplements his clinical acumen with bountiful experience. He also presents a case for cultural differences that impact disenfranchised grief and styles of disenfranchised grieving (Doka & Martin, 2001). These important points are pertinent to our conceptualization about officer-patient's presentation of complex trauma and grief. Doka's insight aids in understanding that how officers are allowed to mourn may be affected by the "culture of counseling." How that culture of counseling deals with issues of social embarrassment and anxiety about grieving is influential. For example, while mourning a fallen fellow officer is a legitimate grief, mourning the loss of a partner with whom one may have worked with for years is often considered disturbed. Mourning a disability granted for a line of duty injury at 75% of one's pay is considered madness. Mourning the loss of a vagrant on one's beat is considered weak, unprofessional, and suspect—at worst an officer is labeled "shaky." Considering that many losses are disenfranchised, we are best served by listening to what Doka says so well in his model of disenfranchised grief. I will illustrate with an example for each point of reference.

Doka's Model of Disenfranchised Grief (Doka, 1989, 2002)

1. *There is a lack of acknowledgment that a loss has taken place.* For example, Mary, an FD medic, has achieved a friendly relationship with the local alcoholic, Larry, who, as Mary puts it, "Is kind of a nice guy." Larry got seriously injured during his latest drinking binge and was found in critical condition. Mary was called by local police and EMT units and administered first-aid rescue. She realized Larry suffered from severe injuries in what appeared to be an accidental fall. After administering first-aid rescue, Mary returned to home-base, Battalion X. She was met by her peers, most of whom were acting in accord with standard operating procedure (SOP). That SOP is similar to what Doka called "sociological legitimate mores," in this case, gallows humor, which delimited Mary's support in a way that demeaned her. Mary's sorrow and feeling of despair at the loss of Larry was met with ribald humor. Mary felt upset at her peers, yet she moved on in silence, suffering alone. Mary's loss was not acknowledged and even less sanctioned by her peers.

2. *There is a lack of recognition of the relationship.* Mary had the courage to take a risk and mentioned to some of her closer peers that she felt bad. She wanted to do something for Larry. In return for her plea for support, Mary received jibes: she put on a smile to avoid being spotted for what was in reality a stolid social display. Some jibes were, "Mary, what do you want to do? I suppose you'd like us to help you put him in a gold hearse?" Then, the putatively helpful emendation with, "Mary, oh Mary. Come on Mary, get real, sweetie! That dude was a scuz, he was a lowlife alkie, who gives a shit less?" The anger, shame, and feeling of humiliation was very real for Mary. It was compartmentalized in silence.

3. *There is an exclusion of the griever.* Mary wondered about what Larry's life was like before alcohol, and how, if any way, she could help. Yet, Mary learned her lesson well. She kept to herself. She felt his family would exclude her from attending Larry's funeral. She thought many times of making a ceremonial with her peers. She rejected this wish. She said, "It was just too weird to do something for a stranger, as her peers said." During this time, Larry was brought to the morgue to rule out foul play. Mary had not only experienced a silencing of her views, she was led to disenfranchising what was meaningful in her own view. The context of cultural and ecological pressure achieved the influence of enforcing silence in Mary.

4. *The context is a disenfranchisement of death itself.* Mary wanted to see Larry one last time. She pined away about it, and two days later she chose to head down to the morgue. She realized upon her arrival that Larry was taken out for burial in an unmarked grave in Potter's Field. No one had come to claim his body. When Mary tried to approach one of her peers, her peer said, "Are you for real, Mary? Come on. Don't waste your time. There are real victims who can use it. He's not a real person. Come on, I can see a *real victim* like some kid. You know that guy was a smelly rotten drunk. Shake it off. Remember you really got to develop a thick skin. That's good and healthy, so develop it, okay!" That pressure to disenfranchise one's genuine loss has a heavy cost in developing a festering wound without drainage. That is what complicated grief is all about. The drainage that is built up is evidenced for what has been called, *complicated mourning.*

Dr. Theresa Rando—Complicated Mourning

Rando has presented a number of important works on grief (1984, 1993). She defines grief as being uncomplicated or, in other cases, becoming complicated. We will look at her presentation of complicated mourning and grief. Rando suggests loss may be unacceptable from a specific cultural perspective, mythology. Such loss may not have an acceptable definition that allows its expression. Rando suggests these unacceptable losses are best observed from a relationship of the patient to himself, unacceptable losses in relation to others, and unacceptable losses in relation to one's culture or a dominant culture (1984, 1993).

Rando's focus on complicated grief and unacceptable losses is especially relevant to police and public-safety loss on a cultural, ecological, and sociological level. Her explication of loss includes unacknowledged, unsupported loss in which grieving is viewed as less than legitimate for certain situations. Readers are well advised to refer to Rando's later opus (1993) on complicated mourning. Some examples of those "certain situations" may be conceptualized as relevant to public-safety populations.

Unacceptable losses and complicated grief relevant to police and public safety are evidenced. Some examples include a correction officer who witnesses a fellow correction officer commit suicide; or a police officer experiences the loss of a partner who is incarcerated, suspended, or interrogated; a tenured detective in her homicide squad starts to feel painful and confusing loss for people who are considered unworthy of being truly grieved, such as prostitutes junkies, alcoholics, and homeless people. Manifestations of complicated grief may be related to self-blame and guilt schemas. This is exemplified by officers who may have guilt about actions in the field, where they view themselves as incompetent, unworthy, cowards, or fearful. Examples of some actions subject to these distortions are accidental discharge of a firearm, retreating during a public-safety action where other members are seriously injured, being beaten or injured in the line of duty or off duty, and losing safety equipment.

Rando points out multiple losses that may be overwhelming, sudden, and affecting many areas of the patient's life. In conceptualizing these multiple losses, Complex PTSD and dissociation may come into our focus. Rando shows how idealized loss may reflect a deep and profound loss. Idealized loss can lead to many other losses related to the ideal and all the investment lost in time and human space in the officer-patient's life.

Let us look at an example of a similar complicated loss. Captain Joan lost her dream of becoming a Deputy Inspector (DI). She served her Department for 41 years without any further political appointment and now faced mandated retirement. She dreamed of making her *wings*, that is, becoming a full Inspector, or Deputy chief. Captain Joan explains to you, "Politics and charm are not part of my repertoire, but excellent production and creativity is." Having bucked the political stream, she never became a favorite. At 62 years of age, she never achieved her "ideal image" of where she should be. Pursuit of that goal developed and was nurtured in what she felt earlier was an excellent choice of putting off marriage and having children to facilitate her moving up the ranks from Captain to Chief of Police. Achieving her life goal of getting to the top "has meant the world to me, but no big deal. That's life." You can hear massive denial in that sentence. If Captain Joan gave a life of investment to that goal, sacrificing pleasure and other desires, that loss *is* a big deal. It's the loss of many years of her life and living. Grieving that idealized loss comes with all the losses associated with her pursuit of that ideal. Those losses include a litany of other losses embedded in this occupational loss: wishes, dreams, and years invested in her pursuit of the Inspector's and even Chief's shield. None would be realized.

Captain Joan was forced to retire based on her age, which, although biased, was complicated by peers who told her, "Joan, I bet you're thrilled. Wow, it's your golden years. Are you in heaven or what?" Others say, "Joan you made it two times over your terms of service." In addition to traumas you start to uncover, Captain Joan brings up her recently receiving a possible detection of squamous cells in her breast region. She had never dealt with her fear over her own mortality. This example of Captain Joan's complicated and unmourned loss needs to be addressed. That loss is now presented in the context of an emerging and potentially pernicious form of cancer—the big C at the time of her retirement. Rando's ingenuity lies in many areas; locking into the least obvious may yield the greatest returns in the therapy hours. One return in our understanding of loss leads us into the subtle genius and contributions of Dr. R. R. Ellis, psychologist, artist, writer, jazz musician, and professor extraordinaire. I have learned a great deal from him and will now try to do some justice in presenting his work.

Complicated Thanatological Trauma
Anxiety and Dread

Dr. Richard R. Ellis, psychologist, scholar, and expert in thanatology and grief therapy, has made original contributions to the vocabulary of assessment and intervention in the area of loss. One of those doctoral students indebted to his incisive understanding and ability to teach and relate his extraordinary wisdom in clinical practice is this author.

Dr. Ellis suggests we pay keen attention to the patient's descriptions, chosen words, and attitudes toward grieving, loss, and death as well as acknowledging patients as individuals. This means we should look into the unique patterns of language the patient utilized and figure out how words are used, what words are chosen, and in what context they are used as a focus for our attention. That attention deliberately helps to guide our understanding in assessing whether or not a patient has understood that death really occurs and is part of everyone's life process. What fears does death hold for the patient?

This does not imply the obvious; with auras of loss, death-related topics are subtleties often neglected during the process of assessment, which may find the patient appearing anywhere on a continuum ranging from mature realization to extreme denial. This is an important point, because there are many paths that feed into thanatological-trauma anxiety or dread that are not death anxiety and dread. The difference is that thanatological-trauma anxiety is felt emotionally and psychophysiologically as trauma related to death, dying, or grieving. When this type of trauma comes into consciousness, anxiety emerges. That trauma includes the patient's intrusive memories in which the threat of death, witness to death, and relationship of the patient to the victim or survivor had some level of investment.

Thanatological dread of trauma reveals itself as extreme avoidance and massive denial in the patient. The question is, how can you hear thanatological dread of trauma? Dr. Ellis suggests that listening carefully can help you hear the subtle gradations of thanatological dread of trauma on a continuum (Ellis, 1992, 1994; Rudofossi & Ellis, 1999). The point on the continuum where the therapist may encourage the patient to openly discuss death in a meaningful way may be countered by the other extreme dread, avoidance and massive denial. Ellis suggests that at the core of extreme avoidance lies a complicated thanatological dread of trauma. While veridical understanding may be elusive, a closer approximation to truth may be facilitated by actively attuning your ear to the patient's descriptions of death, which include the patient's depictions of the value given to life, living, and his own mortality. It may be easier for the patient to ease into talking about death through the experiences of "important others."

That, too, gives you information that is useful about the way patients may need another significant person to validate their own choices or attitudes about death. However, it may help you develop a hypothesis about how the officer-patient needs to distance herself from death through the descriptions of other people. In another way of looking at this tendency, you may observe an inroad for support and motivation for autoexposure to thanatologic dread of trauma by the officer being able to come in to engage in therapy. That exposure may enhance actual coping with equally effective cognitive reassessment of the thanatological dread of trauma. On the other hand, Ellis (1994) suggests the officer-patient's attempt at autoexposure to this type of trauma may support an avoidance, rather than mastery of thanatological dread of trauma.

Supernatural Beliefs After Experiencing Complex Trauma

Another of Ellis's contributions is identifying supernatural beliefs in a patient's presentation that are superordinate to cultural and religious beliefs (1994). Supernatural beliefs may support irrational schemas that support consequent emotional distress, which may be hidden because the patient may not express them directly or even indirectly as part of resistance to disclosure, which may be a fear of you labeling him. Ellis also suggests that resistance may be due in part to the therapist's desire to see the patient as a rational, educated professional, not as a person who still may abide by superstitious beliefs. Ellis (1994) accepts a theory of hidden supernatural beliefs as helping in assessing complicated grief. His conjecture is compelling and insightful.

Applying Ellis's (1994) insight into understanding supernatural beliefs as being a relevant factor in some officer-patients denial of grief is helpful as is assessing the officer-patient's supernatural schemas as a factor in creating emotional distress. That emotional distress may be a mix of terror of "approach and avoidance" about some ritual behavior, and the outcome being feared as having catastrophic consequences. It may be that those distortions may escalate and accrete as cumulative trauma where violent death is part of that experience as adults. Officer-patients who have experienced long periods of trauma may have superstitious beliefs that they believe may have caused the tragic event. Actions or inaction may be misinterpreted as related to supernatural beliefs. Resistance about any disclosure of these beliefs is fueled by fear the therapist may degrade, humiliate, or withdraw from the officer-patient for that belief. It may be hard to detect supporting irrational beliefs leading to terror and extreme anxiety, which may become obfuscated or dismissed before the therapist gets a handle on how deleterious these beliefs are. How can this happen?

In the case of an officer-patient with a graduate education in mental health, the therapist might not consider supernatural beliefs. The supernatural beliefs may or may not be cultural beliefs, but may result from a supercultural belief in supernatural aspects that leads to trauma, loss, and influences prior to that officer's education and training. It can persist in the officer-patient, which can be very disturbing to her patient. The supernatural belief may be far from a religious or spiritual foundation of patient's faith. The belief in that superstition ensures a denial of death, and the officer-patient may induce trauma when her behavior follows a stereotypical performance. Perhaps what Ellis proffers to us as clinicians is a prescription that is a proscription against precogitating how patients must deal with loss.

Ellis's approach suggests an aphorism for our approach to complex trauma which I express as follows: *if we can tolerate that a veridical understanding of trauma is as elusive as Elysian fields with marshmallow strawberries, then we can see a clearer vision that captures some glimpses of the patient's evolution in therapy and outside of therapy. That acceptance may help us lead to an encounter with the officer-patient made genuine by accepting that we cannot reach a complete understanding of the trauma and grief of someone else.* That subtle but poignant truth brings us to another helpful inroad with officer-patients suffering from trauma. The words chosen and the way patients speak to you about other people's perspective about life and death is a way of gauging their own traumatic thanatological anxiety and dread. This important distinction offers a new insight and approach to C-PTSD and dissociative disorders when put in perspective with police and public-safety populations. An avoidance and excessive discomfort with the experience of thanatological dread can be due to excessive exposure to trauma and loss. Conversely, a desire followed by behavior that the officer-patient presents in wanting to be near death, becoming immersed in death investigations, or the morbid details of death, may be an attempt to numb the intrusive symptoms and fears associated with thanatological dread. As in the defense mechanism of "reaction-formation," the patient may present the opposite unconscious motivation of what she truly desires, which is not only dynamic, but existential and involves the loss of meaning in suffering experienced as despair.

Another variation may be that silence in response to death and loss is indicative of how far removed a patient may be from loss, and that includes loss related to traumatic experiences. The ability of an officer-patient to talk about death without feeling and experiencing its meaningfulness may indicate numbness, intellectualization, and denial. In approaching death as a therapist, being aware of your own mortality and acceptance of your own mortality helps you by conveying your sensibility and attitude to the patient by your own toleration of death situations about which the officer-patient speaks. This is not suggesting that death is easy to accept for anyone, including you and me, but it is important to be able to tolerate this part of life. Our therapeutic task is working on understanding the superstitious foundation patients believe. We will now look at some other tasks that Worden has presented as important in understanding four variations of complicated grief.

DR. J. WILLIAM WORDEN: CHRONIC, DELAYED, EXCESSIVE, MASKED—COMPLICATED GRIEF

Dr. Worden's prodigious background includes advanced degrees in theology, a doctorate in psychology, as well as research and clinical work that spans three decades. I will present his layout of complicated and pathological grief. Worden defines mourning as the more general process people experience after a loss. However, grief refers to the individual's reaction to the loss. Worden advocates, along with Freud, that mourning is an active process (Worden, 2001) and includes the patient's active involvement with what Worden calls tasks of grieving, which are objectives the patient fulfills, not outcomes that time passively brings forth as so much therapeutic manna.

The patient successfully mourns the loss if she achieves the four tasks of grieving (Worden, 2001):

1. *To accept the reality of the loss.* Keep in mind loss can range over a broad variety of types and in different contexts.
2. *To work through the pain of the loss.* When the actual feelings are facilitated through being able to express what one is feeling and to accept those feelings.
3. *To adjust to an environment in which the deceased is missing.* When the patient can feel and understand that the deceased is not coming back, that the person has died. This is not without respect for the religious and spiritual beliefs of patients. It is a situation in which the bodily form of the deceased will not come around the corner one more time.
4. *To emotionally relocate the deceased and move on with life.* In this task, the dead person is not hidden somewhere nor forgotten, but remembered

in a very human way as the real and fallible person was. The deceased is no longer an ever-present influence in the life of the griever. Moving on with life means integration and investment in one's own life and goals without the deceased.

Of course, loss of a person to death is not the only loss one can experience. The list of other losses we can grieve for is almost endless: status, ideas, health, wealth, body parts, relationships, possessions, hope, faith, etc., etc., etc.

FOUR VARIATIONS OF COMPLICATED GRIEF REACTIONS

1. *Chronic grief reactions* are longer than cultural and social norms suggest for relatives, cohorts, peers, and people with the same background. The patient may not continue with living meaningfully. One may mourn "what might have been, but never was to be."

That loss may be expressed through intense hope and searching for the lost relationship and person. Intense despair may follow at times when the lost person or other, such as a pet, does not return. Although a healthy level of ambivalence exists in all relationships, Worden (2001) addresses the unhealthy ambivalence of excessive hate and love toward a significant other, which, in the context of PPS-CPTSD, may be part of chronic grief reactions and disso-ciative splitting.

Noteworthy is a high level of dependence and attachment to the person now lost. An example you may see in your practice is a shattering of the relation-ship between police partners. Often they had shared years together in many life-threatening situations. The loss of the partner may create an unhealthy ambivalence (disenfranchised in the culture), which may result in chronic grief reactions (Rudofossi, 1997).

Let us look at the case example of Irving, a seasoned patrolperson, who took the promotional exam and was promoted a year ago. Irving briefly let his partner of three years, Sally, know he would miss her. Their last night together on the job Irving had dinner with her. They shared war stories and cajoled each other about job-related thinly veiled sexual innuendos in a tasteful way (not uncommon between male and female officers). He never expressed to her that he enjoyed working with her. Instead, he departed with a gruff nod and exhorted her to "Take care of yourself, Sally." While more verbal, Sally was as emo-tionally stolid. They both moved on. Sally got a new partner, and Irving moved on to his new position as sergeant.

I became Irving's therapist. At first, Irving denied feeling any loss associated with his losing his partner Sally. As far as his promotion, he said, "Doc, it's the best thing that could have happened to me." Stopping, he looked at me as an officer will when he gets into his command presence mode, and stared at me saying, "Like I said, it was the best thing that happened to me. I mean it. I really do, you know?" I was far from convinced by his presentation. I thought and conjectured as a hunch. If Officer Irving truly felt "promotion was the best thing in the world," then why did he choose the words he did, repeat them and look down at me from his command stance? Police officers will do this. Had he really felt that way, he most likely would have said only, "The best thing that happened to me" period. He would not follow up with the clear disavowal, "I mean it. I really do, you know?" followed with the stare to convince me. It gave me a hint of how important being a police officer was in his life rather than his promotion to sergeant.

I was partially correct in my hunch. He had ambivalent feelings toward being promoted. He started many reminiscences about Sally: how she was, and what she was doing. Other losses in regard to his buddies in the precinct platoon emerged with less intensity. As he put it, "I enjoyed pounding the beat. You know my partner Sally. You know that feisty, shrewd, argumentative, yet highly capable street cop she was. I miss her, you know." That was followed by tears. That was the beginning of our work.

2. *Delayed grief reactions* may be inhibited, suppressed, and postponed. Although the possibility of emotional expression maybe expressed, it is not intense enough for a real mourning and grieving process. This is especially true when the culture says that expressing loss and grief is not appropriate because of someone's responsibility and position. For example, in public safety, first responders just do not mourn the loss of people who commit suicide, substance abusers, or the mentally ill (disenfranchised loss). This may be evidenced with peers in a situation where an officer took his own life and possibly another's. The loss expressed by one officer may receive ridicule because that officer is perceived as no longer being worthy of the shield. That is, the deceased went beyond the boundaries of police mores and is now unacceptable as an appropriate officer to be mourned. The loss may be compounded by influences within and without the department. Guilt over what the former partner may have done to reach out and help that officer can become overwhelming if unspoken. Let us look at an example. Tommy's former partner and friend, Bobby, died of a self-inflicted gunshot wound. What had transpired in a reconstruction of the suicide/homicide was that Bobby confronted his significant other and a third party assumed to be part of a love tryst. Bobby shot and killed all parties. Tommy was feeling numbness, anger, shock, guilt, and overwhelming sadness and fear about Bobby's murder/homicide. Some of the other members of the command said they would simply neither go to the funeral nor give any funds to Bobby's family, but would only donate to the significant other's family. Bobby, they said, "Lost his shield, never deserved it, and had become no better then a perp." Upon hearing this, Tommy closed up like a clam and kept it bottled up. It emerged 15 years later while he was discussing his new initiative in an antibias public-safety program for victims of assault.

3. *Exaggerated grief reactions* are associated with a patient whose symptoms may be expressed in an excessive way. Behaviors, cognitions, and emotions related to grieving may become excessive and disabling. As Worden (2001) points out, this excessive expression can indicate comorbidity with other disorders, which may be illustrated with depression coexisting with exaggerated grief reactions. Serious clinical disorders may develop after a loss, which can act as a catalyst. One example is Correction Officer (C.O.) Pam whose partner Shawnique was assaulted seven years ago.

C.O. Pam felt she should have acted differently and felt guilt related to her role in the attack. Pam felt she could have thwarted the assault by inmates who tried to take over the cell block. We explored guilt, including a variant of survivor guilt when officer-patients believe they have contributed to some injury, although not death, of the surviving partner. As we explored her loss and associated thoughts about her role in the trauma, Officer Pam expressed symptoms consistent with unipolar depression (premorbid) and PTSD. The assessment of Officer Pam included a comorbid diagnosis of depression mixed with delayed PTSD and complicated grief.

4. *Masked grief reactions* may be experienced as symptomatic presentation, which can cause difficulty in the officer-patient's life. However, that officer-patient does not see or recognize the fact that symptoms are related to the experience of loss. An absence of expressed grief may be as pathological as excessive reactions in time and intensity.

The key here is insufficiently developed ego strength to deal with the loss through the work of mourning, which does not go away but lingers underground. Masked grief reactions can be expressed through symptomatic presentation or through some maladaptive behavior.

Let us look at an example of masked grief through one traumatic loss of Firefighter Officer Y, who presented many high-risk behaviors. He shared dangerous risks that developed about three years ago, such as bungee jumping, driving in collision derbies, and parachuting in rough terrain. During a thorough assessment, FF Officer Y gave a detailed account of his firehouse buddy, whom he could not save after finding himself trapped and needing to get out or be burned alive. While Officer Y said, "I made it home without incident. My best friend did not," he assured himself and his peers he had brushed off the loss as forgotten and done, his avoidance was matched with feelings of "being alone" and "numbing out" when he thought of his buddy, who was buried in a closed-casket funeral. FF Officer Y did not attend because he said he had gotten sick at the time. He shared that he had many days off when he had a "strange bug." The doctors could not find a medical cause.

We eventually understood the emergence of that strange bug presented as an illness about a week before, during, and about a week after the anniversary of his best buddy's death (another clue of a conversion disorder related to unmourned loss). Officer Y never visited the gravesite (another clue of massive denial). He expressed how he felt better with his great new energy that allowed him to take more risks. During one session, he told how his risk-taking enabled him to do the right thing. After my Socratic follow-up in a gentle, but persistent probe of "What was doing that right thing?" an answer emerged. Risk taking served as an unconscious compensation for imagined failings as an officer. Officer Y said to me, "If I had real privates, I could have prevented my friend's death." When I responded how difficult it must have been for him, he replied, "No, not at all!" Officer Y continued, "Now I know myself, what I have to continue doing is make sure that no one would die again over my inability to do what I had to do." His latest attempt to "undo" his overwhelming guilt in this masked grief reaction was diving off Montauk, Long Island, where he would face a white shark in a steel cage. His other major defense was somatically to experience the weird bug, which consisted of itching and burning pain that predictably came at the anniversary of the original traumatic loss. It may be the officer acted out what he could not express. Once the loss was identified, the somatic symptoms and the excessive risk-taking was no longer necessary to undo Officer Y's loss. Picking up the clues is an important task in your assessment of complicated grief.

Fortunately, Worden presents clues to aid us in identifying complicated grief.

WORDEN'S ELEVEN CLUES TO HELP IDENTIFY COMPLICATED GRIEF (2001)

Clue 1—The patient may not be able to speak about the deceased without experiencing intense and fresh grief anytime the person's name is mentioned.

Clue 2—Even minor events trigger an intense grief reaction, which is related to the patient's losses.

Clue 3—During your sessions, the patient presents themes of loss.

Clue 4—Material possessions of the deceased are left in their original position, preserving the environment as it was at the time of the death.

Clue 5—Physical symptoms may mimic the illness or injury the deceased experienced.

Clue 6—Radical changes in the patient's lifestyle accompany the loss, which may include significant relationships being ignored or ended abruptly.

Clue 7—The patient exhibits guilt and lowered self-esteem through subclinical depression or false euphoria.

Clue 8—The patient exercises a compulsion to imitate the dead as a way of gaining restitution and forgiveness.

Clue 9—There is indulgence in self-destructive impulses.

Clue 10—Unaccountable sadness occurs around certain times of the year without awareness that this is in sync with the anniversary.

Clue 11—A phobia about illness or about death is often related to the illness that took the deceased.

Worden's (2001) clues leave us with a practical and conceptual framework for approaching complex grief reactions.

R. R. Ellis reminds us,

> Any of these eleven clues may, in milder forms be present in uncomplicated grief. Usually in uncomplicated grief the clues eventually diminish significantly or disappear. Complications exist if any clue persists unabatedly at a high level of intensity for an inordinate amount of time. Remember that no one knows what would be a so called normal length of time; it depends on the individual case. (Ellis, 1994)

The branch of complex trauma we have reviewed has served its purpose if you have a working knowledge base for recognizing the complicated grief in PPS-CPTSD.

DISENFRANCHISED AND COMPLEX GRIEF AND DISSOCIATIVE DISORDERS: PPS-CPTSD

As we have observed, death and thanatological trauma are prolific in police and public-safety populations. Consider that disenfranchisement of traumatic loss may have put off mourning and grief work for a career spanning two to four decades of an officer's life. Officer-patients have developed persistent personality styles in response to the experiences of field trauma. A career of the typical officer-patient is from 10 to 40 years, averaging 20 years.

During this time, the cumulative experience of secondary trauma by moribund, gallows humor and structural foundations are likely to fall apart when the officer-patient attempts to assimilate into the mainstream culture. Officer-patients who have developed very sophisticated skills within their ecological niche may experience their darkest hour upon their retirement. That may also occur when restless activity ceases because of reassignment to modified duties or placement on sick report; perhaps because the restless activity and defenses to ward off a bombardment of unacknowledged losses and multiple traumas emerge all at once. *That conspiracy of silence becomes deafening in its thunderous exclamation in the swells of the grief of trauma.*

Once again we are challenged as clinicians in our attempts to understand this phenomenon. It may be a perceptual shock, which is a structural displacement into a niche unsupported by experience, which we will address as the last branch of complex trauma. That psychomedical sequella of stress and maladaptive resistance toward "working through" is predictably related to hypertension, diabetes, heart attacks, strokes, and ultimately premature morbidity.

The prevention of any of those deleterious outcomes begins with responsible treatment of PPS-CPTSD syndromes presented as complex grief, trauma, and dissociative disorders. Often in these instances the defenses are placed in a context that facilitates a sensibility as well as an applied approach within what I have developed as the eco-ethological approach.

ECO-ETHOLOGICAL EXISTENTIAL ANALYSIS: FOUNDATIONS IN LOGOTHERAPY

Before we approach PPS-CPTSD through the ecological and ethological approach, we will first review salient points in Frankl's existential analysis/ logotherapy (Frankl, 1978, 1988, 2000). A modified existential analysis is critical to a theory and intervention-based therapy with traumatized officer-patients. There are four reasons why this is so: The existentially informed perspective offers a solid boundary that accepts drives and their derivatives as influences within a human ecology. Second, an evolutionary perspective that guides an ecological-ethological perspective of human perception of trauma and loss may be best balanced by a meaningful basis of what is ethically sound in a perspective that acknowledges conscience and choice, which, when exercised responsibly, is responsive to a police and public-safety culture and perspective. Third, conscience and ethics as a conscious choice are preeminent in the scientific approach. By extending and making that choice explicit, we are extending what exists through our approach as clinicians. Without ethics and conscience, one cannot conduct science, including applied biological insight and its larger science of applied psychology. Fourth, to speak about human evolution and drive derivatives without a human context is to not speak about human evolution at all. But it may be a reified superstition of what humans are supposed to be like abstractly. Perhaps we can call that bias "animal morphism."

Suggesting that, human evolution is best seen only in terms of progress and perfection of the human race. That bias may be a step toward reinforcing social Darwinism, and that has been chillingly tried already in the Third Reich. It is a misunderstanding of human evolution as we are imperfect and will always be.

While these four reasons may be my own skewed view, I believe we have evolved as therapists to realize that the existential meaning in our lives is best complemented by a humility and commonality in the human condition, which includes acknowledging the drive derivatives without excusing away our ability to choose. It is our choice that remains primary in our view of human development. If not, civilization itself may be threatened. *While cultural competence is critical to this approach and all effective approaches, including those of trauma and grief therapy, we serve no benevolent outcome when we condone bigotry or bias in the name of any cultural, ecological, or ethological influence, including political correctness.* However, we can better understand what occurs with the hope of connection, which is what the existentialists contribute in encounter and engagement at the deepest level of being genuine. I have therefore presented what hopefully expands Frankl's contributions to my own eco-ethological approach to loss in trauma in ambulatory and traditional assessment and treatment with officer-patients.

In keeping with my stance, we cannot separate what initially and theoretically emerged as two distinct and parallel paths: the existential as Frankl applied it, my modification of his approach for use with traumatized public-safety officers, and the eco-ethological approach I developed. My approach remains balanced by keeping the existential insight and method Frankl posited as an indispensable component of trauma within the reality of the human condition, which includes the drives and conflicts where unconscious and conscious move in ever-increasing complexities; suggesting drives and their derivatives have evolved in what has created "existential vacuums," which exist in and are inseparable from ecological niches of trauma and loss. We may dare to embrace existential foundations in which meaning converges with drive derivatives and ecological niches on perpendicular intersecting planes rather than two parallel planes never meeting on finite landscapes of experience, such as grief in trauma. The convergence may be where meaning is derived when drive derivatives are placed within an ecological system with ethological influences that evolve with meaning, or the rejection of meaning, in life itself.

Frankl makes a point that suggests a historical truth in a creative wish. He suggests the Holocaust, in which millions died, was related to one person who acted as a catalyst for the most aggressive acting out of destructive instincts: Adolph Hitler. Frankl suggests that if Hitler had confronted his demons in an existential way by means of not repressing his own voice and conscience through a will to meaning, his monstrosities may have been turned around into a socially useful avenue. How that may be achieved is interestingly couched in Frankl's fictional role as a psychotherapist with Hitler as his patient.

> It follows a psychotherapist must not impose a value on the patient. The patient must be referred to his own conscience. And if I am asked, as I am time and again, whether this neutralism would have to be maintained even in the case of Hitler. I answer in the affirmative because I am convinced that Hitler would never have become what he did unless he had suppressed within himself the voice of conscience. (Frankl, 1988, p. 66)

Whether or not we agree with these implications, Frankl's imaginative suggestion has a compelling resonance. Propaganda and terrorism are the greatest threats to choice and conscience. If viewed from our conceptual framework of trauma and loss, they are a motivating force to choose well. Frankl writes,

> Man is pushed by drives. But he is pulled by values. He is always free to accept or to reject a value a situation offers. Values will still have to stand a test, the test of man's conscience unless he refuses to obey his conscience and suppresses its voice. (Frankl, 1978, p. 57)

In a succinct message, George Santayana says it all: "those who cannot remember the past are condemned to repeat it" (Santayana, 1906). The history of interest here is that of the officer-patient's experiences of loss and trauma. The clinician's task is helping him to speak of it in his own voice.

THE ECO-ETHOLOGICAL APPROACH TO TRAUMA IN AN EXISTENTIAL PERSPECTIVE

Like other types of trauma brought before the clinician, public-safety trauma is acute, sudden, and usually beyond control. Further, it is not one static event but multiple influences that merge as an experience, and may be nested within one event in relation to multiple other events. The context is one of an active participant, whose selective attention is changing in the different pick-up of information. The imposed roles are ever-changing within the flow of public-safety experience—no less than the river of Heraclitus, and as complex as Lucretius elements.

In fact, that perpetual change may be a strong indicator of where the dilemma lies. In many cases, the officer-patient believes, "There is no real retreat. I will be back in the bag (pounding the beat), so why bother thinking twice about it. If I try to retreat, I'll be labeled a crybaby. No thanks. Onward and forward." Sadly, onward and forward, as we have already observed, is likely to become untoward damage, which emerges like a volcanic eruption, when it can no longer be contained in compartments or states of unconsciousness as in dissociation.

The countertransference of disgust, revulsion, fear, and anxiety for the therapist can unwittingly collude with the officer-patient's despair. Psychoanalytic therapy sheds light on not only conceptualizing this resistance, but in working through it. This is accomplished through making conscious the conflicts of transference and countertransference and compromise formations that emerge over time (Brenner, 1976, 1982).

In addition, logotherapy addresses the different problems of despair, anguish, and existential angst addressed by exploration of meaning in the patient's life. That meaning is what may be the most important inroad to whether or not an officer-patient chooses life or, on a continuum, chooses to embrace self-sabotage. Yes, the choice is his.

Self-sabotage can destroy an officer-patient's life on a conscious and unconscious level. Our understanding of this choice may be life saving when we can facilitate insight of why and how to change this self-sabotage. Only by our understanding and consistent attitude of interpreting the conflicts of the officer-patient can we hope to share that perspective with him.

A DIFFICULT EXISTENTIAL CHALLENGE:
TO DISILLUSIONMENT AND LACK OF TRUST

At times you may experience an officer-patient's challenge to his choice of coming forward and trying out therapy. Some of these challenges are drawn from my practice: "Hey, Doc, why the hell should I bother with therapy? To get better and then get thrown out on the streets again?"; "What can you really offer me that a bottle of booze and a warm chick can't?"; "What is meaningful in a life full of death and misery and day-in-and-day-out warfare, even though you've been a cop? What do you know right now about the war on the streets?"; "Who understands my pain? Who will take a fall for me and with me when all the shit hits the fan? Will you?"; "Can you blame me for feeling so self-reliant? I've read Emerson and I trust only my buddies. I need time to trust you. 'Till then, I'm going to check you out."

As a Cop-Doc, I have been stopped in my tracks by officers who challenge my intentions and empathy, attempting to engage them. *It is important to understand that some officer-patients simply will not be motivated, regardless of your skill.* For example, no matter what attempt I made to break through the resistance of some officer-patients, I could not. My attempts were rendered futile. The officer-patient you get to know may present initially as narcissistic, hostile, anxious, raging, sarcastic, withdrawn, and self-deprecating all, in various permutations and dosages.

The majority of officer-patients eventually will accept that you do have something to offer them, as happened in my own experience time and again. I believe, in retrospect, that development occurred because I had the attitude of toleration, confidence, and optimism in that officer-patient's ability to find meaning in his life. I was able to relate that attitude to the officer-patient.

However, the officer-patients first needed to tell me the facts of their stories before any such relationships could develop. *In fact, many had pummeled their beat with too many disappointments and did not want to add yet another one—me!* After years of disappointment and disillusionment, their scoffing at my attempts to open their walled-off space of defense through resistance was understandable. The officer-patient's walls were shaped through perceived self-preservation. They would not be torn down by my direct confrontation. I understood these defenses. They made superb sense. That sensibility included a defensive constellation built around complicated, disenfranchised trauma and loss understood through a psychodynamic, cognitive-behavioral, eco-ethological, and existential perspective.

Put in sharper perspective, the day-in-and-day-out ecology of trauma and loss may have imposed a stronghold of defenses, which is better understood in the context of resistance, which, as we have reviewed, is a defense against disclosure. Distortion about feelings and ideas about the therapist abound. While well known, that is very hard for you and me to tolerate. Understanding that the destructive impulse and aggressive tendency is not neutralized through a maturational and environmental process is bound to repeat itself in the forging of many relationships. The relationship that is ripe for the picking falls on us as the counselor, therapist, facilitator, doctor, or master of the healing mind. Still, hardship follows when your toleration of maintaining a professional and empathic stance as therapist is challenged to the edge. Indubitably, no matter how capable and sophisticated you are, that challenge is likely to be presented on a number of fronts, as illustrated in the examples above. That front of resistance can derail you if you're not aware of the vacuum that complex trauma and grief can shape. *After all, in the officer-patient's frame of reference, I am at best, as you are, a well-meaning stranger; at worst, another disappointing relationship in the making.* It is important to realize that our commitment for doing our type of work will be challenged up front. Preparing for that does not require alarm, but you are required to have on hand your strategy for initially engaging the officer-patient on his own terms, without losing your own.

Often, with time and your tolerance, what follows your persistent attitude of toleration is a positive payoff, the fruit of which is a clarification of defenses that you can expose meaningfully and insightfully. That exposure may be the deconstruction of walls that have served the purpose of maladaptation, a situation impermeable to outsiders.

It is important to realize that you are not the officer-patient's object of ridicule, but you may be the subject of an officer-patient's expression of scorn. From a psychoanalytic perspective, as Brenner reminds us, transference is ubiquitous, as is the expression of an internal conflict between unmourned losses and compromise formations (Brenner, 1974, 1976, 1982). I suggest that if the officer-patient can accept that outlook, he may gain a new perspective. A transference to other disappointing authority figures can reemerge as disappointing. Rediscovering the motivation for becoming an officer in the first place can lead to redemption of energy displaced in the dysphoria of trauma.

That redemption of energy also may be viewed as complementary to the cognitive-behavioral approach (Beck, 1985; Ellis, 1962, 1985; Freeman & Reinecke, 1993; Lazarus, 1972), which suggests that allowing creative impulses to be enjoyed and committing to meaningful work will help to increase happiness, pleasure, and finding meaning in life. The psychodynamic approach suggests increasing the ability to find intimacy, pleasure, and mature expression with another human being. Bringing out the unconscious struggle and compromise formations of the patient gradually leads to increasing the conscious ability to embrace pleasure, meaning, and intimacy.

Although the means to achieve these ends are different, the commonality lies in the goal. In all approaches, the goal is actually to find meaning, pleasure, and creativity in one's life. In the existential perspective, the officer can regain meaning in his life. That also puts in perspective the threats of terrorism officers endure, as Frankl (1988) points to his experiences in the death camps, where, as long as he had a reason to live, he could, and did bear any suffering. If we ever needed this message from a courageous human being who embraced the meaning of Arête, it is now. What is relevant to our understanding now is specifying a problem related to resistance toward life itself. If you stare into the abyss from a precipice that has no clear boundary, and you intend to etch an experience of meaningful engagement, "You may find that abyss staring right back at you," as Nietzsche suggested (1888/1985).

The abyss of cynicism, burnout, and stress of public-service professionals epitomizes what Frankl called the *existential vacuum* (2000). He defines existential vacuum as the "frustration of the will to meaning" (1988, p. 24). He elaborates on the disparate consequences of the existential vacuum in comparison with finding meaning in life.

> The most important need, however, the basic need for meaning, remains more often than not ignored and neglected. And it is so important because once a man's will to meaning is fulfilled; he becomes capable of suffering, of coping with frustrations and tensions. On the other hand, if man's will to meaning is frustrated, he is equally inclined to take his (own) life. . . ." (1988, p. 22)

Multiple trauma and loss that are dissociated, complex, and disenfranchised may defy the therapeutic tasks at hand. When Freud coined "working through" (1924a), he meant working through the traumatic losses. Energy can hardly be spared and even less likely expended wastefully. Yet, that is what happens if one's own choice of meaning is frustrated. But how does that frustration on an existential level come about, and how is it likely to be expressed to you?

Unheard Disenfranchised Grief and the Cry for Expression

Sadly, disenfranchisement of the very trauma and loss experienced may often lead to a rejection of life on an existential level, because it seems meaningless and frustrating. As one officer, who had written her sketch of grief on her flysheet of a patrol memo pad shared, "I swim in a cesspool of human tragedy, who am I to think I can clear the refuse? Besides, that has become my source of inspiration and desperation. Which pool will I dip my future in?" While eloquent and poignant as a razor's slice, that level of disillusionment is all too common.

Many officer-patients you will see are hurting badly, suffering from that "psych-ache" that Schneidman so aptly described and reviewed in my earlier publication (Rudofossi, 2007; Schneidman, 1996). These projections may be and are likely to include very early life conflicts and vulnerabilities unique to his history. Some are infantile in origin, although evolved through altered presentations. What may be projected onto you is a reflection of reality as the officer perceives it: a reality of disenfranchised trauma and grief that have been heaped into unrealized loss, aching for expression.

That aching for expression of unrealized loss may be expressed if you as a therapist believe there is a meaning in life and living. While some existential therapists point out that existential tenets are best received without ultimate meaning, I would agree with Frankl in the title of his classic, that "ultimate meaning" is integral as a motivation to move on (Frankl, 2000). The will to find what is meaningful in the daily lives of officer-patients defies description, yet it suggests finding meaning in work, creativity, and worthwhile investment in life as critical. The challenge of resistance is in defiance to your well-timed and empathic interventions.

Keep in mind, a consistent empathic and tolerant attitude (including empathic failures: not intentional, but subject to idealized distortions as well as demonized distortions) may help create a new response in the officer-patient to openly disclose to you. However, this is by no means likely to be achieved with ease.

Whether the valence is exacerbated more by "tendency/endogenous" or ecological-ethological influences in the formation of that distress, an over-whelming critical mass has been reached, the threshold has been experienced. The stance that the officer-patient makes may influence his commitment to therapy, which relevant to our population of officer-patients, in which depersonalization, derealization, suffering, anomie, and existential despair can set in due to the apparent void of an abyss where meaning once was. That may be the thread linking the somatic and psychic healing through other means and techniques that complement this clinical approach, in which meaning is explored, not prescribed. Insight is supported by each officer-patient finding meaning in the suffering through loss in the trauma he presents to us as therapists.

Our Attitude Facilitates Choice: Existential Meaning or Despair?

You may be pondering why I have chosen to place the importance of the therapist's attitude in the context of a conceptual foundation of police and public-safety Complex PTSD. That good question is answered in part with our conceptual background, which has been achieved at this point in our conversation. Realizing what is not spoken, unrealized, and unidentified may be the most important work we have to focus on to be effective. This realization requires genuine compassion on our part, which is a component of our attitude. Conveying your attitude with compassion is informed by your preparation of the fundamental groundwork. Compassion can be delivered from a number of stances, including one that is supportive, neutral, active, and a combination of all three. Choosing life is a fundamental choice that demands our attention.

Choosing Life: A Fundamental Choice, Responsibility, and Will to Meaning

The context of the basic motivation to choose life, and to engage in healing through therapy, is so fundamental that it may be forgotten in our approach to what we take for granted in our officer-patients. That assumption can lead even the best of therapists to miss the SOS call from our patients, which will likely be infused with all the difficult manifestations of resistance you will encounter.

What may remain unexposed is the crucial pivot of motivation and commitment toward choosing life. Without this fundamental, we cannot begin our work at all. The motivation that may fuel the officer-patient's ability to embrace choice is making the choice explicit, that is, to choose life over death and its destructive and self-sabotaging drive derivatives. These can include drinking oneself to death, taking risks so great that flirtation with death is played out on a daily basis, accidental death whereby conscious awareness was blocked in one's choice for self-preservation, and the more obvious choice of direct suicide.

Considering that an officer-patient's lack of trust and belief may have emerged in an ecology of deprivation and disappointments on the beat, which is of the worst type: an officer-patient is treated with indifference when trying to express the meaning of his suffering. Prior to the officer-patient gaining a perspective of meaning, your understanding that his meaning may be lost, may be the first of steps in helping him rediscover what is meaningful in his life. That meaning may be approached on a number of levels and within different approaches. I suggest the existential one offers an avenue that is adequate to meet the need.

Facts Are Not Fate: Even in the Midst of Existential Despair

Frankl offered a living legacy, which ought to stand as his epitaph. It is the gift of wisdom imparted by his genius: "Facts are not fate. What matters is the stand we take toward them. . . . One must go through his own existential despair if he is to learn how to immunize his patients against it" (1978, p. 137).

That inspiration may help us in our work. Our stand includes the suggestion of choice and validation of an officer's experiences. Those experiences cumulatively may have precluded any mutual dance, having been staged in a stadium constructed of voids, perhaps culminating in a sense of futility and despair. That despair about a life-long investment in an ecology of violence and suffering may spur the triad of the existential vacuum that Frankl presents as the context of existential despair: *addictive behaviors*: alcoholism, indiscrete sexuality, gambling and high-risk taking; depression, self-sabotage, and suicide; and aggression as moments of rage (Frankl, 1988, 2000; Graber, 2003). That toll of unrequited loss in the vortex of trauma in a majority of public servants is evident by this triad of the existential vacuum (Ainsworth, 1995; Barnes, 2007; Benner, 1991, 1998, 2001; Ker Muir, Jr., 1977; Kirschman, 1997; Lambert,

1986; Lifton, 1973, 1980; Mitchell, 1988; Mitchell & Everly, 1996; Neiderhoffer, 1967; Reese, 1991; Rudofossi, 1997; Southwick, 2007; Thorpe, 2007; Toch, 2002). The triad of the existential vacuum suggests the symptomatic despair, cynicism, and pessimism experienced by public-safety and police officers, which includes the noncommissioned and commissioned soldiers.

The ability to function may not be an adequate measure for weighing existential despair. Your clinical skills may be the best measuring tools of all. Varnishing the exterior of an oak tree does not lessen the unseen inner decay. The husk is not without the seed of what may be reborn in the crucible of therapy that seeks to find what was lost. Trauma cannot exist without loss; it always holds a wound and emptiness. Logotherapy is one therapy that embodies meaning. Logotherapy suggests life is meaningful—even when the worst has occurred, as in the Holocaust. Officer-patients can relate to Frankl, who was a real thriver, who responded to massive and repetitive trauma and loss himself.

While a massive trauma can be denied, it will leak out. If we pay attention, we will see that ooze. Trauma is defined as a wound; an open wound is one that has not healed. Where healing has begun, raw scars of psychic tissue appear. Grieving the disenfranchised and complex trauma is a painful journey. Withered clichés on the calloused skin of overuse today can lead to the officer-patient's leaking out his denial. "I'm okay, it's standard operating procedure to deal with death." That is a hint about how deep the acculturation follows the ecological demands. I suggest that no apology for identifying existential despair is needed. What humans are capable of reaching usually falls below the zenith, and above the base of our potential. In strong part, understanding choice and commitment may make the difference.

Clinical understanding is framed by the mettle of practice and the lives of officer-patients. Understanding the effect of trauma and loss on public-safety officers means consistently engaging the officer-patient where meaningfulness lies. That may be achieved by your facilitating how and what each officer-patient's reality entails. Each officer-patient presents her history of suffering. Some present the worst of war zones and the real depravity that they witness. Senseless violence and misery is the staple that many officer-patients experience. Validating that trauma is a way of providing an environment conducive to working through the trauma and loss. The holding environment of therapy engages the officer-patient and therapist in response to deprivation that is hardly heard and even less understood. In a way, you become part of a new bridge that includes a meaningful direction, eliciting hopeful optimism that what is suffered is not meaningless.

A suggestion from Frankl helps this way of conceptualizing trauma:

> Freud has taught us to unmask the neurotic, to reveal the hidden unconscious motivations underlying his behavior. . . . Unmasking has to stop at the point when confronted with what no longer can be unmasked, simply because

it is authentic. If some unmasking psychologists do not stop when confronted with something authentic, they still are masking something. That is their own hidden motivation, unconscious desire, to devalue, debase and depreciate what is genuine, what is genuinely human, in man. (1978)

Frankl's (1978) perspective affords him profound insight into those who suffer repetitive loss and trauma.

Giving up the will to find meaning in life is tantamount to giving up on life itself: there are many roads to self-destruction. That may be true whether we are looking at accidental deaths provoked by extreme risk taking or alcoholism and substance abuse, legal or otherwise. This existential vacuum is poignant in the development of Complex PTSD in public service, the antidote of a modified existential analysis is indispensable.

Frankl suggests the existential vacuum is the frustration of the will to meaning. His view is similar to what Durkheim called anomie (norm-less-ness, devoid of value and related to some forms of suicide) (Durkheim, 1897/1951; Frankl, 1988). Frankl defines his existential vacuum as a sociogenic neurosis. A situation with the demands of conformity or totalitarianism threatens to swallow up man's ability to choose for himself (Cardoso, Davis, Goldberg, Herschkowitz, Niehoff, & Restak, 2001; Frankl, 1988; Graber, 2003). Frankl suggests, "the perception of meaning, as I see it, could be defined as suddenly becoming aware of a possibility against the background of reality. . . . It goes without saying we cannot tell a patient what a situation should mean to him. Even less is it possible to tell him wherein he should see the meaning of his life as a whole. *But we may well show him that life never ceases to offer us a meaning up to its last breath*" (Frankl, 2000, p. 141, emphasis mine). Reaching an officer-patient way before his last breath is our goal.

A Triad of Existential Hope

To counter the triad of existential despair, Frankl presents a positive triad in three fundamental areas of the patient's humanity, health, and healing:

1. *The freedom of will.* "Man's freedom is no freedom from conditions, but rather freedom to take a stand on whatever conditions might confront him. . . . Man is and always remains capable of resisting and braving even the worst conditions" (1988, p. 16).
2. *The will to meaning.* "Rather than being a substitute for depth psychology, height psychology is only a supplement—(which takes into account the 'higher aspirations' of the human psyche: not only man's seeking of pleasure and power, but also his search for meaning)—but it does focus on the specifically human phenomena—among them man's desire to find and fulfill a meaning in his life, or for that matter in the individual life situations confronting him. I have circumscribed this most human of all human needs by the motivation term, will to meaning" (1978, 2000, p. 139).

3. *The meaning of life.* This brings us to the level of the "noological-dimension" where life has an inherent meaning in itself. Frankl suggests the anthropological aspect of *man qua man* in a unique view of *logos* or meaning. Optimism and choice to confront trauma become apparent when there is a purpose and meaning in each person's life itself—a *telos*. Frankl elaborates: "What matters is not the features of our character or the drives and instincts per se, but rather the stand we take toward them. And the capacity to take such a stand is what makes us human beings" (1988, p. 17). In that emphasis, I would disagree with Frankl that the drives and their derivatives do matter as very important influences in our lives, as do the cognitions we have about them and any other event in our lives. One may even say that the functioning of a persons tendencies [drive derivatives] underscores the traits and personality style of that officer-patient. However, I would agree wholeheartedly that the ultimate and decisive importance lies in *our human stance* and ability to confront those features, character, and influences through our own choices as human beings.

Frankl extends his anecdote to the toxicity of the existential vacuum. "To be sure if man is to find meanings in an age without values, *he has to be equipped with the full capacity of conscience . . . in an age of the existential vacuum.* The foremost task instead of being satisfied with transmitting traditions and knowledge is to refine that capacity which allows man to find unique meanings. *A lively and vivid conscience is also the only thing that enables man to resist the effects of the existential vacuum, namely, conformism and totalitarianism*" (1988, p. 66, emphasis mine).

The task of the clinician to uncover in redeeming what is meaningful in the officer-patient's life experiences with trauma, I suggest, is a cornerstone of mental health. The frame within the ecology of trauma and loss may also optimistically bring out despair, doubt, questions, and resolution leading to a renewed or rediscovered vitality hitherto buried in the heap of denial of losses. That vitality may be choosing a different path that builds on the crisis precipitated by the eco-ethological influences of trauma. It is our stance of realistic optimism that can be conveyed in the moments of therapy; ultimately it is the officer-patient's choice to make his mark in life.

Frankl put it straight: "Man will not cease to hate as long as he is taught that it is the impulses and mechanisms that do the hating. It is he who does it!" In speaking about the ability to choose life, Frankl views as decisive the patient's "response his reaction in turn will basically depend on whether or not he sees in survival something meaningful—even if it is painful" (Frankl, 1988, p. 34). It is the ecological niche and the ethological influences in trauma that provide the unique understanding of surviving the impact of suffering complex loss in trauma—it is the existential analysis of the meaning that may be rediscovered that is not only healing, but motivational toward achieving and maintaining resilience. In furthering two techniques that help the healing process along, Frankl developed De-reflection and Paradoxical Intention.

De-reflection and Paradoxical Intention

In Frankl's approach, it is the attention to one's self—one's behaviors, one's thoughts, one's achievements, one's material possessions, and one's physical and mental appearance—that can become the subject of a hyperintention. For instance, a grasping for pleasure, satisfaction, material, or psychological demands by hyperintention (an overexaggeration) of focus on self-gratification can lead unwittingly to its opposite. The hyperintention may "evoke hyper-reflection where the person is watching him/her self, too intensely (unhealthy narcissism) by doing so the patient detracts from him/her self, rather than focusing in on what is meaningful in life" (Frankl, 1986). Extreme idealism is one causality of officer-patients with this tendency, the demand for perfectionism makes an ideal into an elusive mirror with no real reflection for the beholder.

Hyperreflection in the context of the ecological demands and ethological motivation to deny loss is likely to exacerbate a toxic accumulation. Much of that loss is likely to be internalized. What is the process that supports internalization? Police and public-safety officers often attempt to deny, suppress, and avoid (multiple and disenfranchised) loss in trauma. Invariably, defensive constellations emerge through repeated attempts to flee from loss in trauma.

Depending on the officer's vulnerabilities, emotional regulation, and biological predisposition, it makes sense that the various manifestations of these defenses are compromises to loss in trauma. Hyperattention to one's own behavior as a police and public-safety officer provides a sense of control and mastery. It also acts as a general defense against expression of loss and grieving. This may offer a selective advantage during combat and in keeping a social distance intact, including one's own peers. Anxiety fuels aggression as much as fear. Loss is offset and, I suggest, is manifested through five core personality styles expressed in large part as a defense against loss. The Controlling Hyperfocused Style; Addictive Hyperexcited Style; The Sadistic Hyperaggressive Style; The Idiosyncratic Hyper-intuitive Style; The Adaptive-Intuitive Style.

Grief syndromes are channeled in large part through hypervigilance, hyperfocus, hyperaggressive, and hyperexcitability; all as styles that keep the officer distant from her own processing of loss. Keep in mind Frankl's addiction, aggression, and depression as branches rooted in the loss and despair over that loss. This diversion from loss may lead the officer-patient to focus on his behavior in police and public-safety roles and identity where negative judgment, hostility/rage, depression, and addictions thrive in an ecology of trauma that suppresses loss as an ethological advantage in a quasi-military hierarchy.

This massive denial of losses in the ethological demands of survival may overpower and harness the officer-patients intention toward extreme self-judgment in light of peer approval, situational demands, status, and extremely romanticized versions of how one should have acted. The hyperintention becomes the hyperattention to demands reflected in the ecology of one's development within their niche: the officer-patient's position, status, and survival within the unit. Optimism may be reduced to one's own survival and one's unit's survival. Hyperattention varies by the officer's style and niche. Attempts at reparation are evidenced in each account from all officers. The aspect of trauma that remains most troublesome clinically is the focus of the officer-patient on his behavior in terms of undefined identity modes, situational demands, conflicts, and defenses, which has not been articulated adequately in this book, if at all in the context of personality styles. Behavior by omission or commission, real or imagined, becomes magnified and individualized in maladaptive hyperreflection. The compromise as a defense against loss is one of harsh and punitive self-judgment or through aggression directed outward against others.

The ability to see oneself in a realistic view is paradoxically and myopically closed to the narrowest focus that trauma provides. Such a narrow focus may disrupt the expression of loss through healthy grieving while provoking defensive constellations through maladaptive patterns.

A solution is given in part by Frankl, who suggests dereflection and paradoxical intention. This approach is helpful with the officer-patient. He explains,

> Logotherapy is out to pull into play centrifugal forces instead of striving for hyper-reflection on one self, it is by forgetting oneself. Instead of hyper-reflection it is through de-reflection and paradoxical intention. That is self-transcendence. De-reflection from the pursuit of pleasure, happiness, or even power. Self-transcendence cannot be pursued, but letting it ensue as a side effect of fulfilling a meaning or fulfillment through another person. (1988, p. 72)

Paradoxical intention is achieved by seeking to do exactly what one is suffering from in anticipation of the worst of fears becoming realized—anticipatory anxiety. In our situation of thanatological dread, traumatophobia, and the fear of expressing the loss, paradoxical intention may help initiate the grieving process.

Dereflection is the intentional reflection away from oneself onto another person or meaningful purpose in one's life. We will see how we can use these wonderfully effective techniques with other therapeutic approaches in the chapters to follow. In his own summary of logotherapy as an integrative approach, Frankl asserts,

> It is true, logotherapy deals with the logos; it deals with meaning. Specifically, I see the meaning of logotherapy in helping others to see meaning in life. But one cannot give meaning to the life of others. And if this is true of meaning, per se, how much more does it hold for ultimate meaning? *The more comprehensive the meaning, the less comprehensible it is* . . . (italics added). As

to logotherapy, it is not a panacea. It therefore is open to cooperation with other approaches to psychotherapy; it is open to its own evolution. (1988, p. 136)

With Frankl's suggestion in mind, the evolution he points to, I suggest, may hold promise in my eco-ethological existential analytic approach to PPS-CPTSD. Now that we have traversed Complex PTSD, dissociation, complicated, disenfranchised grief, and the Existential Triad, we are ready for the final component of our conceptual model of PPS-CPTSD.

Qualification of PSS-CPTSD—
In the Context of an Eco-Ethological Approach

A qualification is in order at this point. We can add to our clarity of PPS-CPTSD first and foremost by acknowledging that no simple formula exists. If we can accept that fact with humility, realizing the complexity of complex trauma and dissociation, we may resolve to construct tentative working hypotheses.

In at least one perspective of how science operates, working hypotheses are all we have. They may help us understand the "blinking moments" of the therapeutic hour. Our realization may be that while blinking moments may be lost, they may be rediscovered. Did you hear that? Our working hypotheses may slowly paint the canvas of any disorder—impression by impression—yet, the picture that emerges may not resemble our initial hypothesis. Blinking moments suggest encounter and ambiguity.

By accepting that ambiguity, along with our experiential understanding, we eventually can meet the officer-patient's clinical problems via the flux of his genuine presentation. I suggest that if we force the paint-by-symptom approach to the disorder, as some envision being scientific, we may not observe, assess, diagnose, and ultimately treat the officer-patient appropriately. The ambiguity and change evidenced in Complex PTSD and DID evolve as the treatment that forms in response to it; that is, as a psychodynamic, cognitive-behavioral, gestalt perspective is guided by a modified existential analysis. I, for one, cannot offer you a step-by-step approach: I cannot do that since the patient cannot fit into such a paradigm. He is as unique as his situation, which is interpreted in the light of his individuality. However, with the aforementioned qualifications in mind, I am confident you will be an informed therapist who can be ready to achieve a working relationship and understanding of the officer-patient before you. Some initial facts are necessary to establish that understanding. Let us move on and review some of them.

PSS-CPTSD—In the Context of an
Eco-Ethological Understanding

The populations of individuals who experience frequent and multiple trauma on a regular basis are police and public-safety officers (Benner, 1991; Hirsch,

Katz, & Cohen, 1998; Kirschman, 1997; Reese, 1991; Rudofossi, 1994, 1997; Rudofossi & Ellis, 1999; Spielberger, Grier, & Greenfield, 1982; Toch, 2002). The fact is, events police officers experience on a cumulative level are traumatic stressors for the general population. To date, these events occur with high frequency in police populations. In my research on my police officer patients, the frequency of events, per individual patients, that can be classified as traumatic ranged from 10 to 900 plus. Many of the officers expressed disenfranchised loss, complicated grief, and anxiety over the traumatic events.

LIST OF BULLET POINTS ON ECO-ETHOLOGICAL EXISTENTIAL ANALYTIC RESEARCH

The mean number of known traumatic events per officer was 30. Some frequent experiences were outside the acknowledged triggers for trauma. Disenfranchised losses repeatedly reported by officers include:

- Being on the scene of a dying assault victim
- Witnessing the crime-scene victim and then having to do all the legal and technical work involved
- Providing death notifications to victim's families
- Rendering aid to a heart-attack victim or a child choking to death
- Not knowing the outcome of cases the officers were highly invested in, such as an elderly person's suicide
- Witnessing the assault against a partner
- Handling sudden change in increasingly sophisticated and disparate identity modes as officers (see Rudofossi, 2007).

Although any one of these events can classify as disenfranchised trauma and loss, they are largely unidentified in public-safety populations.

The public-safety population includes veterans and active soldiers, firefighters, special agents, medical officers (paraprofessionals to doctoral-level educated), correction officers, emergency service technicians, medics, and civilian emergency-communication operators. The experience of even one would be cause for attention with other populations, yet are not even moments for pause when a safety officer experiences these events. Why?

My research indicated that the type of trauma and the environmental conditions are major factors in the development of Complex PTSD. I suggest one riot or gang war may be perceived as multiple and layered events rather than the awkward categorization of one traumatic event. How and where to place traumatic events have added to the complexity of intrapsychic ethological and physiological visceral responses along with the ambient ecology of environmental cues, such as blaring sirens, blood and body matter, and the screams of victims. All this adds to the complexity of deciphering what is ecological and ethological in influence in the context of dissociation, complex trauma, complicated grief, and existential despair, which is what I call the core of PPS-CPTSD.

As we reviewed earlier, dissociative states may emerge in the survivor of C-PTSD. That is of interest in our population of public-safety officers and police. It appears that officer's multiple roles and experiences of trauma may be more similar to survivors of sexual, political, and physical trauma than one may superficially dismiss in a discursive manner. The officer typically has to not only witness but to intervene in situations that would be overwhelming for most people.

I suggest most of the officer's expectations are reinforced on multiple levels of the culture, as well as institutional rules and regulations. That reinforcement may provide the officer with a sense of failure and consequent loss since assimilation and accommodation to these traumatic events remains incomplete because the officer seldom knows what happens to the victim and is thrust into multiple and contradictory roles, often in direct opposition to each other. This may induce a psychobiological change in emotion and defenses, which are ethologically determined. Many ideas and feelings related to one's roles remain guarded and unexpressed because of the fear of legal exposure and prosecution that is objectively transmitted through institutional and grassroot culture. The use of your unconscious in attuning to the officer-patient's positions may help create empathic successes that are psychoanalytically informed.

A criticism heard from some colleagues deserves clarification: validation of the traumatic event may take away the ability to resolve the painful emotional suffering and hidden anguish. To the contrary, that validation of the ecological and ethological development of trauma facilitates the work of any of the effective therapy approaches, including EMDR, existential, cognitive-behavioral, and psychodynamic approaches.

Your achievement is enhanced by appreciation of evolutionary mechanisms underlying maladaptation in the patient's behavior, emotional expression, and cognitive appraisal. That appreciation is at the level of conscious and unconscious countertransference, with the help of your balanced perspective to mobilize your own healthy interest, and creativity rather than avoidance, withdrawal, and complicity. Those are the very real toxic and negative visceral reactions. As a good therapist, you will actively listen for and clarify their appearances, which furthers the likelihood of your ability to relate genuine empathy for the officer-patient.

Our review in this chapter of PPS-CPTSD illustrated the commonality of certain antecedents for this syndrome, which are initiation rites in the experience of public-safety and police professionals, who are likely to experience repeated trauma as massive and unexpressed loss. That overwhelming and compartmentalized loss triggers dissociation between demands of survival as an adaptation, which includes multiple and complex interactions. The context of development in police and public-safety officer populations may parallel combat experiences and social demands of daily reintegration into civilian society. It is with this foundation in mind that I presented in an earlier publication operational definitions related to PPS-CPTSD (Rudofossi, 1997, 2007).

Adaptive skills and maladaptive responses are shaped in part by ingenuity in processing, coping, and defending against trauma and loss, which is in part learned through intragenerational cultural transmission. That intragenerational cultural transmission in a police and public-safety agency is imparted and conditioned, learned and reinforced in verbal and nonverbal ethological aspects of transmission as to what is acceptable and what is not. The eco-ethological niche affords certain behaviors, thoughts, and emotional responses as adaptive, some which are extinguished over time.

Being aware of these influences can help your ability to value the reality that shapes officers' selective advantage in establishing coping strategies and defenses, including emotive, cognitive, and behavioral repertoires within an evolutionary context. Overall, these findings support PPS-CPTSD in public-safety officers as a developmental syndrome.

A developmental syndrome of PPS-CPTSD is made comprehensible when a consistency exists between events experienced as traumatic and a stability in the context of an officers persistence in his style of adaptation and maladaptation in strategies of defense and approach to that event. One such consistency exists in the phenomenon that I call "telescoping of traumatic loss."

Telescoping of traumatic loss is a spontaneous effect of repressed past trauma emerging in the here and now of the encounter between therapist and patient. Telescoping was initially defined in 1971 (Kohut, 1971, 1977) as original trauma from infantile development resurfacing in the transference relationship. The source of this theory is found in Freud's original theory, including his famous 1924b paper on working through and repetition compulsion. Repetition compulsion was conceived as "acting out" through a reenactment of what is unprocessed through unconscious determination in daily living in lieu of being remembered and expressed. This process gets reenacted in the relationship with the therapist (transference), who rather than responding to this reenactment, takes an analytic stance by iterating insight through interpretation based on ongoing conjecture about intrapsychic conflict in the patient (Brenner, 1976).

Clarification may lead to what was originally traumatic. While the trauma therapist does not ignore childhood trauma, telescoping may be spontaneous recovery of long lost memories. Those lost memories expose the frozen layer of what was conscious at one time, has become consciously suppressed, and eventually unconsciously repressed and compartmentalized. In a way, the repetition compulsion may be observed when the patient is seen in a dissociative state, which is when the telescoping may occur.

I offer a complementary modification through an existential analytic eco-ethological perspective. Traumatic emotional abreaction of original trauma emerges spontaneously, or through therapist direction when past trauma is alluded to in the session. Original trauma is defined as an adult safety officer directly experiencing trauma in light of field adaptation, relationships, and personal meaning of that layered trauma. Original trauma refers to an active and earlier frame that later traumas relate and are compared with. It is a yardstick for gaining a perspective on the impact later traumatic events have in the accompaniment of earlier trauma. Often it is this past event that is more complicated than one that may be presented as problematic.

For instance, a patient narrating a current trauma in a fleeting moment makes a reference to an earlier unmentioned event, perhaps in a mumble. The therapist responds empathetically by direct clarification: "why the far and lost look; what are you seeing right now?" (see chapters 3 and 4). Focusing on the nonverbal transference through your own countertransference feelings and observations of the officer-patient's dissociation is helpful. Your well-timed clarification of officer-patient's dissociative states, delivered in a warm, genuine, and empathic style communicates where the defense explicitly will take therapist and patient alike. This inroad supportively opens up earlier events.

Exploration into where, how, and when the original trauma was experienced is optimally processed in terms of visceral, emotional and cognitive experiences in the ecological niche it occurred in. Original trauma is primary compared with the current trauma, consciously verbalized as secondary. The original trauma of an officer-patient may be clarified along with telescoping that leads to earlier childhood trauma, tendencies, and vulnerabilities. However, the goal here is to optimize working with the trauma and loss associated with being a police and public-safety officer.

If we look at each situation of trauma as a telescope through the lens of ethology, it makes superb sense that the ecological demands of the quantum psychic moment of trauma once experienced initiates a new schema. That new schema has consequences on an unconscious level of preparedness and evolved physiological tracks that help adaptation through specialization to similar situations, which initiate the pick-up of invariant information in response to situational demands that evoke the formation and development of new schema. The discrimination of a noxious situation, from a nonnoxious situation may not be clear in the active participant.

That nonnoxious situation would be moving from the war zone to the peace-time domestic situation. From an ethological perspective, the specialization that is invested with survival value may stay with the officer-patient when they leave the beat, which may not be on a conscious level. The forcing of switching on and off as part of the larger cultural demands is one level of stress and strain, the larger the difference in ecological demands the more the pressure on the officer. The response to multiple trauma and perceived invariants lends insight into the sensibility of the defense constellation of dissociation. That reality may include multiple experiences the officer-patient may attempt to process at once.

The disruption that may occur to an officer-patient's social support after repetitive trauma may be exacerbated by a number of problems, such as attempts at self-soothing: addictions, along with acting out and consequent legal difficulties. Aggressive drive derivatives that were neutralized may revert to earlier modes of direct aggression that are supported by the ecological niche.

Numbing, massive denial, and traumatophobia, along with the defenses of depersonalization and derealization may create the illusion of being okay. Addiction to trauma as "counterphobic responses" may lead to the officer-patient saying, "I'm okay," while increasing risk-taking, satisfying aggressive expression through legitimate rites: increasing addictive behaviors in a loop that spirals downward without notice, until the risk or the aggression goes too far. In the ecological niche of the officer-patient (his unit and the demands exacted), the addictive behaviors may be accepted and even reinforced until one's behaviors are met with punitive consequences by outside agencies. When these consequences occur, he may be left disenfranchised not only from one's social support network, but from the larger culture of the police and public-safety world based on the specialization and the psychological demands of that specialization.

As discussed in an earlier work (Rudofossi, 2007), identity modes are an unusual strain, coupled with traumatic dissociation as a means of adaptation. Identity modes are understood as not only modes of responsiveness, but integral in identity development. They can sensibly be understood in terms of an adaptive functional dissociation.

For example, a hostage situation, or a woman being pinned under a car, or a person attempting suicide is a situational demand that becomes ethologically embedded in memory and emotion. That imprint of ethological survival value is an adaptation in the situation as well as others that are similar in the invariant ecological niches they occur in. The other side of that adaptation is the maladaptation in the transition from one of trauma to one of civilian life. The abuse to the human psyche from the demands of reequilibration from a primacy on an eco-ethological dimension to one of societal standards takes place several times a day and at minimum once a day.

With this in mind, let's go back and reconsider identity modes in the context of what Dr. Putnam in his magnum opus on multiple personality disorder explains as etiology in some cases of DID. In some patients, MPD may emerge as a response to witnessing repeated traumatic experiences of murder by terrorism (Putnam, 1989).

The point is that witnessing near-death experiences that are violent and manmade is associated with development of multiple personality disorder (Putnam, 1989). That relevance begs our attention to an inexhaustible harvest of hidden dissociation in police and public-safety population. Consider that officer-patients are most likely to be witnesses to murder in their late adolescence to early adult years, when they are most vulnerable, which is when they are appointed to their public-service positions. I will share with you the development of clinical examples to follow: In chapters 3 and 4, this harvest may be understood in the thorny bushes of trauma that prick each officer-patient's life and identity with the force of loss and variations in defenses against that loss.

The persistence of one's identity is important to adaptation, as well as health in personality development. However, there are ecological niches in which this consistency in one's personality may not aid adaptation, but decrease the likelihood of survival. On the other hand, certain distasteful and mercurial presentations via adaptation may increase the likelihood of survival. One such presentation may be likened to a chameleon. Nietzsche offered an interesting philosophy of "as if" persons in the context of historical, sociological, and political influences (Kaufmann, 1966). However, Helen Deutsch was the first to write of such personality disorders. She called people with this disorder "as-if" personalities in 1942 in regard to what was interestingly framed in the context of borderline and schizophrenic syndromes (Deutsch, 1965).

We have all heard of the chameleon-like ability of certain notables who employ adaptation by changing their own style to accommodate the demands of a given situation: examples include some actors, infamous criminals, and some politicians. That response is believed to be negligible and indicative of a person with an underdeveloped ego. Yet it may have an adaptive purpose that eludes its superficial dismissal as a simple weakness of character. It is well known that this personality is associated with the borderline character. I suggest a very different perspective in the context of police and public-safety officers.

From the perspective of ethology and adaptation, this response may be an endogenous vulnerability: as an ability to dissociate at times. Some officers may experience identity dissociation that exemplifies the chameleon predisposition. This may result in the ability to mimic as an adaptation with survival value, rather than any atavistic character trait. That is, to survive overwhelming trauma, a chameleon response may be shaped by ecological demands. The survival value is embedded in ethological influence, and that starts with mimicking and persists in part through operant and classical conditioning.

It also persists and is modified by the unconscious wishes underlying one's image of being a police and public-safety officer. The defenses against the losses, guilt, shame, and violations of ideals, including fantasies related to these ideals, generate conflict. Here I am modifying the genius of insight as first suggested by Freud (1924), modified by Hartmann (1958), and refined by Brenner (1974, 1976, 1982) in his formulation of compromise formations: I suggest these compromise formations may be in response to identity modes that emerge in response to the repetitive trauma that evoke cumulative losses. These losses are experienced as a threat to the satisfaction of the aggression-drive derivatives, which serve an evolutionary function for the officer-patient as described earlier.

One example is deep cover, narcotics, intelligence, detective work, as well as other situations, in which the officer has to blend in to the ecological demands his niche affords. Alters in identity may originate as *functional adaptive-dissociation* within the context of the ambient environment of violence, and antiaffordance of multiple trauma within the officer-patient's ecological niche. In place of alters identity modes suggests the intense survival value with the dynamic meaning in ethological, ecological, and unconscious terms. It is also normalizing the eco-ethological influences and reintegrating the officer-patient's dissociation by the clinician at first understanding the very adaptation as healthier in a very toxic situational demand without conspirators. Within that context of trauma and loss, that is too threatening, one's survival depends on the ability and skill to dissociate.

That persistence of one's ability to maintain a consistent self-concept over time and different contexts may be altered as much as brain chemistry through the ecological demands in situations where roles are switched, like a chameleon's hue. This eco-ethological reality may exist for tens of thousands of officer-patients, one of whom may be the one who walks into your office. The idiosyncratic hypervigilant officer is likely to be most vulnerable to this level of adaptive functional dissociation (see chapter 3).

Moving on in our conceptualization: it appears that some situations relevant to the etiology of MPD/DID are the repeated witnessing of death and misery, the present threat of terrorism, and the lack of cultural validation in an ecology of violence. I suggest in police and public-safety officers that contradictory and often rapid psychological, physiological, and chemical changes evoked by situational demands may alter the perceptual and physiological tracks when the officer-patient's attention modes and memories change in response to each distinct situation. The conflicts in these identity modes, each of which push the officer's survival skills in simultaneously opposing directions for flight *and* fight, may result in what we will call "police experimental neurosis." The neurological evocation for such intense and oppositional stress and strain may have a very high cost biopsychologically. It is the actual events of traumas that shapes and interacts with the officer's emerging police personality style, which includes cognitive, behavioral, and emotional strategies shaped by the ethological-emotional selective advantages within the context of his ecological niche (unit in the command). The ambient background of violence in each trauma event demands joint exploration between the recounting by the officer-patient and the clinician who listens with his "third ear."

THE AMBIENT BACKGROUND OF VIOLENCE IN THE FORMATION OF DISSOCIATIVE IDENTITY MODES

Dissociation may entail behavioral, lingual, memory, and neurological substrates that effect emotional and cognitive processes. In my conceptualization, that intensity may become more like character features, or identity modes, when the officer-patient attempts adaptation to assimilate and accommodate to the invariant aspects of antiaffordances in multiple traumatic events. Those invariant aspects of antiaffordances may afford the "ambient background" of aggression. Examples are the experiential aspects through repeated assaults, witnessing murder, and repeated violence on a number of levels to which the officer-patient attends. The ecological demand to express oneself in the language of violence and force may become, through the antiaffordances of multiple experiences of traumatic events, a way of acceptable living with all the distortions in mores and rituals that may accompany the ethological influence of survival value. Through the experience of random violence, the participants may gain a tradition through the motif of rituals, ideals, and symbols shaped by the persistence of what is reliable—the ecology of violence. That ecological reality of public-safety officers may be the cumulative experience of sudden threats of danger in inner city neighborhoods. These neighborhoods may be perceived as ecological niches of political and social unrest, where exposure to riots and gang wars may contain multiple traumas and losses in officer-patients whose responsibilities, roles, and tasks may change without preparation. Ecological niches may create an ambient environment where feedback loops develop in response and are shaped by the relative context of the loss in trauma. That relative influence bears insight into what is perceived as loss and resilience and how, on a survival level, functional dissociation develops. That ecological niche is surrounded by the defensive rituals and ideals of each unit within the larger context of the overall culture.

From an evolutionary perspective, what has persisted has offered a selective advantage to the unit and its members survival. In an ethological sense, that may reinforce the intransigent aspects of bonding among military and police buddies. However, that functional dissociation may not be a healthy one, but one that is forged on survival as the prime motivation. It is not healthy because survival is a base approach to life, yet it is fundamental as a basis for life and living. But a basis for survival may replace what is meaningful outside of that context and permeate every aspect of that officer's life. One aspect of that survival is reconnected in a meaningful way with you as a therapist in the "working through" process with the officer-patient.

LOSS AND THE DISTORTION OF HUMAN TIME: EMOTIONAL CONSTRICTION AROUND THE HELIX OF IQ

Approaching what can be very difficult countertransference in complex trauma is your working through the loss in trauma, which includes the toxic and visceral descriptions you will hear. In our work with patients, examples of difficulty we encounter along that emotional constriction include the persistence of relating to why and how the patients distort time. That distortion of time may be reconceptualized as a freezing of time in the space laid out by a traumatic event.

That space is laid out by the repetition of patterns of behavior that initially are adaptive and responsive to survival value, which does not dissipate because of the awareness and intelligence of the officer-patient. The higher the intelligence, perhaps the deeper the self-doubt and maybe compulsion to reenact the trauma. There also is resistance to the encounter of discovery of that very repressed loss of one's self, and more so with one's therapist. Without the loss being acknowledged emotionally and experientially, it is bound to be reenacted through other means. It is within the resistance that the reenactment takes place and why the therapeutic alliance may be the most important aspect of neutralizing that very resistance. In fact, within an eco-ethological therapy, the prediction is that those most impacted by trauma and loss are those with higher levels of intelligence and commitment to ideals in their identity as officers.

My hypothesis from experience with scores of hundreds of officers is, the higher the intelligence, the more profound the pain. I think a clearer question is: Who suffers from trauma syndromes more severely than their peers and why? I suggest it is those who are emotionally strong or intellectually perspicacious who are more capable of dealing with stress. Vulnerability, including dependent personality traits, may exacerbate trauma. The converse perspective may be posited on anecdotal evidence: An officer's ability to bond with fellow officers may be the product of a higher level of emotional intelligence. The officer-patient who experiences the deepest and most repressed trauma may be the one with higher levels of intelligence, including an ability to functionally dissociate in one's niche. The loss, when taken out of that niche, may trigger the PPS-CPTSD, similar to taking a fish out of water. Hence, a significant and disenfranchised loss may be centered in those officers facing or living in retirement. The officer-patient with the idiosyncratic hypervigilant and hyperfocused police personality style has the most increased likelihood to use adaptive functional dissociation to cope with overwhelming loss in trauma (see chapters 2 and 3).

A Reconnaissance of the Quantum Moment of Loss in the Officer-Patient

While PSS-CPTSD has been the adhesion of the conceptual spires of complex grief, dissociation, trauma, and existential despair, the hub from which complex trauma emerges is nourished by loss. Consider a cornerstone of my work with police officer-patients: One can experience loss and grief *without trauma*. But the converse is not true, that is, one cannot experience what is defined as a traumatic response *without having experienced loss*. That is elusive, but clearly based on a physical, psychological, and mental level by logic and observation of evidence: the twin pillars of science (Christensen, 2001; Kerlinger & Lee, 2002).

Put another way, an officer-patient must experience *a mental appreciation and experience of loss of security, loss of predictability* in their own assumptions about one's world, as Janoff-Bulman (1989, 1992) posited. In addition, that same officer must experience the subjective distress of anger at violations of what was, and now is not (loss of reliability); anxiety as abandonment separation (loss of other, status, or prior level of functioning); and the mental/cognitive (helplessness/hopelessness) that is a loss of one's confidence and outlook. And that officer-patient experiencing behavioral manifestations (avoidant and withdrawal phases) also loses contact with his environment and other people. If the officer-patient does not experience each of these components of trauma, he does not have PTSD. According to the Diagnostic Statistical Manual of Mental Disorders (DSM-IV) (1994) operational definition, loss is not an important aspect of PTSD.

I contend that loss is the hub of trauma. Our conversation of trauma would be bereft, yes, bereft without integration of *loss* on a firm clinical and research foundation, which some of the finest researchers and clinicians have devoted their lifetimes to building.

As I have suggested throughout this chapter and in an earlier book (Rudofossi, 2007), the culture of public safety has its own mores, traditions, customs, and rituals. Some are written, and some are not. However, it is not only cultural, but ecological and ethological influences in an evolutionary context that shape the impact of repetitive trauma and loss on the individual public-safety and police officer's experience. That is still not the entire picture.

I suggest these influences have three directions, which have multiple and complex interactions. The first direction is intrapersonal, the second is interpersonal, and the third is interaction within adaptation to the culture of policing and public safety. Yet, what is cultural is neither ecological nor ethological.

I suggest the ecological and ethological influences of the ambient environment of the officer-patient's niche have a multidirectional feedback loop with the macroculture of policing and pubic safety. That loop has evolved within the context of individual vulnerabilities and tendencies each officer brings in their biopsychosocial experiences. While it may seem at this point that the clinician must have an extensive perspective to effectively treat the individual officer-patient, that is not the case I am making. The point is to understand that the complexity and the impact of loss is not only multidimensional, but equally individual as is your application of what is presented.

In our conceptual focus, survival is primary. Being numb and dissociating is a great strength when one is thrust into the midst of situations that may emotionally overwhelm even the most highly trained officer. The myths of the public-safety culture are functionally connected with survival. The value of existential numbing through addictions, aggression, or depression supports the antiaffordance of not mourning the losses while reinforcing numbing, extinguishing attempts to grieve. This is especially certain for losses not accepted in the dominant culture as really normal.

As we have observed in police culture, anger may be acceptable and projected on legitimate objects of derision such as perpetrators and those who are viewed as exploitative. This displacement of loss thwarts grief and solidifies denial in what we will examine as the "righteous anger" many officers express openly while the loss and grief that is unmourned remains repressed.

What remains repressed is liable to be reopened at a time of trauma, which is a consistent staple of experience in police and public safety. In terms of anticipatory scanning of what may happen in the ecology and ethology of loss in trauma, the hypervigilant, hyperavoidant, hyperfocused, and hyperexcited styles of officer-patients become sensible ways in which adaptation has led to maladaptation within a broad continuum. I will give you a fleshed-out perspective in chapter 2 that addresses that issue.

For now, thinking about massive denial as resistance may shed light on the evolutionary function of numbing, which may be supported as a means of adaptation becoming impervious to pain may be learned through imitation of veteran officers and conditioned by ecological and ethological influences in the struggle for survival value where emotional expression of pain and loss is devalued. That function for survival value may be adaptive in the heat of enforcement preparedness, and I suggest may be prolific in public-safety and police ethology. It is the type of denial that strikes at what is so meaningful— being ignored, disenfranchised—which is loss at its peak.

It is the attitude toward such trauma that may be addressed via the realization of what meaning that trauma has evoked in the evolution of the officer-patient as an individual. I suggest that although the aphorism that ontogeny recapitulates phylogeny may in part be true, then phylogeny can be redirected by ontogeny. Nowhere is this more possible than in the survival conflicts nested in an ecology of terror threats and compromise as unique ethological adaptations capable of being confronted in the ubiquitous nature of transference and the existential analysis that emerges in collaboration between therapist and officer-patient.

Within this context, the experience of psychic trauma becomes more tangible rather than elusive. I suggest that by realizing the blinking moments of trauma by stringing together the different strengths and formidable understanding each perspective brings to our work, we may better explicate trauma and grief processes as we enhance our trauma and grief therapy in the next three chapters, based on the applied synergistic theory we have established here.

REFERENCES

Ainsworth, P. B. (1995). *Psychology and policing in a changing world.* New York: John Wiley & Sons.

Barnes, B. (2007). *Discussion of Logotherapy goal's during World Wide Logotherapy Conference at Dallas Texas.* Dallas Texas.

Beck, A. (1985). *Cognitive therapy and the emotional disorders.* New York: International Universities Press.

Benner, A. (1991). *The changing cop: A longitudinal study of psychological testing within law enforcement.* San Francisco, CA: Saybrook Institute Publication.

Benner, A. (1998). *The challenge for police psychology in the twenty first century: Moving beyond efficient to effective.* Paper presentation and lecture at conference held by the Federal Bureau of Investigation, Washington, DC.

Benner, A. (2001). *Suicide and law enforcement.* Washington, DC: Federal Bureau of Investigation.

Braun, B. (1988). The BASK model of dissociation. *Dissociation, 1,* 4-23.

Brenner, C. (1974). *An elementary textbook of psychoanalysis.* New York: Doubleday/Dell Publishing Company.

Brenner, C. (1976). *Psychoanalytic technique and psychic conflict.* New Haven, CT: International University Press.

Brenner, C. (1982). *The mind in conflict.* New Haven, CT: International University Press.

Benjamin, L. (1993). *Interpersonal diagnosis and treatment of personality disorders.* New York: Guilford Press.

Bowlby, J. (1975). *Attachment and loss: Loss* (Vol. 1). New York: Basic Books.

Cannon, W. B. (1914). The emergency function of the adrenal medulla in pain and the major emotions. *American Journal of Physiology, 3,* 356-372.

Cardoso, S., Davis, P., Goldberg, C., Herschkowitz, N. E., Niehoff, D., & Restak, R. (2001). Dying to kill: The Mind of the terrorist. *Cerebrum, The Dana Forum on Brain Science, 3*(3), 12-38.

Chu, J. (1998). *The responsible treatment of complex post-traumatic and dissociative disorders.* New York: John Wiley

Christensen, L. (2001). *Experimental methodology.* Boston: Allyn & Bacon.

Cohen, L., Berzoff, J., & Ellin, M. (1995). *Dissociative identity disorder.* Hillsdale, NJ: Jason Aronson Publications.

Deutsch, H. (1965). *Neuroses and character types.* New York: International Universities Press.

Diagnostic Statistical Manual of Mental Disorders [DSM-IV] (4th ed.). (1994). Washington, DC: American Psychiatric Association.

Doka, K. (1985). Expectation of death, participation in funeral arrangements, and grief adjustment. *Omega, 15,* 119-129.

Doka, K. J. (Ed.). (1989). *Disenfranchised grief: Recognizing hidden sorrow.* Lexington, MA: Research Press.

Doka, K. J. (2002). *Disenfranchised grief: New directions, challenges, and strategies for practice.* Champaign, IL: Research Press.

Doka, K. J., & Martin, T. L. (2001). *Men don't cry, women do: Transcending gender stereotypes of grief.* Philadelphia: Brunner/Mazel.

Durkheim, E. (1951). *Suicide.* Glencoe, IL: Free Press. (Original Work published 1897.)

Ellis, A. (1962). *Reason and emotion in psychotherapy.* Secaucus, NJ: Lyle Stuart.

Ellis, A. (1985). *Overcoming resistance: Rational-emotive therapy with difficult patients.* New York: Springer.

Ellis, R. R. (1992). *Young children: Disenfranchised grievers.* In New York University School of Social Work Personality Development. New York: Ginn Press Publications.

Ellis, R. R. (1994). *Supervision of goal's of grief work during practicum at New York University.* New York: New York University.

Ellis, R. R., & Williams, M. B., & Zinner, E. S. (1999). The connection between grief and trauma: An overview. In E. S. Zinner & M. B. Williams (Eds.), *When a community weeps: Case studies in group survivorship* (pp. 3-17). Philadelphia: Brunner/Mazel.

Figley, C. (1985). *Trauma and its* wake: *The study and treatment of post traumatic stress disorder and its treatment.* New York: Brunner/Mazel.

Frankl, V. (1978). *The unheard cry for meaning.* New York: Washington Square Press.

Frankl, V. (1988). *The will to meaning.* New York & London: Meridian Book Publishers.

Frankl, V. (2000). *Man's search for ultimate meaning.* Cambridge, MA: Perseus Publishing.

Freeman, A., & Reinecke, M. (1993). *Cognitive therapy of suicidal behavior: A manual for treatment.* New York: Springer Publishers.

Freud, A. (1936). *Ego and the mechanisms of defense.* New York: International University Press.

Freud, S. (1924a). Mourning and melancholia. In J. Strachey (Eds.), *The standard edition of the complete psychological works of Sigmund Freud in collaboration with Anna Freud* (Vol. 2, pp. 336-376). London: The Hogarth Press.

Freud, S. (1924b). Recollection, repetition and working through. In J. Strachey (Ed.), *The standard edition of the complete psychological works of Sigmund Freud in collaboration with Anna Freud* (Vol. 12, pp. 366-376). London: The Hogarth Press.

Freud, S., Ferenczi, S., Abraham, K., Simmel, E., & Jones, E. (1921). *Psychoanalysis and the war neuroses.* London & New York: International Psycho-Analytic Press.

Fromm, E. (1973). *The anatomy of human destructiveness.* New York: Holt, Reinhart, Winston.

Gabbard, K., & Gabbard, K. (1987). *Psychiatry and the cinema.* Chicago & London: Chicago University Press.

Gabbard, G., & Western, D. (2003). Rethinking therapeutic action. *International Journal of Psychoanalysis, 84,* 823-841.

Gibson, J. J. (1966). *The senses considered as perceptual systems.* Boston: Houghton Mifflin.

Gibson, J. J. (1986). *The ecological approach to visual perception.* New Jersey: Lawrence Erlbaum Associates.

Gibson, J. J., & Gibson, E. (1955). Perceptual learning: Differentiation or enrichment? *Psychological Review, 62,* 32-41.

Giller, E. L. (Ed.). (1990). *Biological assessment and treatment of post traumatic stress disorder.* Washington, DC: American Psychiatric Press.

Goleman, D. (1992, January). Wounds that never heal. How trauma changes your brain. *Psychology Today,* pp. 62-68.

Goleman, D. (1994, October). Emotional memory of trauma: Cahill's study. *New York Times, Science Time Tuesday.*

Gottlieb, R. (1997). Does the mind fall apart in multiple personality disorder? Some proposals based on a psychoanalytic case. *Journal of the American Psychoanalytic Association, 45*(3), 57-74

Gould, S. (2002). *The structure of evolutionary theory.* Cambridge, MA: The Belknap Press of Harvard University.

Graber, A. (2003). *Viktor Frankl Logotherapy.* Wyndham, NY: Hall Press.

Hartmann, H. (1958). *Ego psychology and the problem of adaptation.* New York: International University Press.

Hartmann, E. (1984). *The nightmare*. New York: Basic Books, Inc.

Helson, H. (1964). *Adaption-level theory*. New York: Harper and Row.

Hendin, H. (1983). Combat never ends: The paranoid adaptation to posttraumatic stress. *American Journal of Psychotherapy, 38*, 121-131.

Herman, J. (1992). *Trauma and recovery*. New York: Basic Books.

Hirsch, R., Katz, R., & Cohen, D. (1998). *Cop to cop: A peer support training manual for law enforcement officers*. New York: The Peer Support Training Institute.

Horowitz, J. M. (1974). Stress response syndrome: Character style and dynamic psychotherapy. *Archives of General Psychiatry, 31,* 177-198.

Horowitz, J. M. (1976). *Stress response syndrome*. New York: Jason Aronson.

Horowitz, J. M. (1998). *Cognitive psychodynamics: From conflict to character*. New York: Wiley Press.

Horowitz, J. M. (1999). *Essential papers on post traumatic stress disorder*. New York: New York University Press.

Horowitz, J. M. (2003). *Treatment of stress response syndrome*. Washington, DC: American Psychiatric Press.

James, G. (1994, March). An officers painful trip to the edge and his long journey back. *The New York Times*, p. B1.

Janet, P. (1907). *The major symptoms of hysteria*. New York: Macmillan.

Janoff-Bulman, R. (1989). Assumptive worlds and the stress of traumatic events: Applications of the schema construct. *Social Cognition, 7,* 113-136.

Janoff- Bulman, R. (1992). *Shattered assumptions: Towards a new psychology of trauma*. New York: Free Press.

Kardiner, A., & Spiegal, H. (1947). *War, stress, and neurotic illness*. New York: Hoeber Press.

Kaufmann, W. (1966). *Basic writings*. New York: Meridian Book.

Kelly, W. (1985). *Post traumatic stress disorder and the war veteran patient*. New York: Brunner/Mazel.

Kerlinger, F., & Lee, H. (2002). *Foundations of behavioral research*. Sydney, Australia: Wadsworth.

Kernberg, O. (1984). *Severe personality disorders*. New Haven & London: Yale University Press.

Kernberg, O. (1995). *Love relations: Normality and pathology*. New Haven & London: Yale University Press.

Ker Muir, W., Jr. (1977). *Police: Street corner politicians*. Chicago & London: University of Chicago Press.

Kirschman, E. (1997). *I love a cop*. New York & London: Guilford Press.

Kluft, R. (1986). High-functioning multiple personality patients. Three cases. *Journal of Mental Diseases, 4,* 722-726.

Kluft, R. (1992). Discussion: A specialist's perspective on multiple personality disorder. *Psychoanalytic Inquiry, 12,* 139-171.

Kohut, H. (1971) *The analysis of the self*. New York: International Universities Press.

Kohut, H. (1977). *The restoration of the self*. New York: International Universities Press.

Krystal, H. (1968). *Massive psychic trauma*. New York: International Universities Press.

Krystal, J., Kosten, T., Perry B., Southwick S., Mason J., & Giller, E. (1989). Neurobiological aspects of PTSD: Review of clinical and pre-clinical studies. *Behavior Therapy, 20,* 177-198.

Lambert, J. L. (1986). *Police powers and accountability.* London: Croom Helm.

Lazarus, A. (1972). *Behavior therapy and beyond.* New York: McGraw-Hill.

Lifton, J. R. (1973). The sense of immortality: On death and the continuity of life. *American Journal of Psychoanalysis, 33,* 3-15.

Lifton, J. R. (1980). The concept of the survivor. In J. Dimsdale (Ed.), *Survivors, victims, and perpetrators: Essays on the Nazi holocaust* (pp. 113-126). New York: Hemisphere Press.

Linehan, M. M. (1993). *Skills training manual for treating borderline personality disorder.* New York & London: The Guilford Press.

Loftus, E. (1979). *Eyewitness testimony.* Cambridge, MA: Harvard University Press.

Lorenz, K. (1971). *Studies in animal and human behavior* (Vols. I & II). Cambridge, MA: Harvard University Press.

Lorenz, K. (1972). *King Solomon's ring.* New York: The New American Library.

Lorenz, K. (1973). *On aggression.* New York: Bantam Books.

Lorenz, K., & Leyhausen, P. (1973). *Motivation of human and animal behavior: An ethological View.* New York: Van Nostrand Company.

Manchester, W. (1979). *Good-bye darkness: A memoir of the pacific war.* New York: Dell Publishers, Inc.

Marmer, C. (1980). Psychoanalysis of multiple personality. *International Journal of Psychoanalysis, 61,* 677-693.

Masterson, J. (1976). *Psychotherapy of the borderline adult.* New York: Brunner/Mazel.

Masterson, J. (1988). *Search for the real self: Unmasking the personality disorders of our age.* New York: The Free Press.

McNally, R. (2003). *Remembering trauma.* Cambridge, MA: Harvard University Press.

McNamara, J. (1967). Uncertainties in police work. In D. Bordua (Ed.), *The police: Six sociological essays.* New York: Wiley Press.

Meek, C. (1992). *Post traumatic stress disorder.* Sarasota, FL: Professional Resource Books.

Mersky, H. (1992). The manufacture of personalities. *British Journal of Psychiatry, 160,* 327-340.

Mitchell, J. (1988, July 24). Hero burnout. *Chicago Tribune.*

Mitchell, J., & Everly, G., Jr. (1996). *Critical incident stress debriefing: An operations manual for the prevention of traumatic stress among emergency services and disaster worker* (2nd ed.). Baltimore, MA: Chevron Publishing Company.

Morris, D. (1967). *The human zoo.* New York: Doubleday and Company, Inc.

Morris, D. (1969a). *The naked ape.* New York: Dell Book, Inc.

Morris, D. (1969b). *Primate ethology.* New York: Doubleday and Company, Inc.

Morris, D. (1971). *Intimate behavior.* New York: Random House.

Morris, D. (1977). *Man watching: A field guide to human behavior.* London: Cape Press.

Morris, R., & Morris, D. (1966). *Men and apes.* New York: Random House.

Myers, C. (1940). *Shell shock in France 1914-1918.* Oxford: Cambridge University Press.

Neiderhoffer, A. (1967). *Behind the shield: The police in urban society.* New York: Anchor Books.

Nietzsche, F. (1985). *The use and abuse of history* (A. Collins, trans.). New York: Macmillan.

Pavlov, I. (1941). *Conditioned reflexes and psychiatry.* New York: International Publishers.

Peterson, K., Prout, M., & Schwartz, R. (1992). *Post traumatic stress disorder. A clinicians guide*. New York: Plenum Press.

Postman, N. (1994). *Amusing ourselves to death*. New York: Basic Books.

Putnam, F. (1989). *Diagnosis and treatment of multiple personality disorder*. New York: Guilford Press.

Rado, S. (1939). Developments in the psychoanalytic conception and treatment of the neuroses. *Psychoanalytic Quarterly, 8,* 427.

Rado, S. (1956). *Psychoanalysis of behavior*. New York & London: Grune and Stratton, Inc.

Rando, T. (1984). *Grief, dying and death: Clinical interventions for caregivers*. Champaign, IL: Research Press.

Rando, T. (1993). *Treatment of complicated mourning: Clinicians guide*. Champaign, IL: Research Press.

Rappaport, D. (1971). *Emotions and memory*. New York: International University Press.

Reese, J. (1991). *Critical incidents in policing*. Washington, DC: U.S. Department of Justice, Federal Bureau of Investigation.

Richards, A., & Willick, M. (1986). *Psychoanalysis: The science of mental conflict*. Hillsdale, NJ: The Analytic Press.

Rudofossi, D. (1994a, February). Affective differential profiles of police officers. In T. Smith (Chair). Northeastern University. *Affective Education in Applied Psychology*. Symposium conducted at Eastern Education Research Association, Sarasota Florida.

Rudofossi, D. (1994b, December). *The effects of repetitive trauma in adulthood and dissociation*. Talk given at the New York Society for the Study of Multiple Personality and Dissociation. Columbia University, NY.

Rudofossi, D. (1997). *The impact of trauma and loss on affective profiles of police officers*. Bell Harbor, MI: Bell & Howell Company.

Rudofossi, D. (2007). *Working with traumatized police officer-patients: A clinicians guide to Complex PTSD Syndromes in public safety professionals*. New York: Baywood.

Rudofossi, D., & Ellis, R. (1999, August). *Differential police personality styles use of coping strategies, ego mechanism of defenses in adaptation to trauma and loss*. Symposium conducted at American Psychological Association, Boston, Massachusetts.

Santayana, G. (1906). *The life of reason: The phases of human progress*. New York: C. Scribners Sons.

Schneidman, E. (1996). *The suicidal mind*. Oxford & New York: Oxford University Press.

Schwartz, H. (1994). From dissociation to negotiation: A relational psychoanalytic perspective on multiple personality disorder. *Psychoanalytic Psychology, 11,* 189-231.

Schiff, W. (1979). *Perception: A text book*. New York: New York University Press.

Shapiro, D. (1965). *Neurotic styles*. New York: Basic Books.

Silverstein, R. (1992). *The correlation between combat related trauma processing and male ego development*. Ann Arbor, MI: Bell & Howell Company.

Smith, R. D., Buffington, P. W., & McCard, R. H. (1982). *Multiple personality: Theory, diagnosis, and treatment, a case study*. New York: Irvington Publishers, Inc.

Solomon, H., & Yakovlev, P. (1945). *Manual of military neuropsychiatry*. Philadelphia & London: W. B. Saunders Company.

Southwick, S. (2007). *Discussion of Logotherapy goal's during World Wide Logotherapy Conference at Dallas Texas,* Dallas, Texas.

Spielberger, C., Grier, K., & Greenfield, G. (1982, Spring). Major dimensions of stress in law enforcement. *Florida Fraternal Order of Police Journal, 18,* 30-50.

Styron, W. (1997). *Darkness visible.* New York: Vintage Books.

Terr, L. (1990). *Too scared to cry.* New York: HarperCollins.

Thorpe, J. (2007). *Discussion of Logotherapy goal's during World Wide Logotherapy Conference at Dallas Texas,* Dallas, Texas.

Tinbergen, N. (1948). *The study of instincts.* Oxford: Oxford University Press.

Tinbergen, N. (1969). *Curious naturalists.* New York: The American Museum of Natural History Press.

Toch, H. (2002). *Stress in policing.* Washington, DC: American Psychological Association.

Vaillant, G. (1977). *Adaptation to life.* Boston, MA: Little Brown.

Van Der Kolk, B., Greenberg, M., Boyd, H., & Krystal, J. (1985). Inescapable shock, neurotransmitters and addition to trauma: Toward a psychobiology of posttraumatic stress disorder. *Journal of Biological Psychiatry, 20,* 314-325.

Van Der Kolk, B. (1987). *Psychological trauma.* Washington, DC: American Psychiatric Press.

Van Der Kolk, B. (1989). The compulsion to repeat the trauma. Re-enactment, re-victimization, and masochism. *Psychiatric Clinics of North America, 12,* 389-411, Washington, DC.

Van Der Kolk, B., & Saporta, J. (1991). The biological response to psychic trauma: Mechanisms and treatment of intrusion and numbing. *Anxiety Research,* 4, 199-212.

Worden, J. W. (2001). *Grief counseling & grief therapy.* New York: Springer Publishing.

Wolpe, J. (1952). Experimental neurosis as learned behavior. *British Journal of Psychology, 43,* 243-268.

Yehudi, R., Resnick, H, Kahana, B, & Giller, E. (1993). Long lasting hormonal alterations in extreme stress in humans: Normative or maladaptive? *Journal of Psychosomatic Medicine, 55,* 287-297.

PART II

Emerging from PPS-CPTSD: Unmasking Five Police Personalities

CHAPTER 2
A Primer on Police Personality Styles as Adaptation to Complex Trauma

> A relevant and intriguing parallel may be drawn between the phylogenic evolution of a species genetic composition and the ontogenetic development of an individual organism's adaptive strategies ("its personality style"). . . . These distinctive ways of *adaptation, engendered by the interaction of biological endowment and social experience comprise the elements of what is termed personality styles* . . . (emphasis added). Theodore Millon, PhD, Dr. Sci. (1990)

This chapter is a brief introduction to the theoretical and methodological basis for the utility and justification of different public-safety personality styles as they emerged in response to complex losses hidden in trauma syndromes. The original hypothesis, methodology, and empirical derivations of the distinct clusters and clinical refinement that led to the five police personality styles is summarized here (Rudofossi, 1997; Rudofossi & Ellis, 1999).

What will follow for the remainder of the book, excluding the final chapter, is a detailed summary of each distinct personality style laid out in the next chapter. The actual composite profile is presented in the unadulterated words of the officers themselves, where possible. The existential-analytic eco-ethological approach in assessing, clarifying, and confronting schematic distortions and irrational beliefs are suggested for each separate style presented.

The initial core schemas are presented with specific resistance and defenses that you are likely to encounter within that personality style. The strengths of each style are highlighted to maximize the inroad for active cognitive and behavioral change, with consequent improvement in affective and emotional expression. For each profile, the first and most unique trauma chosen directly enlightens a boundary to each distinct police personality style.

One of the original approaches I developed is to highlight the *why* of behavior and cognition for each unique personality style in the context of eco-ethological influences. Each of the five police personality styles illustrates how the therapist can explore, clarify, and confront with maximum efficacy where schemas have become (mal)adaptive from composite case officer-patients. This range of presentation from mild to severe symptoms underscores my approach to emotional disturbance as a continuum that exists within each specific style presented. This presentation highlights an optimistic attitude that therapy can almost always help, even if it is the modest goal of relating support and establishing self-care through harm reduction, in addition to curtailing a premature discontinuance of sessions. I take the stand that maladaptation itself makes superb ecological sense in terms of ethological adaptation specific to that officer's style. Maladaptive behaviors would likely become extinguished, if they were not repetitively reinforced consciously or unconsciously. The reinforcement is achieved via a self-selected level of what these behaviors consistently offer the individual by way of affordances in their relative niches. What is afforded in the ecology of the units is invariants primed for survival in the geographic public-safety area of concern.

It is not stupidity or disavowal of what appears to be maladaptive or culturally insensitive to the larger society in which the unit or even precinct is placed, but the desperate clinging to what has helped maintain a style of *adaptive functional dissociation* (Rudofossi, 2007) that needs to be actively and empathically explored: part of the therapist's task is to clarify and actively confront an existential analytic eco-ethological perspective through self-help assignments, experimentation and *in vivo* experiences that lead to self discovery and owned responsibility by the patient.

The eco-ethological existential analysis component of learning one's own ability to numb oneself, avoidance through withdrawal, dissociative states, or immersion in repetitive risk taking is than to shift the focus on how and where the officer learned her style. By learning the how and why of maladaptation including the sensibility of how this pattern of behavior and cognition became established and what keeps it durable and resistant to change in the here and now a normalization emerges. This focus helps prevent secondary anxiety and depression by not insisting on overly optimistic goals of immediate change simplifying the complexity and impact of residual effects of repetitive trauma. Rather, the clinician willfully facilitates normalizing what hopefully will become clear as an attempt at adaptation in part to an abnormal environment of multiple experiences of trauma and loss. The experiences of trauma and loss, be they endogenous, exogenous, learned and conditioned, biochemical and genetic, drive motivated, or existential are actively explored. However, the question of accuracy in pinpointing whether the disturbance is exclusively one domain or another seems to be a waste of energy and efficiency for therapist and patient alike in the shared delusion of finding any precise solution.

The humbling reality is the complexity of trauma and loss will never be fully understood in its entirety. Meaning whether it is apparently all of these aforementioned constructs, and exactly what precision is veridical in terms of ascertaining the correct measurement of any one of these, and the myriad interactions of these variables in one single human being in a perceptual context appears to be an impossibility to answer scientifically.

However, working with the officer-patient on finding commonalties through heuristic exploration of what has brought an individual to historically (bio-chemical and genetic in an ecology with ethological motivation); socially (conditioned and learned) in the context of her history of trauma and loss experiences and style of coping in terms of endogenous emotional volatility, rage escalation, violent, passive or deescalation tendencies (innately motivated) illustrating where choice and responsibility are possible, all lead to realistic reappraisal of a humane and effective solution without capitulation to pessimism and labeling that is dehumanizing. An eco-ethological existential analysis provides a clinician with the skills to exchange a general psychoeducation about trauma and stress for a heuristic exploration achieved with an officer- patient anew.

In other words, rather than creating more complexity without solution, it is more up to the human task of therapist and patient to work on the goals of accepting the limitations in understanding the etiology of complex trauma without forsaking the impact and work of partial understanding and change.

THE BLUE WALL OF SILENCE: AFFORDANCE FOR MANY STYLES OF ADAPTATION TO A MALADAPTIVE ECOLOGY

The most poignant question is, why bother to read this chapter and perhaps this book? Isn't a single general inclusive picture of law-enforcement officers adequate for healthful change through intervention and therapy? Why offer five distinct personality styles of intrapersonal cognitive, affective, emotional, and existential schemas expressed through interpersonal styles of coping through patterns of behavior, social relationships, defensiveness, and resistance?

Isn't an integrative method of treatment that effects growth in emotional and mental health through change in the patient enough without creating a new personology and yet more classifications for the clinician? Finally, is the term "police personality styles" an accurate description for the different styles of coping and (mal)adaptation to the culture and ecology of law enforcement, including multiple experiences with repetitive trauma and loss?

Well, yes. I wholeheartedly endorse the implied bottom line that a patient who has an improvement in healthful and happier living through motivation and change is a clear measure of good therapy, regardless of modality. However, insight alone rarely changes embedded perceptual patterns without hard work at probing what cognitive, affective and behavioral patterns and how and why they continue operating intra- and interpersonally. Not only is this hard work for the patient, but hard work for the therapist, when dealing with law-enforcement officers who are hard at task to break what is called "the blue wall of silence." The blue wall of silence is maintained on an existential level and an eco-ethological sensibility primed by survival value.

It is motivation that is also directly targeted in my new approach. How? In part, it is also knowing the why of behavior, thoughts, feelings and emotional overload that deconstructs and normalizes the secondary anxiety, anger, guilt, and depression over why the officer continues to react in the same patterns even after finding out the roots of her style. It also helps toward self-acceptance of her style as a way of being, yet would be very helpful in repositioning and reconstructing what may be a new way of self-efficacy through "ones' will to meaning" by modifying Frankl's existential approach in acceptance of the sordid situations law-enforcement officers are forced to cope with without denial, capitulation, or projecting superstitious entities that disempower one's ability to chose one's own path—in becoming.

For a therapist to gain a working understanding of an individual law-enforcement officer's potential to act out violently with self or others, an extra effort is necessitated. The heart of this effort is the intra/interpersonal style of resistance and defensiveness in light of prior repetitive trauma and losses forged in the socialization process and investment for survival in their identity as a humane being and officer.

The quote at the beginning of the chapter by Dr. Ted Millon, perhaps the foremost personologist of the twentieth century, uses the term "personality styles" interchangeably with "adaptive strategies." He goes on to clarify the "distinctive ways of adaptation, engendered by the interaction of biological endowment and social experience comprise the elements of what is termed personality styles" (Millon, 1990). In a later magnum opus, he refines the use of personality style/ disorder as fundamentally "an ideal reference point to compare a person to, for conceptual and heuristic purposes," not as a categorical imperative (Millon, 1996). The implication is personality style is not used as a pejorative label (Goffman, 1967; Ryan, 1972; Szasz, 1961), but as a conceptual framework for applied psychotherapy in a developmental and evolutionary perspective (Millon, 1990, 1996). This operational definition of personality styles, and its application in psychotherapy is qualified as a pragmatic construct for clinical and research purposes (Millon, 1990, 1996; Sperry, 1995) in this chapter and elsewhere.

Millon's model operational definition of personality styles has four levels: The first is the Behavioral level, which consists of the domain of expressive acts and interpersonal conduct. The second is the phenomenological level; the domain consists of cognitive style, object representations and self-image. The third is the Intrapsychic level; the domain consists of regulatory mechanisms and morphological organization. The fourth is the Biophysical level; the domain consists of mood and temperament (1990, 1996).

In the chapter to follow, I limit each personality style (profile) to be inclusive of all four levels, as Millon suggests. Due to the scope of this book, the profile is limited to the most salient and discriminative presentations empirically. This helps distinguish one profile from another for clinical and assessment usefulness, regardless of therapy approach. It is not a definitive presentation and to iterate a focal point. I am presenting a heuristic model for effective understanding of individual differences. Trauma and loss are the most germane experiences officers are impacted by, and yet the most neglected is the hub of each profile presentation in this guide. This understanding is offered briefly in a clinically useful way in the next chapter as a working guide of the various personality styles, and how to approach each patient within a developmental context. In essence, this original and empirically based knowledge of personality styles can effect a change in the experienced and credentialed psychotherapist attempting a rational and responsible approach with public-safety officers.

Using the eco-ethological existential analytic approach with public-safety officers offers an effective approach even if you are used to working in a different modality. It is important for you to understand how and why the patient developed certain behaviors in a complex pattern of relating, affective displays, situational roles, emotional expressiveness and existential paradigms of meaning. This is done through an active heuristic hypothesis-driven approach, which at the core is scientific and humane in probing and searching with the patient for the schemas embedded in a paradigm exhibited uniquely in each personality style. Patiently and actively relating your understanding achieves the goal of normalizing the how and why in a complementary active directive challenging of irrational beliefs and psychodynamic compromises embedded in each stylized paradigm. I suggest this is real empathy from any perspective.

At the core of the eco-ethological existential analytic approach is the active change through dialogue and challenging one's way of thinking, relating, and behaving with others, self, and the world in the here and now. An elegant scientific approach begs an inclusion that is sorely needed by sorting through the etiology and the dynamic interplay of complex interactions and intra- and interpsychological processes with insight, but not for insight alone. Active altering of maladaptive patterns on all levels is enriched by knowing the how and why of thought and behavior in the context of your patient's unique public-safety personality style. The words used by patients in a dialogue with you are not accidental and nearly always relay meaningful communication about their deep-rooted beliefs, which can often times clash with their espoused knowledge. The context of the use of words in attempting to communicate, or avoid communicating—self-report addendums added on to questionnaires, poems, or even little invectives used in the session—is informative and has as different meanings as much as the individual using them. Yet, the semantic texture of the words chosen is nested in the personality style as the most reducible and discrete anchor that the therapist can use in modifying his own initial approach in the therapy experience (Fromm, 1951). An active approach here may be effected by the therapist modifying his semantic approach to different personality styles in a well-timed intervention. This will be illustrated with examples for each composite profile.

Lastly and most importantly, the approach to one patient, with certain resistances, inhibitions, and styles of relating and feeling toward others, puts the therapist squarely in the hot seat. Unlike other populations, law-enforcement officers are unique in usually having lethal force in firearms readily available, the power to incarcerate another, and are trained to take action against others when a threat is perceived. It is unlikely the therapist will be the recipient of open aggression. However, responsibility lies in trying to achieve a more accurate assessment and intervention when feasible in ameliorating impulsivity and acting out with self or others violently. Psychotherapy interventions presented in this guide in dealing with daily stress, trauma, and loss are informed by understanding the personality style they are embedded in. This ability in discrimination helps increase the likelihood of a sound clinical judgment.

However, I refer to Irving Yalom's, MD caveat to clinicians to not take so seriously the validity of nosological precision in personality diagnosis as a worthy critique. After all, precision fits nicely with chemical reactions, yet it is speculative at best when combined with the classification of people into fixed categorical imperatives. Attempting to reduce an ever-changing fluid, complex, and humane being into a fixed category eludes a rational approach and is as likely as fixing Heraclitus's River. Yet, for purposes of a guide for an assessment and treatment approach that is flexibly structured and empirically based, distinguishing one style of personality from another is an elegant and rational approach. Yalom (1989, 1996) himself has implicitly used this approach in many of his informal rich presentations of patients without resort to reductionism. Having articulated qualifications and emendations to my approach, let us enjoin a brief overview of the foundations of Public-Safety Personality Styles to follow.

ORIGINAL STUDIES AND FOUNDATIONS FOR PUBLIC-SAFETY PERSONALITY STYLES

I conducted my first study with police in 1992-1993 as a pilot study. After quite a few informal interviews with my peers, I set up a few small-scale structured interviews of self-reports, including risk-taking behaviors and attitudes, anxiety levels, and need for excitement. In an experimental research design in a controlled setting, a simulated auto designed for proprioception and braking responses to simulated risk factors through a series of interactive videos were measured by choice reaction times. In sum, the results were not large enough for any scientific generalization. Yet, my hypothesis was bolstered by observations that law-enforcement officers interpreted events discriminatively within group and between group in emotional, measured behavioral responses, and cognitive styles.

One comparative study recorded the frequency of NYU students who crossed at stop signs without stopping and looking for traffic. I made a comparative observation of police recruits doing the same thing two blocks from the Police Academy. The results of my handwritten chi-square analysis was statistically significant in establishing differences in higher-risk taking by officer candidates.

Due to obstacles, including a lack of any demographic information except student status of both groups of participants, I made a mental note of my findings, which fueled my passion to refine my hypothesis and put it to the rigor of scientific testing.

This was followed by a large-scale pilot study in 1994 with a population of 60 participants, which yielded significant results for a valid and reliable instrument for research.

In a large-scale study, 576 volunteers were selected randomly. One of the original hypotheses was presented verbatim as follows:

> Differential affective profiles will emerge as a result of distinct (sub)groupings of police participant's based upon stress responsivity as measured by the scales of anxiety, anger and sadness and the self report section of the cumulative police trauma scale. (Rudofossi, 1994)

METHODOLOGY FOR DERIVING CLUSTER ANALYSIS

In choosing what type of major clustering method to use, the research problem of classification of cases framed the solution. A method that would not force the data, but rather merge the similar cases through minimizing the distance of cases based upon the similarity of cases through an agglomerative method was desirable. A visual dendogram was chosen for clear boundary formation. Furthermore, the preferred technique of agglomeration combined cases by similarities through maximization of the least distance between two cluster points, diminishing the probability of overspread through artificial inflation of distances, which led to choosing the hierarchical agglomerative cluster analysis by using the single-linkage bottom-up technique.

FINDINGS IN A NUT SHELL

The original research in detail that was conducted from 1994 to 1995, codified, quantified, and written up in 1996, and published in 1997, can be found by the researcher and clinician who desires more detail, including statistical operations (Rudofossi, 1997). The original findings were expanded and defined with an in-depth protocol through extensive interviews, assessment, and interventions by the author from 1996 to 2000 (Rudofossi, 2001).

The reliability of the piloted research clinical instrument was an alpha coefficient of .84 for the initial pilot study, with 60 participants (Rudofossi, 1994, Appendix D). The actual research study with 576 participants separate from the pilot study yielded acceptable levels of validity through inferential statistical operations as follows: First, the internal consistency of the scale's 33 items of the three subscales of anger, anxiety, and sadness was .89. Second, the internal reliability formula yielded a mean of .42 for each item-whole coefficient and an overall alpha of .89 (see Rudofossi, 1997). The acceptable standard has been set at .70.

One out of five returned instruments was appropriately filled out and returned to the researcher. The population of assessment was over 2% of the entire NYPD population. The financing of the research was independent of the NYPD and the police unions, diminishing the confounding of obligation and constraint, increasing the likelihood of bias in reporting results and conclusions.

In the first hypothesis, separate and unique factors emerged in discrimination between different events depicted through vignettes of actual police experiences as measured by the cumulative police trauma scale, and confirmed through the technique of factor analysis (Rudofossi, 1997).

The second hypothesis was predicated upon the first being confirmed. Having been confirmed, the statistical technique of cluster analysis was warranted and yielded confirmatory evidence of differential affective profiles of police participants based upon stress response as measured by the scales of anxiety, anger, and sadness and the self-report section of the Cumulative Police Trauma Scale.

The original findings delineated nine clusters and five subclusters that were later reduced to five clearly defined and renamed profiles of law-enforcement officers. This was done by coalescing clusters into profiles that were first defined in terms of events experienced and cognitive, experiential, affective, and emotional differences in response. By affective I mean the feelings expressed or inhibited by the participants. Emotions is used in relation to an evolutionary and survival value of the expressiveness and responses of that participant. A review of my protocol and more findings can be found by the clinician and researcher (Rudofossi, 1997, 2007; Rudofossi & Ellis, 1999).

The goal in this parsimonious reduction was to highlight sensitivity as well as specificity of each style by discrimination of each, as compared with the other. I struggled with the best means of presentation and concluded one actual case example for each cluster would present a gestalt that had genuine meaning and realism, which can help the clinician as well as the researcher. Each case presentation will focus on the unique role trauma and loss have contributed to the prominent display of symptoms.

The frame of each personality style is based upon and modified from Millon's model, which in judgment, offered the most comprehensive approach to the researcher and clinician (Millon, 1996). The content of material is presented as it was first observed and disclosed, with the qualification that each patient has been protected from identifying variables. It is important to highlight that in presenting these case profiles in a style that is unavoidably candid, it was and is a great privilege to work with the unique individuals who have opened up a universe of rich and varied experiences. I have been privileged to listen to and learn a great deal from each in the process of crisis intervention, assessment, and the therapeutic process in public and then private practice with countless officer-patients.

The differentiation from one profile to another is not only based upon Euclidean space, but the commonality of experiences and equally important responsive and unique levels of intrapsychic defensiveness for survival (ethological motivation in an ecological niche and contextual paradigm); biophysical level of mood and temperament (ethological demands and selective adaptation in an ecological niche); behavioral levels of expressive acts and interpersonal conduct (ethological motivation shaped and modeled in unique ecological niches); and phenomenological level of self-image, cognitive style, and object representations. The phenomenological differentiation from one profile to another is modified and uniquely built upon an existential analysis and a logotherapy foundation.

The section for each profile I present is titled, "Discussion of Personality Style Development" and is a summary of many clarifications and confrontations during assessment and therapy sessions with officers, which helped understand the how and why styles developed, as well as the evolutionary value in etiology covered in the other sections. I have integrated evolutionary theory, largely developed from my introduction to this area of science through the disciplined tutelage of my former graduate professor, Irving Brick, PhD [Embryologist and Evolutionary Biologist] at New York University, Graduate School of Arts & Science, and the reader of my MA Essay (1987), Dr. Terry Jordan [Medical Psychologist and Measurement Expert], and Dr. William Schiff [Psychophysicist and Ecological Psychologist] for bringing to me the possibilities of this fascinating field without hyperbole. Theodore Millon's PhD, Dr. Sci. seminal works contributed to my modified approach to personology in a pragmatic application for public-safety officer-patients.

Theoretically, Millon (1990) deconstructed Freud's nascent model of a three-tiered paradigm of the mind based upon polarity of subject (ego), object [external world] *as the real,* pleasure-pain [economically] and active-passive as the [biological]. Millon offers his model as a revised strategy of behavior, thought, and emotion that maximizes success in three different major areas that Freud first postulated. However, he postulates a bipolar component that separates dimensions of each pole. For example, in the context of separate bipolar dimension's of pleasure pain and also, self (subject)-others (object) Dr. Millon asserts,

> *Pleasure and pain are bipolar,* that is, *separate dimensions:* a person can be high or low on either or both, for example, Schizoids experience little pleasure and little pain. Pleasure and pain are conceptual antitheses or opposites; *each end has its own significance rather than exhibiting merely different levels of degrees of the same phenomenon,* for example, pleasure is not a low or high level of pain, nor is pain a high (or low level) of pleasure. . . . As with pleasure and pain, *self [ego] and other [objects] are bi-polar,* compromising two independent and antithetical dimensions; persons may simultaneously be high or low on either or both. For example, avoidants typically express little interests nor gain much pleasure from either self or others; by contrast,

to be focused on the welfare of others does not preclude self-interest. *Passivity and activity* represent a *unipolar dimension* that is *they correspond essentially to quantitative differences in degree on a single continuum* or gradient of motion or performance. In other words, a person cannot engage in both minimal passivity and minimal activity the less they do of one the more they do of the other. (Millon, 1990, emphasis mine)

The above quote suggests the importance of discrimination in regard to assessing a clinical problem that is one of not only degrees of quantity, but qualitative differences. Identity modes forged in the field of combat, whether domestic or foreign terrorism (see Rudofossi, 2007), are understood in this context of individual differences officer-patients present as antithetical and yet interdependent modes of adaptive functional dissociation. The adaptive functional dissociation exhausts front line officer-patients in resisting losses impacted by repetitive trauma and the defenses that continue to evolve in the combat ecology of survival in the ethological motivation of life and death struggles.

Differential diagnosis highlights discrimination for assessment between profiles with similar content that can be mistakenly identified. This section also underscores the work of personology in elucidating this profile in the specific context of public safety.

The roots of psychopathologies or healthy adaptiveness need be primarily descriptive in groundwork, rather than secondarily interpretive, which is true in trauma and loss research as it is in all other clinical work. *Without basing clinical descriptions through the words and behaviors of the individuals who are experiencing the trauma and loss, in their own eco-ethological niche, one is in danger of creating chimeras in ivory towers rather than depictions as the officer-participant experienced it.* However, judgments of police officers who are blind (unconscious) to the developmental context it occurred in is judgmental and can lead to social distancing, dehumanization, and creating barriers to bridges in relating and understanding the individual officer-patients struggles. To ignore and gloss over the reality of trauma and loss, or deny the impact of its intensity in shaping the human psyche is to dwell in the realm of ignorance, if not arrogance. That ignorance and arrogance can be a blind spot in the analysis of clinician and officer-patient.

The antidote in part is offered by the richness of clinical data amassed and coalesced for these profiles and will allow a view of police that has been hitherto shielded from public scrutiny, despite the profile of sociopathic and sadistic behavior, cognition's, and traits emergent through ones prior disposition and the focus on style, not disorder (Millon, 1990, 1996; Sperry, 1995). I firmly believe, along with Sigmund Freud, that one ought not court mediocrity by watering down one's findings for political, economic, or superficial conformities to popular notions, but rather go forward in realistic presentations of one's findings for the advancement of science and authentic comprehension of human complexities, regardless of modern pressures for political correctness or intellectual fascism insidious and modern forms of tyrannies (Freud, 1894/1963; Fromm, 1951; Rudofossi, 1997, 2007).

Creating a foundation for further controlled and naturalistic observations is a clear, critical, and important component of effective-treatment in understanding this unique minority in dire need of professional assistance, I have been advocating for this research since 1992 as a participant observer. It is time for an effective, responsible treatment of a very traumatized and marginalized population by serious and committed clinician-scientists. In order to ameliorate the anguish of trauma and loss, the clinician needs to understand the structure of this universe, which has been laid out throughout this book.

The other pressing solution-focused approach involves a treatment plan that incorporates the different types of enduring characterological traits of the specific officer-patient presenting in the here and now. The therapist is ill-advised, unless she knows how this behavioral and cognitive pattern developed, and the utility in terms of ecological and ethological significance before rushing to normalize the impact of traumatic loss. This apolitical approach is most likely to be met by suspending judgment or one-sided adherence to any treatment modality; on the other hand integration needs to follow a rational disciplined approach. What I am asserting is more than a tentative theory: An empirical and pragmatic approach that moves clinicians to appreciate the reality of officer's lives and their actual coping mechanisms within a personological perspective. The evidence of research highlights a complex interdynamic of personology development that is endogenous in potential, and impacted and shaped developmentally by repetitive and complex interactions of the traumatic events experienced within an ecological and ethologic context.

In order to protect the identities of the actual officer's who were part of the original research and the officers who had courageously volunteered for mental health services, an agglomeration of traits and defense mechanisms, coping strategies, and genuine accounts are presented for the reader; whether researcher, scientist-practitioner, psychiatrist, psychologist, or other scientist, the clinical material is real and the composite characters are real. I hope the reader can take the following chapters not as an interesting piece on individual psychopathology, but as part of an eco-ethologic (mal)adaptiveness to a world of trauma and loss far above the normal experiences by a representative sample of men and women who represent the police population in terms of age, race, ethnicity, intelligence, and culture.

Many of the officers within these clusters have been able to, through therapy and pharmacologic interventions, ameliorate and channel their endogenous levels of aggression, impulsiveness, depression, and various manifestations of mental and behavioral symptoms to the point of going beyond functioning in movement, with gains in genuine motility and strengthened resilience and more mature defense mechanisms than when first seen within the eco-ethological niche they were established in, after extensive and intensive psychopharmacologic and psychotherapeutic interventions.

My research and experience with police participant's, which is extensive, thus far has led to the conclusion that it *is the traumatic experiences and loss that officers experience that leads to the devastating mental health problems we encounter in our professional practice of psychology, not administrative, internal bureaucracy or politics.* Although all play an important role in psychopathology maintenance, it is not born from these common stressors to all bureaucracies. What really differentiates these police participants are not only the highly charged experiences encountered, but the differential affective style of personality, in part endogenous endowment, and in larger part exogenous experience. The existential analysis is incisive when these differences in personality styles are laid out as the contextual basis to move forward with securing meaning in the gap of multiple losses inflicted in the wounds of traumas.

Hopefully, if you, the clinician or researcher, walk away with one axiom from my research and clinical work, it is that genuine and meaningful differences endure in patterns of (mal)adaptation taking on characterologic styles in the police population; and that, indeed, police officers are a marginalized minority that needs a great deal of empathy and support as well as intervention, that traumatic events are extremely variable, there is no accident or fortuitous recounting of an event, it is almost always meaningful, contextual, and rich in the eco-ethological meaning for that individual officer.

Officers are neither villains nor saints, but they are human, with all that implies. When an officer says, "I am O.K." and nothing bothers him, do not take it for granted that is the case; the skeptical approach is the healthiest; you might say all trauma is only the exposed tip of the iceberg: without proper navigation and awareness of what to probe for, one might miss it only to have it arise suddenly and devastatingly for clinician and patient alike. Finally, I suggest that in listening to the words spoken by these participants, omissions of the overt words of trauma and loss in each profile by no means ought to be interpreted as nonexistent trauma and loss. Further, there is much more excavation into the conscious and ecological determinants of trauma and loss that exist, but are not yet picked up due to the difficulty of research with this population. This is once again an imperfect, rough-hewn sketch of the composite case examples I am privileged to introduce. All have signed a waiver to allow their material presented without identification; it is to them I owe a large debt of gratitude. Finally, it is hard to admit, but honestly, this work itself is the first tremor of an avalanche with much yardage and depth encrusted under the surface.

Suggestions for inroads for a therapy alliance and maintenance for each profile, offered at the conclusion of this book, increases your chances for an initial successful approach to broadening the rational discourse of growth and healthful living that is meaningfully defined with the public-safety officer—responsibly, respectfully, and within their level of development in the here and now. It is not fact written in stone, but exist on buoys that shine in the anonymity of a dusk-gray sea, illuminating the context of the style in the wonder of the individual officer sitting with you for shared exploration—an activity. *That is the hub of existential therapy that is secure in its center; where officer's emptied canteens of precious water of life litter the shores like a vacuum filled anew from the wells of unique and individualized sources of reenfranchised meaning.*

My final qualification prior to the presentation of the following original profiles is that I am solely responsible for this work, including all the foibles—that is all too human. You would be well advised to view this section as hypothetical constructs that are empirically and clinically supported at this time.

REFERENCES

Freud, S. (1894/1963). *Therapy and technique.* New York: Macmillan.

Fromm, E. (1951). *The forgotten language.* New York: Grove Press.

Goffman, E. (1967). *Stigma.* New York: Simon and Schuster.

Millon, T. (1990). *Toward a new personology.* New York: John Wiley and Sons, Inc.

Millon, T. (1996). *Disorders of personality: DSMIV and beyond.* New York: John Wiley, Inc.

Rudofossi, D. (1994, February). Affective differential profiles of police officers. In T. Smith (Chair), Northeastern University. *Affective education in applied psychology.* Symposium conducted at Eastern Education Research Association, Sarasota Florida.

Rudofossi, D. (1997). *The impact of trauma and loss on affective profiles of police officers.* Ann Arbor, MI: Bell and Howell Publication.

Rudofossi, D., & Ellis, R. (1999, August). Differential police personality styles in adaptation to trauma and loss. *Symposium at American Psychological Association,* Boston, Massachusetts.

Rudofossi, D. (2007). *Working with police officer-patients: A clinician's guide to Complex PTSD syndromes in public safety professionals.* New York: Baywood.

Ryan, W. (1972). *Blaming the victim.* New York: Vintage Books.

Sperry, L. (1995). *Handbook of diagnosis and treatment of the DSMIV personality disorders.* New York: Brunner/Mazel.

Szasz, T. (1961). *The myth of mental illness.* New York: Hoeber Medical Division, Harper and Row.

Yalom, I. (1989). *Loves executioner.* New York: Basic Books.

Yalom, I. (1996). *Lying on the couch.* New York: Basic Books.

CHAPTER 3
Toward Achieving an Effective Eco-Ethological Existential Analysis with the Five Varieties of Public-Safety Personality Styles

> It is more important to know what sort of person has a disease than to know what sort of disease a person has. Hippocrates. (Heidel, 1941)

Forged in the crucible of my experience as a participant observer (uniform psychologist and sergeant), I present five police personality styles in this chapter. The purpose is to enhance the skills of the therapist, with the emphasis on intervention. However, as this chapter offers a tentative model, it is not written in stone and makes no presumption of such a claim.

What the chapter does offer is a guide. That helps the therapist understand differences each officer-patient presents and will ultimately provide a focus for intervention. Each presentation includes the officer-patient's personality styles, traits, features, tendencies, behavior, cognitions, affect, and emotions (ethological states). Change may take place through different means, but the one of interest here is the process of grief and trauma therapy. Joint exploration of the present works back to the hedge stones of the traumatic past. Our task is to expose ungrieved losses to the light of today. The clinician may achieve this task by gaining a better understanding of patterns, features, and traits of each officer-patient through examination of his personality style.

Each personality style comprises core beliefs/schemas, specific resistances, and defenses you are likely to encounter. The strengths of each personality style are highlighted to maximize insight and cognitive-behavioral change through consequent improvement in affective and emotional expression of loss. Clinical case examples guide exploration, clarification, and insight for the therapist seeking to structure interventions. In my presentation of the five personality styles, individual identities and integrity of each participant is protected. Therefore, keep in mind that each personality style I present is a composite of many participants. The composite yields a clear description without revealing the identity of any individual officer-patient.

USING POLICE AND PUBLIC-SAFETY
PERSONALITY STYLES

Describing psychopathology, maladaptation, or healthy adaptation helps provide some structure that may lead to refinement of sophisticated clinical use. Without clinical descriptions, including the words and behaviors of individual officer-patients who are experiencing loss in trauma, a danger exists in clinical practice. Therapists may create chimeras that become ever elusive, rather than the earthy experience of the officer-participant. Therapist responsiveness toward officer-patients may become unintentionally blind to the context of an officer's personality style and how it developed, which may lead to impasses in the therapeutic relationship.

The motif that has threaded and bonded the pages of this entire book, and no less in my presentation of the five personality styles, is the multidimensional losses experienced in trauma. If the therapist unwittingly glosses over the intensity of loss once, twice perhaps, the likely outcome is that the therapeutic alliance will not be fractured. However, a sigh of relief is not yet warranted. If the therapist repeatedly does not attend to the officer-patient's loss, trust may rupture and impede the ability to grieve. If a therapist unwittingly develops a pattern whereby the officer-patient experiences a denial of loss, it is likely that disenfranchised loss may become reburied in all the maladaptive defenses with vehemence and recalcitrance. That bleak outcome is far from the therapists conscious desire.

I suggest a helpful means of dealing with this impasse lies in the therapist understanding the resistances and the promise of alliance each of the five personality styles presents. By understanding the developmental context of the officer's personality style the therapist may facilitate expression of grief in an officer-patient. *The humbling reality may be that the complexity of loss may never be fully understood.* However, appreciating these complexities and limitations does not block the search for commonalties through heuristic exploration that leads to an optimistic and realistic reappraisal of an effective solution without capitulating to the officer-patient's pessimism and without dehumanizing him.

The task of therapist and patient, without applying simplistic labels, is to work together on accepting the limitations in understanding the etiology without forsaking the impact and work of partial understanding and change, subject to error, that is the heart of intervention. The task may be served by the therapist's heeding Yalom's caveat to psychologists and psychiatrists not to take so seriously the validity of nosological precision in personality diagnosis (Yalom, 1983, 1985, 1989, 1996). Yalom's is a worthy critique. Attempting to reduce an ever-changing fluid complex, human being into a fixed category eludes a rational approach, and is as likely as fixing Heraclitus river on a microscopic slide.

RESISTANCE FROM AN ECO-ETHOLOGICAL PERSPECTIVE

The persistence of maladaptive behaviors is a serious problem. These behaviors would likely become extinguished if they were not consistently reinforced on a conscious and unconscious level. We may best gain insight by understanding what behaviors offer each individual of what is afforded in his ecological niche. Defenses are viewed in context, specificity, and efficacy; that is, actions that support their persistence.

Learning to focus on how and where the officer's style of adaptation emerged through numbing, avoidance, withdrawal, dissociative states, or immersion in repetitive risk taking is important in focusing your own stylistic approach. Halting secondary anxiety and depression by desisting from overly optimistic goals of immediate change is important in effecting change in the context of differences each officer-patient presents.

In part, ethological motivation supports defenses, their emergence, and persistence. This motivation develops within the ecology of the unit that the officer-patient develops his professional identity. Invariants shape what becomes invested with survival value. I use the term invariants in the context of personality styles that develop, and what these invariants shape in terms of what is afforded within each officer-patient's ecological niche. Persistent behaviors, cognitions, and affect are infused with cultural significance, rituals, and drive derivatives that are sexual and aggressive. Ethological motivation in any living organism includes drive derivatives of a sexualized and aggressive nature. Officer-patients and all humans are so influenced. Influence however is not absolute determination. It is susceptible to therapeutic intervention. Ethological motivation is by no means uniform in the presentations of each officer-patient. As therapists using the eco-ethological approach to trauma and loss we attempt to answer why and make sensible maladaptive and repetitive patterns the officer-patient presents on a conscious and unconscious level.

Normalizing maladaptation to an abnormal environment of multiple experiences of trauma and loss is not easy. The task is to show how these defenses may make superb sense in the context of the individual officer-patient's developmental experience, yet now have evolved into maladaptive patterns. The abstraction of trauma is exchanged for a clear insight into the eco-ethological developmental influence and connecting that to traumatic distress. Trauma and loss is in part endogenous (drive derivatives), exogenous, unconscious, conscious, learned, conditioned, biochemical, and genetic. However, these influences are not only maladaptive responses to loss in trauma but also include healthier adaptation, resilience, and effective accommodation to these experiences. The therapist mobilizes and enhances these healthier responses depending on the officer-patient's willingness to effect changes in his life.

A patient who has an improvement in healthful living through motivation and change is a clear measure of good therapy, regardless of modality. However, keep in mind insight offered once, twice, or thrice rarely changes embedded perceptual patterns without hard work at probing what conscious and unconscious cognitive, affective, and behavioral patterns are operating intra- and interpersonally. The therapist needs to clarify repeated insights while using the full repertoire of his skills. Not only is this hard work for the patient, but hard work for the therapist when dealing with officers who are hard at work holding the blue wall of silence—a very thick wall indeed! (Benner, 1991; Gilmartin, 2002; Schlossberg & Freeman, 1974).

The therapist directly targets the officer-patient's motivation as a mobilizing force in the eco-ethological approach. How? In part, it is knowing the why of behavior, thoughts, feelings, and emotional overload which deconstructs and normalizes the secondary anxiety, anger, guilt, and depression. The why an officer reacts to in similar patterns across situations is key to change within the roots of each officer's personality style. An extra effort is necessary for a therapist to gain an understanding of an individual law-enforcement officer's potential to act out violently with self or others. The heart of this effort is the intra/inter-personal style of resistance and defensiveness in light of prior repetitive loss forged in the socialization process shaped by an ecology of trauma. With this in mind, a tentative framework for the application of how evolutionary influences have shaped each personality style through the lens of losses within the ecology of repetitive trauma is offered.

THE MODEL FOR THE FIVE POLICE AND PUBLIC-SAFETY PERSONALITY STYLES

Millon, perhaps the foremost personologist of the twentieth century, suggests that personality styles are strongly influenced by adaptive strategies.

Millon refines the use of personality style as fundamentally "an ideal reference point to compare a person to, for conceptual and heuristic purposes" (1996, p. 121). While the presentation of the five personality styles in this chapter is not a definitive guide, it does suggest a reference point for further understanding.

A leading psychoanalyst of our time, Dr. Charles Brenner, suggests how important personality traits may be in regard to our understanding and intervention with trauma:

> What used to be called shell shock is the result of an overwhelming influx
> of external stimuli which has then automatically given rise to anxiety. Freud

himself raised *this possibility* and many authors have subsequently appeared to assume that was true, or at least that Freud believed it to be true. *Actually Freud (1926) expressed the opinion that called the "participation of the deepest layers of the personality.* (1974, p. 74; my emphasis)

The beginning of understanding may, in fact, lie within an attempt to understand the officer's personality styles as a reference point from which individualized working hypotheses emerge (Brenner, 1974; Ellis, 1999; Millon, 1990; Scharf, 2003). It is to their wisdom that I suggest we cede in our approach. With these emendations in mind I use Millon's operational definition of personality styles on four levels as follows:

> The first is the behavioral level, which consists of the domain of expressive acts and interpersonal conduct.
> The second level is the phenomenological level, cognitive style, object representations, and self-image.
> The third level is the intra-psychic level of regulatory mechanisms and morphological organization.
> The fourth level is the biophysical level of mood and temperament (1990, 1996).

While Millon's model offers a highly useful personality model, due to the scope of this book, the profiles are limited to clinically salient perspectives. This helps distinguish one profile from another for clinical intervention, regardless of therapy approach. This understanding is offered briefly as a working guide to the various personality styles within a developmental context. In essence, an empirically based knowledge of personality styles offers the psychotherapist a rational and responsible approach with public-safety professionals seeking therapy. I have modified Millon's model as follows:

Intra-psychic level of defensiveness for survival

Biophysical level of mood and temperament

Behavioral levels of expressive acts and interpersonal conduct

Phenomenological level of self-image, cognitive style, and object representations

I have added additional sections to guide practice:

Differential diagnosis: highlights discrimination for assessment between profiles with similar content.

Epitome of why officer joined public service

Verbatim record of a traumatic event: underscoring stylized expression in their own words.

Discussion of personality style development: a summary of sessions with officers that helped understand the how and why styles developed, as well as the evolutionary value in etiology covered in the other sections. Coalescing the importance of the why with a how to achieve change via an eco-ethological existential analysis punctuates the discussion of effecting meaning in the context of trauma.

Suggestions for inroads for a therapy alliance and maintenance: each profile is offered at the conclusion of this book, increases your chances for an initial successful approach to broadening the rational discourse of growth and healthful living that is meaningfully defined with the public-safety officer—responsibly, respectfully, and within their level of development in the here and now. This is also where the core impact of an eco-ethological existential analysis is anchored with a perspective on forwarding healthier goals achieved in therapy.

Clinician's corner: offers you a real feel by giving you one more clinical intervention specific to the style. It is a space where motivation is engendered for you as a therapist and where the doc in the Cop Doc speaks to you in a way that is one-on-one lessons learned in the crucible of effective therapy techniques, without ignoring thwarted attempts and lessons learned.

The five public-safety personality styles to be presented are in the following order:

The Addictive Hyperexcited
The Sadistic Hyperaggressive
The Idiosyncratic Hyperintuitive
The Controlled Hyperfocused
The Adaptive-Intuitive

THE ADDICTIVE HYPEREXCITED PUBLIC-SAFETY PERSONALITY STYLE: INTRAPSYCHIC LEVEL OF DEFENSIVENESS FOR SURVIVAL

This personality style epitomizes what may be loosely called the prototypical interminable adolescent, stuck in the maladaptive belief of invulnerability to danger. Hyperexcitement may be reinforced by the functional value of an excitable extroversion in a quasimilitary setting. An immediate demand for gratification and attention seeking is typically met with bravado, excitement, and a flare for the dramatic. Performance records provide clues in which frequent and intense involvement in rescue is above average. Adaptively, frustration tolerance is very high for enduring pain, inhibiting fear, and successful completion of police tasks. Maladaptive frustration tolerance in delaying hedonic pleasure for genuine relational goals is abysmally low.

The officer-patient with this style is likely to put herself in the hub of all dangerous public-service action and is likely to be characterized by peers as a "cop's cop." Paradoxically, the officer with this personality style has a deep desire to relate to others through taking great risks with her own safety at stake along with the well-being of others. The extraordinary level of trigger-point heroism is markedly extreme, more so than in any other personality style. Trigger-point heroism means running into situations of grave danger without healthy caution and consequential thinking. Manipulating safety and legal guidelines, coupled with taking great personal risks for a commendation is the rule rather than the exception. A need for the approval of peers and supervisors is very high and exaggerated.

BIOPHYSICAL LEVEL OF MOOD

Dissociation and fugue states, as described by Erikson and Rossi (1989), are not uncommon with this style. Altered states of consciousness during excitement at police-related situations may mimic a manic-like state. This is especially true when the officer-patient recounts traumatic events. This has been reliable in interpretation of play-by-play assessment of taped sessions. The patient's self-report of mood was "great," "excited," "elated," and of having "a need to stay high most of the time." A swing from pleasant animation to expansive agitation was common in presentation. An example occurred after 9/11/01, when an officer informed me he was exhilarated by the awesome event. The involvement and the excitement being expressed channeled his low-grade depression into a distraction on one level, and on another it helped him feel needed and have a sense of belonging. This need for excitement as an addiction to trauma may in part be a result of a distraction from depression due to loss, an endogenous addictive craving for trauma, and an exogenous excitement that becomes gradually and biologically supported in neural networks.

PHENOMENOLOGICAL LEVEL OF SELF-IMAGE, COGNITIVE STYLE, AND OBJECT REPRESENTATIONS

This personality style had impulsive, thrill/adventure seeking, and high excitation when thrust in dangerous situations. The highly extroverted orientation toward others portrayed a style of poor judgment, self-sabotage, and inconsequential thinking for self-preservation. This style is similar to combat veterans who become addicted to the war environment (Figley, 1985; Wilson & Zigelbaum, 1983). However, in the case of police and public-safety officers, it is the urban war zones that mold and perpetuate what is afforded in the ecological niche. The emergence of this personality style appears to be developmental, exogenous, and adaptive, rather than innate and incorrigible. Although, as in all the styles there is vulnerability toward the development of one style over another, this is not to say a premorbid psychopathology exists.

The officer's cognitive style is for an immediate release of aggression during police operations. Without reflecting on sound, prudent tactics and consequential thinking, the officer-patients have a style of "do first, then think." While this is not supported formally, it is not unnatural in the context of adolescent thinking and behavior. *In no way is this indicative of a marginal intellect, but it does reveal poor impulse control.* An example of this type of thinking and behavioral response in attempting to solve a problem is as follows: A fellow detective left his keys in the office. In response, the hyperexcited officer, being a cops cop, climbed onto a ledge three stories up, crawled in, and let his peer in. I used Socratic elicitation to gain a sense of whether he had thought of safer alternatives or if he judged the serious danger of his risky behavior. With serious bravado, and lack of self-reflection, he answered without hesitation, "I needed to save my pal from shame, so the boss would not think of us as Keystone cops. All of life is a risk. No sweat."

At the core of irrational beliefs in this officer's style is a belief in one's own invulnerability, the dire need to live up to the perfect hero ideal, and a demand for other's approval. Constant energy and risk is invested and spent in achieving status as the perfect alpha officer in his unit. The risk taking in any conceivable situation follows the irrational belief, "I am invulnerable and will never die." On a less conscious level may be the fear, "I am very vulnerable to death, *but as long as I use these rituals which symbolically reenact death by flirting with it, I control the threat.*" That omnipotent fantasy can be addressed from a psycho-dynamic, cognitive-behavioral, and logotherapeutic approach. Acting out via aggression is legitimized in inverse proportion to the social distance of the victim in relation to the officer's identity. Loss and sadness were acceptable in expression as an attributive projection—to an innocent victim, not a sacred or profane involved victim (see chapter 4).

The self-image of officer-participants focused on what they had done as police, fire officers and emergency responders with little reflection on their personal lives outside of their circumscribed roles as public-safety officers. The appraisal of the officer-participants in this cluster was that aggression was an acceptable means of survival and communication. Many had been involved in the developmental experience of war zones in an ecology of severe trauma. Acting out violently was increased rapidly and likely as the officer's symbolic or real personal space in all its varied facets was violated. This is not a case of brutality; it would be a misnomer, due to the state of intent implied when using these terms. Brutality and sadism as a primary gain is absent. Usually use of force is within legal bounds. The higher risk with these officers is danger to self.

The paradox is that these officers make some of the best public-service officers in terms of standards held primary by peers and the public. Supervisors vary in their reactions to these officers: Authoritative supervisors usually are at logger-heads with them; lenient supervisors are enabling; and authoritarian supervisors are likely to encourage acting out (Baumrind, 1978, 1980; Dekovic & Gerris, 1992, 1994). The reality is peers cover for one another. Sending an officer who is so prolific in arrests precludes looking at high risk as a factor for being referred for psychological/psychiatric assistance. Most supervisors, regardless of style, will suggest or order some rest for a very good and active officer. The likelihood of impulsivity and immaturity in acting out leads to one of the higher threats toward physical, emotional, and mental health.

During the most intense public-safety and police confrontations, these officers take the highest risks and are unusually successful. The need to be there for other officers during a time of crisis, even where it is impossible, is likely to lead to survivor guilt. Even if the officer is on vacation or off duty, that guilt may be severe in this personality style. This internalized guilt may be acted out in a variety of addictive ways without conscious awareness.

What complicates this behavioral pattern are the secondary gains achieved by being an addictive officer. Social benefits unique and insular to what has been popularized as "choir boy practice" (Wambaugh, 1975) include special privileges, being a star player in a unit as a referent for a form of fixated adolescence—immortality—the invulnerable hero.

However, the wake-up to a homecoming of rejection and being cast away when something goes awry may lead to tragedy where the resilience is under-developed. Panic may set in and suicidal risk increased. From a psychodynamic view, this narcissistic injury is reciprocal to the narcissistic inflation that preceded it. Relationships may be romantic, short-lived, and subject to the same type of sabotage, because the officer cannot identify the stressors and adequately verbalize the repetitive traumatic loss, resulting in a displacement of aggression into the domestic situation. That crisis can lead to change and growth if explored therapeutically, not punitively. For example, a male officer may tell his wife she does not understand the police lifestyle. This usually is not due to an intrinsic shortcoming as much as a fear of vulnerability conditioned by traumatic loss. Ambivalence keeps the officer-patient actively using the defense of interminable adolescence. The search for meaning in the war zone may lead to a loss of hope and optimism in life. The peacetime/wartime dichotomy (day in/day out) in an urban war zone may be too intense a split, except for only the healthiest ego to tolerate within a time-limited threshold—an ethereal wish in public service.

BEHAVIORAL LEVEL OF EXPRESSIVE ACTS AND INTERPERSONAL CONDUCT

Constant risk-taking examples in the public-service rescue, pursuit, and arrest role ranges from being the first at a scene (shootout on duty), to off-duty incidents of rescue involvement without waiting for back up by on-duty personnel. This is a pattern and not a one-time situation. Nor is it one in which back up is not possible. High levels of civilian complaints and allegations of use of excessive physical force are usually related to frequent involvement in pursuits and calls for assistance from other officers. Again, this is not when one is in a specialized unit where this is the norm due to revenge tactics by organized criminals such as drug dealers. Off-duty activities are built around the subculture of high-risk behaviors and excitement such as addictive highs, including alcoholism, illicit substances, gambling, indiscriminate one-day sexual relations including orgies, prostitutes, extramarital relations experienced as conquests, speeding at 90 mph, and Russian Roulette. Intoxication to numb one's feelings includes self-soothing attempts through addictive venues that are often destructive. Most of this addictive behavior takes place in subgroups with cultural and eco-ethological significance.

Appointment to specialized details by achieving high-level commendations in which high risk and exposure to dangerous events are noted by superior officers and supplemented by civilians who write and advocate for their hero officers. Behavioral responses to emergency events at times become so hyperexcited that impulse can override constraint with tragic consequences. During these emergency events, expressive acts and behaviors for crime victims are genuine, empathic, and protective, as long as the role of rescuer/hero is accepted by the rescued. But conscious deception through manipulation and exploitation is not present in relationship to victims, which is paradoxical and informative. This officer cares a great deal, but has not gained insight into the high risks and self-sabotage of his approach.

THE EPITOME OF WHAT MOTIVATED THESE OFFICERS TO JOIN A POLICE CAREER

Classic examples of quotes from this personality style were: "it seemed like an amusing idea at the time"; "something different to do that would provide excitement from working in an office or desk-type job. By the way, the benefits aren't bad"; "I always wanted to catch the bad guys."

DIFFERENTIAL DIAGNOSIS

While superficially similar to the hyperaggressive style, this officer's style is distinct. Like the hyperaggressive style, this officer thrives on excitement and getting into frays. The hyperaggressive uses people as pawns consistently to manipulate for gain, destroying any person who gets in their way. In the hyper-excited style, people become intoxicants themselves—reinforcing the officers self-ideal—victims become mirrors for the officer's investment in his own wish for invulnerability.

Behavioral manifestations of high risk exist, but not in a sociopathic manner. This is distinguishable from sociopathy, with genuine feelings of guilt and self-reproach, which exacerbate even more high-risk behaviors as overcompensation in a circle of dangerous and often very costly physical, mental, emotional, and existential damage.

Similarities to narcissistic and borderline traits abound. This may be a pseudo-resemblance where the development of these traits emerges in an environment of constant danger and persistent patterns of survival as resistance and defense against loss. A true concern for other people does exist, not just a shallow reaction. Hyperexcitement may help distance the officer-patient from feeling that pain for others in the loss that trauma brings out.

VERBATIM RECORD OF THE MOST TRAUMATIC EVENT

On 0X/0X/76, the Y Precinct had our annual canoe trip. We had a great time. A lot of drinking, a barbecue, and plenty of laughs. During the bus ride home, the fun continued. About four blocks from the precinct, the bus pulled over and a sergeant said he had an announcement to make. He then told us that PO X was killed that afternoon at xx hours. The bus was silent as we continued to the precinct. We exited the bus and went directly to the bar across from the precinct.

The old timers helped the younger guys. About two hours later, I was drunk and went to my girlfriend. I felt the need to be close to a woman. I was filled with all kinds of feelings: one minute it was anger and then sorrow, then I was fearful and then became guilty. *I felt I should have been there and prevented this. I wanted to be there to help. It was hard to understand how a day that was filled with such happiness, laughter, and so much fun could end in such an unexpected way. After this incident I became somewhat hardened. Not so much shook me up after that as a rookie. Before I was a cop, I never drank. I wanted to fit in and be one of the boys. I started to drink and after a while I got used to drinking. We forgot about all the things on and off the job.*

When I had about five years on the job, my partner and I shared an apartment in the Bronx. He was promoted. The night of his promotion, he asked me for a ride. I was tired and wiped out and drove him to his own car. He drove right under a truck and was killed. I never can forget him, the wild stuff we did together, women, drinking, and all kinds of adventure, most of all that night he was standing in the doorway asking me to wait for him. I was so wasted, I forgot and just left. I killed him by leaving him. I started to drink more heavily. When I would wake up in the morning, I would drink a full glass of vodka. For six weeks, me and another officer drank together and talked all the time about how much we missed Y. During this period, I would cock my gun and put it in my mouth or to my head, but just couldn't pull the trigger. Then my friend, who hung out with us three weeks later after a tour of duty ended, was killed off duty. I saw him that night, and I realized I was joking with him and kind of rough, and it was the last time I would see him. As I said earlier, I don't blame the Police Department, but it was too much for anyone to handle.

I just boozed and went to women for comfort. As my career went on, I became very frustrated with the constant way perps got away with all the crap, and the court system and situations I felt were controlled by politics and the press, not our welfare. The one that sticks in my head most was Tompkins Square Park. When I was there, I felt I did my job and did it well. If it came down to me having to use physical force on a person, I also arrested that person. I felt that the public looked at us as one, and not that out of a large number of police officers who did what we had to, even though only a few made mistakes and were wrong. I also became very prejudiced towards any young guy who would mouth off, and disrespect us. It changed. I went from having fun and excitement to getting all out of sorts. I just didn't even like or know who I was. I started to cut myself with a razor, go to bed with women to ease the pain, just stranger's. It wasn't like the roulette; it was not to kill myself, it was just to stop my fears, my missing my buddies, and focusing on something else. The excitement keeps me going.

DISCUSSION OF PERSONALITY STYLE DEVELOPMENT

How does this officer-patient's style develop when gross denial, functional numbing, attributive projection, and suppression become dominant defenses in addiction to trauma?

At first, extreme anxiety may result from the officer's first experiences with police trauma. The simultaneous conflict of oppositional tendencies (see chapter 4) may stimulate a defensive reaction by suppression of fear and anxiety, which gradually crystallize into repression: Denial of fear, anxiety, and guilt may be assuaged unconsciously by projecting one's normal fear responses onto victims. That defense may ward off self–recrimination about cultural taboos against expressing fear and loss openly. The compassion for victims is remembered in place of one's own loss and trauma. The officer's internalized social distance allows for intense sadness for innocent victims hurt, while hostility for self or peers is safely buffered by being re-directed at perpetrators (see chapter 4).

One's own fear of loss may be overcompensated with aggressive outlets, with little if any emotional expression of loss in socially legitimate and sanctioned outlets. This freezing of genuine expression of loss and trauma for one's self and fellow officers is released by displacement in which the officer may maintain a pseudosense of control and self-soothing in the addictive spiral, which is addressed comprehensively elsewhere (Bishop, 2001).

How might this happen biologically? Psychophysiologically repetitive experience with trauma, heightened anxiety, and the release of endorphins and epinephrine crystallize a physiologically conditioned high. When that high peak experience is reached, it is self-reinforcing and may be hardwired for repetitive thrill seeking to reach that level of excitement (behaviorally through risk taking). Much evidence of this has been obtained for combat veterans (see chapter 4). The instrumental rewards for being an alpha officer are heightened by shared emotional value and higher status in the hierarchy in one's ecological niche, which is a culturally and psychologically legitimate outlet. Emotional contagion (Hatfield, Cacioppo, & Rapson, 1994) for survival accompanies a dehumanization process of perpetrators through this internalized social distance. It serves an adaptive purpose during power struggles.

Still, why does alexithymia—that reported lack of feeling, including fear and sadness for ones own suffering persist? Alexithymia is rewarded via achieving ideal-cop status, where an officer can let all pain, loss, and fear roll off his back. It helps mobilize the officer for pursuit, arrest and custody, and the confrontation identity mode (Rudofossi, 2007).

Levant sheds light on alexithymia:

> Normative male alexithymia is, in my view, a result of trauma—the prolonged insidious trauma of male gender role socialization. After all, a central theme of this process is the restriction and suppression of emotion. (Levant, 1997, p. 19; Levant & Pollack, 1995)

I would suggest Levant's normative male alexithymia be modified to *normative public-service alexithymia* (see chapters 1 and 3), including both genders impacted by a unisex approach to training, socialization, and exposure to trauma in public service. The process of inhibiting expression of fear, guilt, and loss may be through conditioning: instrumental, classical, and intermittent. Impervious armor is overlaid by functional numbness over time. Numbing one's reactive feelings of fear and loss through attributive projection to others, with heightened emotional aggressiveness and hostility *makes superb sense ethologically in terms of survival value.* From a psychodynamic perspective, this is rewarded in the macrocultural mythology of the police department. It is selected for survival value as the participant separates the real risk of death and serious bodily injury from the task at hand. The reward is on many levels through symbolic reinforcement of commendations, hierarchical status, and by getting the bad guy. It enlarges one's sense of narcissistic invulnerability.

This numbing and dissociation comes into play, not only as unconscious (as in intrapsychic forces), but a function of what was once conscious has now become automatic. Reciprocal inhibition of fear of loss is replaced with aggression toward the perpetrator. This consistent reciprocal inhibition extinguishes normative responses to toxic stimuli, such as objective fear and cautious approach. Why? In part, it is plausible to suggest that instrumental and intermittent reinforcement gives the illusion of mastery, which becomes symbolically associated with alexy-thymia and altered states of consciousness where the officer becomes functionally numb. A repetition of original trauma thresholds is achieved with each risk to life and limb. In a sense, repetition compulsion may be evoked paradoxically.

Why then is there a continuity and persistence of this addictive repertoire when the officer is off duty? The addictive behaviors complete the negative cycle while off duty, and in an ecological sense, re-create the environment that is so traumatic on the job. Creation of a buffer between the officer's direct experience of trauma and loss by dissociation from the objective danger and harm is perhaps achieved by re-creating and seeking escape from the highs experienced during actual police events. The officer feels displaced and is likely to resonate on the happenings of the day when a litany of multiple losses in trauma are experienced as extremely painful, as in the earlier verbatim example. That loss is dissolved in further toxic addictions whereby peacetime can be a repetition of wartime. The chaotic aspects are reenacted in life at home with significant others and in some cases, domestic violence may occur. In other cases, a *folie a deux* may occur: the husband or wife is put in the place of the innocent victim with an internalized social distance. *This makes sense of the officer's overprotectiveness of loved members of the family and friends. The danger experienced on the job transfers to situations that are not noxious, but may resemble and trigger the response in domestic situations.* The perception of danger may engender a rigid boundary, and nonrelatedness to those the officer loves most. This situation can lead to poor object relationships and a transmission of intragenerational public service alexythymia into the domestic situation.

This alexithymia may extend the intense bonds in the eco-ethological niches into public service. This tendency to create niches is exclusionary to outsiders when the niche members share a bond invested with sacred animism. An interview with a leading Cop Doc, Dr. Benner, suggests the bond of cops with other cops, and Cop Docs, is deep and enduring, as reported in the APA Monitor (Chamberlin, 2000). Another pioneer Cop Doc, Dr. H. Schlossberg (1974), two decades earlier, suggested the same bond of trust among cops exist. Dr. K. Gilmartin's concept of hypervigilance supports the insulation of officers to "outside-others" perceived as a schematic and socially supported cultural perspective. I peer over their shoulders, and agree.

The daily reindoctrination to a different set of subtle, symbolic, and sacred rules are distinct from the world of non-public-service culture, often interpreted as abrupt and alien to the image of many public officers when functioning for survival within this style. I posit this change between *urban war zones* and *peace home zones* is even more intense and abrupt for officers than, for example, soldiers in foreign constant combat for time-limited events. This displacement triggers complicated PTSD in combat veterans' attempts to acclimate to civilian life (Kelly, 1985). In public service, this is exacerbated when there is no transition or planning for healing and habituation, even less acknowledgment at this time.

The solution at minimum entails law-enforcement agencies using a systematic program of rotations in urban war zones. The processing of disenfranchised grief is unlikely when it is not defined and not accepted as real loss. The re-creation of the ecology of addiction and risks with self-harm and violence becomes more human and understandable.

The balance here is met by the therapist, *not confronting* the narcissism or grandiosity as such, but by valuing the courage and commitment of the officer with cautious optimism. Renarration of the trauma and grief by this officer is often visceral and expressive. An empirical and functional dispute is regarded as valuing the officer. Philosophic and deep insight orientation may be rejected outright. An active directive approach that tackles real issues a patient brings up is highly effective in a Socratic reassessment. By repeating the words and style of the officer, one may gain an alliance into his world, while subtle insights are repeated and owned as the officers are helped along the way. Gaining the confidence of the officer includes a harm-reduction approach. Supporting the value of the adaptive skills as a public-safety officer, while diminishing, if not ideally extinguishing, the high-risk behaviors, helps with a healthier narcissism as a subtle goal of therapy.

Behavioral assignments, role plays, and consequential thinking skills carried into the *in vivo* rehearsals may help integrate some cognitive gains and coping strategies. It offers a less threatening frame to deeper psychodynamic, existential, and cognitive work. Working with this style can be rewarding, challenging, and highly frustrating in the initial stages.

INITIAL INROADS FOR THERAPY MAINTENANCE

The grandiose aspects of this officer's style invariably deflate. Usually a crisis precipitates the shattering of the illusion of invulnerability. Some examples of what may prompt this officer's initial visit include, driving under the influence, being infected with a sexually transmitted disease, injury or assault during a dramatic rescue, legal difficulty as a result of action taken, or survivor guilt after a peer is injured severely or murdered in the line of duty. Impoverished insight is likely and affords gentle clarification, at first through the opportunity of crisis.

It is important, once safety and self-care has been established, to further the drive toward longer-term goals. Be aware that an initial approach that is too philosophical, existential, or dynamic may enable other styles. It is a surefire way of losing the hyperexcited officer style quickly. What is suggested is behavioral assignments, paradoxical and functional disputes as interventions. To lessen resistance, I Socratically use the patient's own words, rephrasing assertions into the right questions. A psychoeducational approach to the centering of attention through positive reinforcement of healthier behaviors and outlets for re-creation works well with a behavioral contingency approach initially. It is important first to get the officer to understand the evolutionary value of self-sabotaging behaviors and cognitions on and off the job, and why it has been used for the purpose of adaptation. This helps ally the therapist with the patient by clarifying the evolutionary context of maladaptation.

This serves three purposes in creating a normalizing process, using positive transference for self-change, and increasing responsibility through a more internal locus of control. It tends to lessen the tendency for resistance by acting out in a desperate need for attention and retribution against the therapist by more risky behaviors. Identifying the different feelings is an important psychoeducational component, before challenging dysfunctional and self-sabotaging cognitions. Behavioral change can reinforce cognitive change through rehearsal and *in vivo* assignments. Identifying disingenuous displays of feelings for real expression helps in verbalizing the cognitions that underlie these affective displays. Encouraging activities that help direct the need for excitement through distraction, though not elegant solutions, are effective. Behavioral assignments can help in exploration and expansion of new ways of socialization, interests, and hobbies with non-police circles, and achieving a sense of self.

Rational recovery and harm reduction techniques may be adapted to many of the mentioned addictions, not only alcoholism (Bishop, 2001). Paradoxical interventions re-create a "healthy narcissism" of self-interest, rather than thoughtless risk taking. A specific inroad is relating back one of the hero stories to the officer and letting her come up with an answer as to why she herself does not count, and yet other officers and the civilian does. You can then work on your technique for getting her to acknowledge the self-sabotaging pattern in her behavior. Following are some questions you, as a therapist, may find helpful:

"I am confused. Why does assistance to another cop not apply to you, just to any other cop?"

"Do you have a double standard, one for you, and another for the rest of the mere mortal officers?"

"What would it mean to loved ones if you really did die in the line of duty?"

A strong motivation in the high-risk behavior in this officer-patient is the wish to be immortalized. One way of achieving immortality is through fame, which can lead to unconscious fulfillment by a line-of-duty death, which guarantees the Inspectors Funeral—a ceremonious rite of passage reserved for the sacred hero.

Making death the quite tangible reality it is can be achieved by demystifying the Inspector's Funeral. This can be approached by assigning the officer-patient the writing of his own eulogy. Equal to this task is confronting the passive withdrawal when frustration is turned toward supervisors, peers, and the job and blaming them for the self-destructive numbing and toxic behaviors, creating a sense of emptiness and despair. The officer-patient presents war stories to the therapists as opportunities to shift external control to internal control.

CLINICIAN'S CORNER—
VISCERAL APPROACH FOR EXTREME RISK-TAKING
REDUCTION, IN VIVO

(*Flirting with death/unconscious suicide or invulnerability*). Note: I suggest not trying this until a relationship is developed with the patient. I frame my approach with the hyperexcited style in mind. This officer depicts trauma with visceral and strong emotions. I use aversive conditioning through flooding, with a counterintuitive approach. I illustrate with the following technique:

> **Therapist:** You know, we have been here before, and it seems like the risk taking is not a big issue. The consequences are: "like, who worries? I'm not going to be a statistic?" Yet, you and I have also figured out, if let's say an accident occurs, and things do not go as planned, then what? Take for example, when you stormed into a street robbery off duty. It could be a disaster waiting to happen, huh?

> **Patient:** Yeah, it could be like (expression of a thousand-yard stare of incredulity). I said, you've been a dinosaur and have not been on the streets for a long time. You know, if you want a gold shield, you've got to work your tail off. I have no hooks, no uncle who is a Chief. You took a lot of risks when you started off.

> **Therapist:** (I did, while some were risky, I do not get distracted). Well, let's get to the heart of it. I want to help you prepare for experiencing what may happen. For example, say you get shot real bad or hurt in a patrol-car accident. After all, it seems you ought to be able to experience some preparation beforehand. So why don't we go there now and bring it to you. [Hesitation in his eyes and facial expression.] Stay with me, do you trust me?

> **Patient**: Yeah of course I do, Doc.

> **Therapist:** Good, I want to help you actually figure out just how high of a risk you would like to take with your life by doing a brief experiment. I am going to ask you to put your trust in me. I will need your cooperation to follow my instructions to a tee, how does that sound?

> **Patient:** Okay, Doc. Why the hell not, what do I have to lose?

> **Therapist:** Exactly, what the hell do you have to lose? Lets start.
> [First, I get the patient to relax, put his feet up and ensure a state of calm. I make a direct request for him to close his eyes. I go on informing the patient to place stopples and his fingers in his ears and hold it (I set the second timer). Then, I am silent, turn off the light and surrounding noise. It usually is within a range of 1 minute to 4 minutes before the patient's eyes open and their fingers drop from their ears.]

> **Therapist:** I noticed you opened your eyes and removed your fingers from your ears.

Patient: I didn't know what you wanted me to do: nothing, no instruction, its strange, Doc.

Therapist: You mean strange in how you felt? Let's say "slightly" is 1, and "freaked out" is 10.

Patient: About an 8, real strange.

Therapist: So, your eyes were closed for 108 seconds. Why open your eyes after only 108 seconds? Why did you also immediately take out your ear stopples?

Patient: It felt like (blank stare). Hey Doc, I just didn't know what to do?

Therapist: So if I got it right, you were so uncomfortable without hearing and seeing me, after only 108 seconds you felt an urge to break away and gain your own sense of control?

Patient: Yeah. It felt like I was suspended in the air, without anything, nothing there.

Therapist: You mean like loss of control—silence with full consciousness— no contact or communication? [Go over the negative affects, anxiety, anger, and confusion, immediately without getting distracted.]

Patient: It felt like hell. I mean like really just strange. I felt I had no control; it got to me.

Therapist: Why hell? Its almost a likelihood if you keep taking the same level of risks you will get your goal achieved, say, traumatic brain injury, loss of sight and hearing, but full consciousness. Imagine now for 108 seconds it feels almost intolerable. The evidence is even in a comfortable setting, being relaxed and with me, whom you trust, your urge for control was overpowering. What do you think about life support or being left conscious if one of your high-risk choices puts you there? [We move on to clarify negative affective consequences.]

Patient: It spooks me out, like all hell. Like that movie *Coma,* or *The Twilight Zone* series. It would be hell.

I go on actively reassessing the value of his courage and efforts with healthy cautious risk taking and the empirical evidence we have discovered. I then review how hard it is to give up control to others. Yet, with his type of risk taking, it is likely almost all control will be lost. This method can and has worked with those with suicidal ideation. After the experiment, I return to a focus on using the experience to deal with the pain, which is a distance between two points, it has already begun and will lessen in time with hard work.

THE SADISTIC HYPERAGGRESSIVE PUBLIC-SAFETY PERSONALITY STYLE: QUALIFICATION FOR THE HYPERAGGRESSIVE STYLE

This personality style is the rarest of all five in police and public-safety officers. However, officers who have this style are in need of the most therapeutic help. The first understandable emotional impulse you will likely feel on an unconscious level is a lack of ease as a therapist. The behavioral activity is to refer this officer-patient out. On a cognitive level, you may think this is above my level of comfort and my acceptable threshold. If you have a high frustration tolerance, your goals in therapy are moderate while hopeful; you may make a lasting impact in this officer's lifestyle. Harm reduction is one such worthwhile goal of therapy. The hyperaggressive officer-patient's style toward others is not a result of overexcitation or hypervigilance, it is infused with a sadistic craving this patient uses to gain control over others. As a therapist I think of my task here as first "Taming the Shrew." This may be an awkward term borrowed from William Shakespeare, but appropriate to our clinical situation. Why this choice? A shrew consumes most of what it gets holds of, so does this officer. Rather than food, manipulation, control, and aggression is the objective. The key may be slowing down the metabolism of aggression to a more socialized and utilitarian purpose in which the officer-patient may learn that serving others brings a higher level of pleasure than the current antisocial tendencies he may exhibit. This initial goal of intervention is a very difficult one, but one that is well worth the effort. Psychodynamic exploration of sadism and excessive aggression may lead to significant gains in character change in long-term therapy. Although it is beyond the scope of this book, it is worth the effort to learn this approach (Ferenczi, 1933; Reich, 1970, 1991; Scharf, 2003).

INTRA-PSYCHIC LEVEL OF DEFENSIVENESS FOR SURVIVAL (BRENNER, 1976)

The extraordinarily destructive potential of this officer-patient is worthy of our attention. This style epitomizes a composite of antisocial, narcissistic, and sadistic traits wherein the officer-patient is likely to exhibit marked brutality, absent a moral and ethical path. The value of other human beings may be based upon fulfillment of his own narcissistic need for amusement, aggressive, and sexual needs, with an omission of genuine empathy. This officer's defensive posturing tends toward acting out: drive derivatives that are aggressive and sexual fuel a predominance of isolation of affect and dehumanization of others (including other officers).

Acting out is marked by an exquisite sensitivity for other's pain and suffering, whether emotional, physical, or mental. I have found this sensitivity is heightened with aggressive zeal: as the expression of pain in other's rise, so does a reciprocal heightened sadism in the officer-patient. An unusual sense of understanding of what one is doing to inflict pain on others is coupled with a sense of extreme moral turpitude. Punishment inflicted on others is viewed in a distorted way as purifying them of their ill-gotten gains. Manipulation of the letter of the law and one's authority may offer a means to manipulate and inflict pain on others. This may be a manipulation of rules, rather than a puritanical belief. Regardless, this manipulation underscores the credo of "might makes right" as the herald for this style. Any tactic is justified as long as one wins.

Securing dominance through the use of power and one-upmanship triggers attention seeking. One may call officers with this personality style the fundamentalists of public safety. Relating to others focuses on distortions as to who is in power. If someone is not capable of being manipulated, they are not worthy of time and effort to maintain a relationship. Finally, there is no desire for the approval of peers and supervisors unless there is an instrumental reward immediately available. Any attempt to really care about the *esprit de corps* of the unit is felt "as if" the officer-patient has relinquished himself to others. In this regard, the problem heralds to a dysfunction of self, including self-soothing skills that remain underdeveloped, which may be developmentally supported through the transference relationship with you.

One red flag for you to watch for is a history of conflicts with authority. This officer acts sadistically in the face of extreme tragedy, not to be mistaken with bravado, indifference, or exhilaration. A clue is the absence of denial, numbing, and dissociation after repetitive trauma is evident. Where there is no fully internalized unconscious sense of conscience of human morality, there may be no need for intrapsychic defenses of guilt, shame, or self-reflection. However, it would be a mistake to believe that no morality exists, as Scharf suggests, (2003); the question may be what type of morality and how to approach that lacunae initially on a behavioral level. Ultimately, if and when enough core ego strength exists, the next step may be relating to others in a more empathic direction (Scharf, 2003).

BIOPHYSICAL LEVEL OF MOOD

Aggression is prominent when this officer's narcissistic enhancement is threatened. Biophysical responses are evidenced as an extreme hostility to threats of, and in some cases actual assault upon the other person when a challenge to this officer's sense of entitlement is provoked; this includes the therapist. Be aware; this can become a volatile situation.

This is not a temporary agitation by a loss of inhibition, but a calculated vengeance. There is remarkable composure when challenged with misdoings and questions involving addictive behaviors, or consequences of one's actions toward others. The level of activity is a restless drive, without the goal of gaining approval from significant others, along with a pattern of control matched by subtle or explicit attack on the general cultural values of the public-safety agency. Patient's self-report of mood description appears to be a subterfuge, with typical responses of "I had control at all times" or "not feeling a thing" along with a verbal description of brutality toward someone because they "dared to disrespect him." Another clue is unlike those in a dissociative state. There is a keen emotional excitement in recounting morbid aspects of critical incidents when pain is inflicted on others. This is persistent and not related to an event in which a fellow officer or he was hurt. Rage follows being wronged or being pushed into doing something against his will. Again, this perception is often a trivial slight.

PHENOMENOLOGICAL LEVEL OF SELF-IMAGE, COGNITIVE STYLE, AND OBJECT REPRESENTATIONS

This officer believes he is the wronged and offended party in almost all cases. Remorse or even self-reflection is neither sought nor accepted. Officers with this style have an impoverished ability for introspection; he is subsumed with other people's sense of vulnerability as a means of exacting revenge. The goal is how to control other's thoughts and behaviors and to elicit pain and suffering. *It is possible that it is their way of establishing a perverse level of relatedness through pain as a medium of communication.* However, in their self-image there is no room for improvement—it could be they have given up hope through repeated attempts at empathic attachment with others. Although this defies a true narcissist, for they have no Echo in a significant other, save there own level of destructiveness. There is an absence of loyalty, commitment to values, and ideals, the stuff that help most of us hold together the social constructs of reality even in the face of pain and struggle. Reality is always mundane, and therefore the quest for excitement is without a telos in and through relating to others. This officer's hostility in cognitive style lies low only when a higher-ranking officer is present. A checkered record of disruption in units with peers and supervisors becomes evident. A staunch irrational belief is that one is always right and entitled to have what one demands. It is also a core of psychoanalytic regression to an infantile state of demanding immediate gratification.

Assaults or excessive use of force are coupled with a lot of relational problems with other officers, who are bound to notice the extreme sadism. Most officers will feel a need to curtail this sadism and may use all kinds of interventions, mostly indirect, due to the cohesion and survival of the unit. To believe and expect more from officers may be unrealistic and too harsh on the officer facing this dilemma.

These individuals, by use of innate intelligence, charm, and manipulation, may make it to top positions. An infantile temper tantrum can be exacted in public service if the person has obtained rank. What is extraordinary is the lack of any sense of remorse, always being right, that the offending party is totally and irrevocably wrong and evil. For example, one officer told me her hero was Herman Goering, who pulled out his own teeth. She held him in high esteem for being a real man. The dribble of racism and anti-Semitism was part of the officer's core complaints. It is this race or that religion that becomes the conduit in which hatred runs deep and ugly. The spirituality, ethical message, and empathy of minorities (in this case, the Jews) forged in the crucible of suffering, may spark the very hatred that mirrors such intense hatred to the distortion of strength as perceived weakness. Contradictions had no impact when clarified or confronted, only a sardonic grin and a lashing back at the therapist in a thinly veiled attempt at reviling and humiliation.

Humor used may be an extreme caustic and abrasive type, not a mature and adaptive type. This public-service officer or supervisor is likely to be characterized as cruel, unusually mean-hearted or a "Gestapo type." Public-service units that specialize in punitive measures for cops are not unusual havens for this style. It is against other officers that sadists may have their heyday with impunity and lack of scrutiny. Consequently, it is here that a psychologist's scrutiny can serve as valuable gatekeeper.

The events of trauma are interpreted as violations of personal injury without the consequent feelings of anxiety, guilt, sadness, or anger that emanate from perceived attacks on the group in varying degrees of intensity in the other styles. This personality style is most likely to use inappropriate physical force mercilessly if they perceive any type of disrespect of their own personal authority. Others are to blame at all times, and the system is always wrong. No supervisor is an ally. Peers are objects to be manipulated.

BEHAVIORAL LEVEL OF EXPRESSIVE ACTS AND INTERPERSONAL CONDUCT

Sadistic behaviors prior to appointment are the norm. Any threat to gratification of narcissistic needs is met with certain, swift, and sadistic retaliation. Verbal challenges to one's beliefs, status, or position are used for legitimization of bias, violence, brutality, criminal behavior, and corruption. Genuine pleasure of even the most severe human and animal suffering is taken as strength. Hedonism is very high, and the delay of gratification is superficial at best. Addictive and high-risk behaviors are typical for this officer. Behavioral indicators are civilian complaints, frequent subjects of internal investigations, driving while intoxicated, and abuse of authority without remorse. The excuse invariably is "the department/my boss/partner made me do it."

Undergirding a cavalier appraisal of danger are opportunities for sanctioned sadistic attacks. Behavioral manifestations exist to dominate over others and prove one's power. If not caught or brought to the attention of supervisors, sadistic behaviors may be reinforced, with graduated risk and escalated violence. This is especially true because many are glib, and the sense of bold action instrumentally reinforces one's ability to go further along. Feigned feelings of remorse, if confronted, become evident in a plastic and social display of expressiveness. The experienced clinician will sense this unconsciously. These individuals seeking excitement and stimulation will recruit more vulnerable and dependent-type officers to join their self-serving causes. In an extremely dehumanizing trait, another clue is a linguistic tendency to speak of other people as "things" or "it."

THE EPITOME OF WHAT MOTIVATED THESE OFFICERS TO A POLICE CAREER

"To be a boss, not a subordinate; 20-year pension. The power of being an officer."

Verbatim Record of the Most Traumatic Event

The one event that I will tell you about occurred on xx/xy/yy. Upon arriving on the scene, we encountered other officers entering a parking garage. We observed a radio car full of bullet holes. As we entered the garage, we observed a male lying dead on the garage floor, a so-called victim; a drug deal gone bad. As we went deeper in the garage to conduct a search, we were fired upon by a perp ducking behind a parked car. We found cover behind cement pillars and other autos and returned fire; it was exciting; I could feel my adrenaline surge. It was gratifying to see the perp dying from our return fire. I placed a flashlight in his eyes and said, "Guess where your going, it ain't heaven." The other cops looked away. I didn't. I couldn't care less. He was a perp. I wish those guys weren't wusses. I did not lose any sleep anytime after this incident. It was a good shooting and that's that. I felt proud one less. I felt this was necessary force and felt no anxiety, anger, or sadness. I was just doing my job. I hope he enjoyed every knot in his last shampoo. [This is not an isolated renarration, but consistent in his style.]

DIFFERENTIAL DIAGNOSIS

Like all styles, this grouping had a range of acting out, from mild to severe. The insincerity and lack of truth was not delusional, confabulation, or motivated by a fantasy life. Unlike the hyperexcited, it is not a quest for approval; here it is for controlling others as if they were instruments for one's own gratification. Relationships are marked by long-term grudges, never ending lists of injustices, and concomitant bloodlust. What is right and wrong is based on what is idio-pathic. The only similarity with the hyperexcited style is the addictive craving for high excitation. However, the hyperexcited style has genuine empathy and is capable of significant change. The sadistic style's aggressive behavior is carried out with a glaring absence of guilt, remorse, or empathy. The hyperfocused style is frightened of their own compulsions, and hence, repress almost any aggressive tendency; the hyperaggressive gloats in his hostility. One is always a pseudo-team player as long as one is on the top of one's own game. Allegiances are quickly made, disbanded, and replaced. These manifestations of defenses and relational style are not isolated but consistent across events.

DISCUSSION OF PERSONALITY STYLE DEVELOPMENT

An innate, genetic tendency of destructiveness may be developed in a fecund ecological and ethological playground, where sadism may be afforded in hidden public-safety niches. This may allow a total abandonment of what would normally be violations of the basic decency we all cherish if not identified and stopped by peers.

Unique to this style is the violence in acting out and sadism rationalized regardless of the social distance or proximity of the victim in relation to themselves. Acting sadistically is situational and contingent on the other officer, the complainant, or even a perpetrator's narcissistic value to the officer's own needs. It appears that the maladaptive value of hyperaggressive and sadistic behavior is the domination, destruction, abstraction, and perversion of some other value, solely reflective of an egocentric perspective. The ego in relation to society, and in the service of the well-being of others, may stimulate growth in some cases. In severe cases, it appears dead, and may in fact be dead beyond our reach as therapists. That may be the outlier in this style, as many have the capacity for growth once motivation is established.

However, motivation is supported by understanding why, the sadistic hyperaggressive officer has an insatiable hunger for power and domination. On some level, it may be the biological, genetic, and socialization process gone awry. The result may be an antisocial flaw in character. In those officer-patients who have gone to an extreme in acting out, guarantees of being reified in perpetual infamy may fuel self-sabotage and self-punishment.

The future holds no allure for the pleasure of the moment. There is an antihedonic level of primitive asceticism and agitation. No feelings of guilt for the most blatant violations of other's rights are forthcoming (Brent, 2001; Freud, 1922; Reese, 1987). The imagination to accept that one may be guilty in some instances is the beginning of caring toward others. The worst of all possible combinations and permutations is the antisocial, aggressive, narcissistic, and borderline rage (Black & Larson, 1999; Cleckley, 1976; Hare, 1993; McCord & McCord, 1956; Millon, 1996; Perls, 1978, 1979; Reese,1987; Reich, 1970, 1991; Samenow, 1984; Toch, 2002; Winnicott, 1984). I posit that officer's endogenous level of hostility and raw aggression may include the fault of ignoring one's voice of conscience. Hardly explicable by any one theory, this style is in part enlightened by all.

It appears an ethologic component, not as an alpha human but as a self-destructive deevolution with an instinctual goal of destruction, may need revisiting. Public service gives this officer power and domination he would likely never obtain through normal competition. *Envy spurs him on in never ending plots and schemes of ever-growing malevolence attributed to others, which all emanates tragically from within.* This violent expression of hatred and envy satisfies what appears to be an endogenous level of sadism inflicted upon others, perhaps in part motivated by envy and fear of any intimacy. That understanding contains the hope and promise of helping this officer-patient redeem what is of value in his soul. The task is twofold: to expose a root of destruction and hopefully to keep these officers in check; and possibly to diminish the harm they inflict. There may be more meaningful and optimistic work that is warranted after these initial and very difficult goals are attained.

INROADS FOR THERAPY
MAINTENANCE

An individual from this style is least likely to be motivated for therapeutic change. The referral of this patient is probably involuntary. Again, for this style, the approach is unconventional. Paradoxical intention is used with a behavioral goal in mind. Moreover, it is done surreptitiously. Change focuses first on persuading the officer that they are in charge and you are there to help them fulfill their need for power. While gaining their alliance, you need to show again and again, subtly, the sabotage aspect of their sadism. They can better meet their needs without inflicting violence and harm.

Using the transference as referential authority may result in a dead end and can create an impasse of egos and will. They are likely to win, as they will resort to using on you every means they use on others. It is equally distasteful for the relational psychodynamic therapist or the most accepting cognitive behavioral therapist. Bribing, cajoling, and pleading with this patient will lead only to more reinforcement and instrumental control over you. Setting boundaries and your own confidence and ability to persevere and not get provoked into giving up are potential inroads. It is still very difficult and may not work.

Loss issues are limited to perceived attacks on the officer's reputation for being dominant, possessing status, or authority. It is this that you target as motivation for behavioral change. Harm reduction through empirical and para-doxical dispute that is constantly driven back to the narcissistic advantage of the patient that is creatively and diplomatically derived from therapy may work.

CLINICIAN'S CORNER—
REDUCING SADISTIC AGGRESSION:
FUNCTIONAL AND PARADOXICAL DISPUTES

I have had little success, with these patients. As an example, in using the paradoxical method after some rapport has been established, however marginal, I focus in on the problem or activating event, including sadistic behavior. In the first unorthodox intervention, I appeal to the mercurial interest and narcissism of this officer-patient to lessen the harm inflicted on others and self.

> **Therapist:** It seems you consider this boss a real thorn. Rather than attempting to get back at him, it seems you sadly have suffered once again. He, so to speak, got over on you once again it seems.

> **Patient:** What do you mean? I got the SOB. Don't you get it, Doc? I win once again; he's scared shitless of me.

> **Therapist:** Yeah, on one hand he is. Hmm, I see what you mean. Yet, supposing I see it your way, each time you threaten to sabotage his work by slowing down and not caring about civilian complaints. Hmm, it seems he gets his way. I mean, the likelihood of other bosses getting involved and limiting your freedom is likely. In that way, I would imagine the other party gets over. I mean, it would seem quite sophisticated if you were even more adept at getting your needs met without him even knowing it.

> **Patient:** What do you mean? I got him riled up and now he knows I'm a force to be reckoned with. Don't you get it?

> **Therapist**: I get it. But how about getting him to act more like you want him to, without resorting to wasting your very precious energy?

> **Patient:** What do you mean, how? Might makes right! He's a no-good sniveling weasel. (Ingratiating laugh)

> **Therapist:** By kind of fogging the dude. I mean by being nice, I mean trying to really act nice. You can laugh all the way to the bank over how you got over and keeping to your way of "might makes right!" You win without ever lifting a hand, or draining your energy. What do you say we try with doing some role plays, right here and now?

[I get some token and superficial agreement. I then go on to illustrate through rehearsal of social skills, assertiveness, and prioritizing goals. The patient believes he has won. He can laugh at how gullible the supervisor may be. This allows sadistic tendencies expression, while in reality rendering the obnoxious and toxic powerless, except in his mind. We then will slowly work on other changes in the same way.]

Another method I use is role reversal. This appeals to his narcissistic pride.

> **Therapist:** I really would like to understand and feel what it's like to be in your place. Perhaps you could play the other person while I get to play you.

Patient: Why should I want to be anyone but me? That's psychobabble crap. Why should I want to be anyone but me? Especially a loser.

Therapist: Well, maybe that's how you see it. But, I really would like to know how it feels to be you. By you being him, you can help me find out how much of a loser he is. Appealing to his narcissism to lord it over (it is hard for him to resist) the paradoxical effect works through the role plays.

A spark of empathy may be fired up and acted upon. I will then model a nonaggressive means of getting instrumental change. I stay away from other disputes and interpretations. I keep it real simple and utilitarian. Why? I am working from two stances: one as a wishful optimist; the other as a technician. Change may occur through behavioral assignments that appeal to the narcissistic fragility you evoke in the patient toward minimizing harm of self. Still, I suggest you hold no illusions that empathy must occur. If you do, you will likely be sorely disappointed, as I was in the few rare instances I tried to gain a core of compassion that was not penetrable, if it was there at all. Sadly, in this instance, I accept my role as a technician, engineering harm reduction rather than a real and enduring therapeutic change. I try my darnedest not to be cajoled into conflict with a patient, making borderline rage look like Southern hospitality. If you have afforded this patient a skill to feel, or understand another perspective, your therapeutic objective is successful. And it is only a beginning.

THE IDIOSYNCRATIC HYPERINTUITIVE PUBLIC-SAFETY PERSONALITY STYLE

Intrapsychic Level of Defensiveness for Survival

How does a creative and highly perceptive officer respond to trauma while having a tendency toward avoiding the emotional expression of loss while exhibiting a style of being overly dependent on others? Complicated loss of original and cumulative trauma is not often expressed directly. Avoidance of emotional hurt parallels maladaptive beliefs of personal inadequacy, shame, and guilt, which remains indirectly expressed and is typically made through an abstract use of language: idiosyncratic metaphors. For instance, in one patient, rather than saying, "I feel overwhelmed," he will say, "I am stuck in the ninth cylinder." In place of saying "the knife soaked in blood of an innocent victim stabbed to death," he will say, "the miasma of the Grim Reaper came back." Amusing and highly intelligent in his use of metaphors as motifs for the grist of therapy, this style presents formidable resistance in a not-so-apparent constellation of defenses.

However, the metaphor or abstract thought that is expressed is not a lack of reality testing (Sass, 1994) or circumstantial thought. Rather, indirect abstract expressiveness may shield this officer-patient from fear and guilt. This undeserved shame is an avoidance of what implores expression: fear, loss, guilt, anxiety, and anger. The symbols become interpretable once the context of the patient's trauma and loss history is disclosed. Functional numbness serves a prominent defense. It may help officers bury disheartened anguish; it also blocks creative expression and productivity. The hypervigilance hides the potential contributions, disavowed healthy competition, assertion of one's own needs, and appreciation of creative potential.

The fact stands that many officers with this tendency make effective and insightful public-service officers: patrol, detectives, rescue, and specialized units. Adaptively, creativity in some situations is owned up to spontaneously and wittingly when trauma and grief is artistically expressed through specialized outlets in public service. Some officers with this style create an adaptive niche without therapy. Allowances for these officer's creative contributions may be afforded by supervisors who are similar or who have psychological sensitivity or awareness.

Biophysical Level of Mood

A mood of restlessness, irritability, and diffuse anxiety is not uncommon. A strong positive transference may develop when boundaries are tested and maintained. If boundaries are not consistent, a dependency that stifles growth of the patient while draining the therapist (projective identification) may develop. Boundaries are gently firmed by a valuing of the patient's ability, not disability in avoidance and withdrawal patterns. This hypervigilance may be provoked by the officer-patient who is attempting to reenact with you (through the transference) his wish for your approval and acknowledgment. The provocation may revolve around a hypervigilance of your attention in figuring out what may be hidden in symbolic, abstract, or metaphorical language. Resolving this by using cognitive techniques with a psychoanalytic sensibility may be useful. Creative fantasy is not always a negative outlet if, all other things being equal, it is not extreme (Freud, 1894/1963; Gilmartin, 1986; Kassinove, 1995; Laing, 1965, 1971, 1985; Perls, 1978; Sass, 1994).

PHENOMENOLOGICAL LEVELS: SELF-IMAGE, COGNITIVE STYLE, AND OBJECT REPRESENTATIONS

This officer's self-image is one that epitomizes avoidance and introversion. This officer presents as less competent in self-descriptions than is usually the case. Safety and trust are issues. Abstraction presented may help compensate for death anxiety and perceived disempowerment. This is related to socialization in public-service agencies where power is expressed through hierarchical structure. This perception of insecurity is offset by a compensation through hypervigilance. As the clinician explores the theme of hypervigilance through thought, affect, and behavioral patterns, trauma experiences in the form of dreams, mental representations, and artistic work may emerge.

Cognitive style in this officer-patient is likely to yield evidence of external locus of control—"the job" (public-service agency)—where choice and responsibility are attributed to others. For instance, changing assignments (horizontal mobility) or promotion through (vertical mobility) are often rejected outright. The paradox is diagnostic; this rejection of mobility is typical of external control, rather than self-initiative. Typical rationalizations I have encountered are: "there is very little danger for me"; "I know the streets, and who would do it if I didn't?"; "The job made me a patrol cop and that's where I'll remain. It sucks though"; "It's all hooks and kissing up. Why bother?"

Underlying this is an avoidant strategy and *hypervigilance* toward danger (Benner, 1991; Gilmartin, 1986), which is fear against internal prosecution such as Internal Affairs probes (this is not without a basis, but nonetheless exaggerated). There are roots the therapist can explore to confirm or disconfirm family dynamics that have led to a fear of personal initiative. The other danger is taking action and being prosecuted by external agencies or being put in the limelight.

Avoidance and withdrawal are also a style of relating to other officers. For example, not being disturbed, getting ones paycheck safely, and retiring was the untoward goal. Uniformed public-service officers represented by this style had problems with that. They vacillated between trust and mistrust of family, friends, and department, which appeared to be more a perceived violation of trust and a fear of vulnerability rather than a paranoid style. The trust and confidence that genuine empathy could be enlisted on their behalf by family, friends, and fellow officers was tested with vigilance in a passive-aggressive approach. These participants sought an angle, at least initially, when a good deed, kind word, or support was proffered. Eventually, the therapist and patient can whittle away at these cognitive distortions; indicating that it is likely learned rather than innate. An effective way may be through clarifying these defensive mechanisms as they arise in the transference.

BEHAVIORAL LEVEL OF EXPRESSIVE ACTS AND INTERPERSONAL CONDUCT

The public-service officer usually presents with an avoidant-introverted style. In a public-safety world of violation of safety and trust, fantasy may help compensate for death anxiety, perceived disempowerment, and a distance from loss and trauma through functional dissociation. In public safety, power and status are expressed through hierarchical structure. A perception of insecurity is offset by a compensation through vigilance.

Behavioral dimensions rated by supervisors often indicate marginal to average performance in an officer who has above-average intelligence and ability. This incongruity is a good area to explore together. Another clue of hypervigilance and avoidance is somatic-symptom proliferation. Symptomatic presentation represents underlying intrapsychic disturbance. Clarification in a nonthreatening manner will usually elicit descriptions of how the patient has avoided challenges and why.

Existential and philosophical challenges may elicit behavioral change when framed supportively. The expression of a creative tendency through appropriate channels brings a liberation of energy and a healing for many officer-patients with this style. They were least likely to use violence as a means of dealing with disrespect by violators of the law. Anecdotally, and paradoxically, this officer was the most likely to be the target of assaults by perpetrators.

THE EPITOME OF WHAT MOTIVATED THESE OFFICERS TO JOIN A POLICE CAREER

"I asked my Dad (a retired detective) for advice about what I should do with my life. He told me, "Become a cop to stop crime, and provide a stable income for a family." My officer-patient paused, reflected, and said, "I did just that, and here I am with the Superman blues."

Verbatim Record of the Most Traumatic Event

I've been involved in many events through the years. Some I remember, but all I want to forget. I've responded to many 10-XX, (calls for assistance by other officers) and made many arrests and seen plenty of hurt and dying people. I'm tired, okay? Tired of seeing it. I don't understand how people can hurt other people for no apparent reason. I've lost friends on the job because of violence, and I'm tired of it. I can do what I have to. Don't get me wrong, I'm a good soldier, and I've always been. I can't take seeing it again and again like pictures that pop up. I've felt confused and weak, and I just want to be able to let it roll off again. I want you and my other doctors to help me get back to feeling strong like I was. I remember working on a midnight shift, 15 years ago August, with my old partner. We were assigned to sector A-D in Red Hook houses. We got a job for a female stabbed. I remember the address. It was in the projects. We had trouble with our car, which I remember was stalling on us. We got there, the ambulance guys, EMT were already there working on her. I looked at her. From my point of view, she was upside down on the floor. I asked her, "Who stabbed you?" She said, "Ms. L." I made the arrest. She was dying right then and there. So I solved my first homicide. Fuck! I would have rather have been able to have stopped my first homicide! I wished so much I could have saved the poor kid from the fuckin' Reaper! I was in all night at the station house filling out paperwork and safeguarding the perp. In the morning, I went with Detective C. to the Kings County Morgue to ID the body. There she was, nude on the table, with that 95 tag on her toe. She hadn't been chopped up yet.

Detective C. asked the doctor to stick a probe into the girls stab wound. It went in all right, all the way in. I remember (at that moment) telling her in my mind: "Hey, please, your only a kid, D. Come on, get up! I was just talking to you. Come on now, what happened?" The probe freaked me out. I remember Detective C. laughed and pointed out that if in the event I got murdered, I'll be on the same table. Talk about freaky, like a miasma leaking out. I felt this wet electricity early in my police career, maybe three years in the bag. Still to this day, I see myself on the project landing, talking to D. upside down. She still looks frantic to me. It makes me feel frantic too. I got department recognition for this arrest. So what?!? People will kill at the drop of a hat. I must be watchful and wary for that possibility. Especially in the work I do. After this, any job coming over in the projects would make me super alert as I saw what happened that night. Between two females, no less! I must be on guard at all times against horror and disappointment because I know either will trip me up if I get caught otherwise. That's why I just do my job and watch my back. And my priority is to collect a check every two weeks.

DIFFERENTIAL DIAGNOSIS

Unlike other personality styles presented, many of these participants prided themselves on being "an odd man" in the unit, agency or department. For example, all public-safety officers have nicknames or handles; many are taken with an air of acceptance. A representative sample is "the precinct house mouse," "firehouse mop," "unit nanny," or "unit pop." A chronic sick record is another clue. The character here is dissimilar to the sadistic hyperaggressive style. The addictive hyperexcited style thrives on excitement and gets into frays; this style, by comparison, avoids conflict. Avoidant strategies may emerge in this officer-patient in his adaptation to an environment where an exquisite sensitivity toward human anguish and suffering is personalized and internalized. In such an internal world, it makes sense to withdraw from others and not to expose himself to vulnerability. Grief and trauma are not worked through.

Similar to the hyperexcited, genuine caring for sacred victims is extant. Sadly, a self-blame and guilt that is unwarranted is accepted as if he is defective and responsible for the multiple losses in trauma experienced. This maladaptation engenders a hypervigilance against making a stand, stating direct assertiveness, and otherwise becoming involved.

DISCUSSION OF DEVELOPMENT OF
PERSONALITY STYLE

Avoiding risk and active participation in public-safety career development is the norm. However, an adequate toleration of discomfort, doing his job adequately and without notice is mastered in an epiphany characterized by a lulling hush.

Why and how this persists as functional dissociation, numbness, and avoidance is a difficult question to answer. I suggest it is selected because it offers high survival value. That lulling hush is a level of self-soothing that is afforded and instrumentally conditioned in his niche. It helps the officer-patient remain at a level that is not personally experienced as overwhelming. It takes creativity to achieve this ambiance in the first place. Ironically the creative impulse is re-directed into the defense of avoidance and idiosyncracy.

But we are back again to the question of why does the officer-patient use abstract patterns of speech and idiosyncratic styles of presentation? Why does such an intelligent and creative person litter the conversation with cryptic and elusive ways of expression rather than a more direct and even presentation?

Expressing discontent through passive indignation may be a safe way of distancing himself. It is also as righteous as it is elusive. A rebellion presented with ambiguity serves the officer's partial satiation of drive derivatives otherwise not satisfied (Brenner, 1976, 1982). It does not disrupt the internal status quo. It is likely tolerated by peers and supervisors alike and can be defended as innocuous if one is accused. Obfuscation through abstract metaphors blunt the edge of owning up, while somewhat directly expressing his pangs of discontent, which is abundant. A protesting voice may be instrumentally extinguished in a hierarchical organization. A passive-aggressive stance that is diffuse will likely be tolerated. It seems as if a counterconditioning is at work wherein the officer maintains, albeit subtly, a distorted sense of power. Yet, it effectively keeps an interpersonal distance that is mysterious, aloof, and intriguing.

That is part of this officer's presentation. Adaptive selection is at work. For example, from the academy training (see Epilogue), street-patrol assignments and keeping a low profile is overlearned and reinforced through some niches hidden in the culture of public service. It is also reinforced on a higher level of police and public-safety culture (Benner, 1991; Gilmartin, 2002). Avoidant strategies are achieved via negative reinforcement when the officer is not recognized or when he is protected from being ostracized. This outcome reestablishes a sense of control for the officer (unlike trauma and loss). Minimal risk means minimal chance of getting involved in any dangerous situation where one can be singled out. This may not be a fear of objective danger. It is with this context in mind that most of these officers are courageous in public-safety actions, but get somatic symptoms with all kinds of imagined fears of prosecution far from the reality of the event. The unconscious potential and conflicts are ripe fields for intervention: the cognitive, behavioral, and emotive strategies equally are not accidental and are likewise ripe for the picking.

Having an idiosyncratic approach creates a diminished likelihood that one will be a team player (avoidant tactic); yet he is still highly dependent on the group for survival. Compensation endures as long as a valued skill is offered within one's group in the eco-ethological niche. A distinct skill is an affordance that pays off in ethological satisfaction. In an advanced hierarchical society like public safety, a specialized skill affords a selective advantage to the officer-patient. The pursuit of what is proffered as a specialized skill is learned and sophisticated. The reciprocity is rewarded by being left alone and by gaining benefits. This is adaptive ethological evolution in action. Ability is coupled with skillfulness serving a need rewarded by adaptation with minimum energy expended. Ethological mechanisms are parsimonious and direct. They may partially satisfy through substitution what is desired unconsciously in sexual and aggressive goals (Brenner, 1974, 1976, 1982, 2003; Richards & Willick, 1986; Scharf, 2003).

The maladaptive consequence may be highly intelligent people who become suffused with apathy and boredom in a retreat from living. It stunts development and the ability to grow through productive competition and genuine cooperation. Although parsimony is good for a tortoise and ergonomics, it hardly suffices for human living.

Avoidant and hypervigilant schemas are revealed through the following statements:

"A good officer understands the least you do, the better."

"Avoid any trouble; the goal is pick up your paycheck every other Thursday period."

"When off duty avoid, crowded areas to avoid being involved with perps."

What was originally a creative impulse, empathic interaction, and investment of a rookie officer in overly optimistic goals is battered through repeated expectations, being shattered into fragmented losses. Maladaptation ensues (Benner, 1991; Gilmartin, 2002; Schlossberg, & Freeman, 1974). The economic solution in a hierarchical structure of power is to create and live in a world of shadows where retreat, avoidance, and hypervigilance tragically replace the balanced substance of healthier assertion, competition, and creativity. In part, this is the weight of trauma, bureau pathology, and stigmatization, not weakness (Goffman, 1961; Ryan, 1972).

This idiosyncratic expression of vigilance and avoidance that becomes exaggerated is beautifully described as *schizos-phrenos,* that is, a broken heart or soul (Laing, 1965, 1971, 1985). Fear and avoidance of existential anxiety stultifies adult development. Tolerating and embracing this existential anxiety may precede adult growth (Fromm, 1951; Lifton, 1993; Yalom, 1983) and creative expression (Buscaglia, 1978; May, 1983). I suggest a purging of the mind and body of toxic accumulation of unspoken, undefined, and symbolic abstraction of traumatic loss may be corequisite to growth. This grief cycles into idiosyncratic symbolism that remains unshared and undiscovered—regardless of how often it is presented—unless your third (analytic) ear picks it up (Reik, 1948).

In conclusion, metaphors and abstractions may be viewed as safety hatches where the patient cautiously treads into relationship building as well as defense building against personal vulnerability. The abstractions you encounter can be reconceptualized as rather awkward invitations for you to engage the officer-patient in trauma and grief work.

Finally, a word of caution: be aware of a problem not uncommon with this style. Freud spoke of "therapy interminable" as a need of the patient to provoke the therapist into transference and countertransference checks that may never end (Freud, 1894/1963). I suggest some officers with this style may explicate such a process. How? A behavioral complement underlying therapy interminable is "symbolism interminable." The presentation of abstractions and over-valued symbols is a counterintuitive conditioning through a form of projective identification/controlling. That is, the officer-patient controls the therapist through an ongoing distraction without clarification as if therapy is a game of chess with interminable checks. This unconscious tendency is rooted in a need to relate circuitously. When I encounter too much abstraction, I suggest the patient may be playing therapeutic chess with me. The very elusive game is, "I show, you seek." The next two sections will illustrate how to confront the problem.

SUGGESTIONS FOR INROADS IN THERAPY MAINTENANCE

The challenge for the therapist is to facilitate a redirection of hyperintuitiveness into a healthier expression of resilience and productivity. It is necessary to normalize the process as difficult, not magical, by making explicit and direct interventions, one of which is to frame behavioral approaches through philosophic and existential challenges elicited Socratically and owned by the patient as his own insight. I suggest such a strategy includes renarration of trauma accomplished by your identifying the idiosyncratic meaning of the officer's personal meaning in symbols presented to you. Overvalued ideas may be recognized through his depiction of metaphors, analogies, similes, and descriptions of sensory material.

Interventions that Move Hypervigilance into Expansion and Inclusion With Others

1. Expand self-vigilance to include wider circles of relatedness first approached by behavioral experiments. The two of you assess experiments jointly on a graduated series of exposure.
2. The experiments may include gradual and successive approximations, targeting risk-taking exposure related to healthy ambition and competition while you dispel likely maladaptive myths.
3. Do *in vivo* rehearsals, role plays, and tangible experiments with patients who directly express creative ideas and involvement in work settings and social events These experiments are presented as puzzle solving and problem identification.

4. As efficacy is gained, peer-support officers may be enlisted in building social circles.
5. Use artwork, diary, and verbal metaphor as a medium to Socratically draw out his solipsistic world. Anchor a realistic confrontation to achieve what may become a real and lasting contribution in the life of the officer.
6. Many of these patients have above-average intelligence and can accept complex and involved existential- and artistic-oriented approaches to express PPS-CPTSD.
7. The essence of all clarification is best achieved by working with the religious and metaphorical leitmotifs without fighting them as irrational, archaic, or primitive.

I remind myself that what is expressed is a desire for relatedness and understanding. You can heuristically shape a reintegration of the broken soul toward spontaneous healing. This repair is a healing process that includes the patient expressing loss. Optimism and investment in life is modeled and guided into lucid expression after emotional release of pain and loss is expressed. An example of how toxic loss that remains built up and not expressed is presented in the inimitable style of Dr. Fritz Perls as an army psychotherapist:

> A soldier was referred after suffering from big welts all over his body and with a deep despair in his eyes. . . . I put him under pentothal and learned that he had been in a concentration camp. I spoke German to him and led him back to his moments of despair and removed the crying block. He really cried his heart out, or shall we say he cried his skin out. He woke in a state of confusion and then he really worked at the typical experience of being completely and freely in the world. At last he had left the concentration camp behind and was with us. The welts disappeared. (Perls, 1979, p. 90)

Dr. Perls may have used a modified heuristic eco-ethological existential analytic approach. Perls' empathy helped the loss to be expressed. In the eco-ethological approach, Dr. Perls worked with the original traumatic loss the patient experienced, which may be described as a quantum psychic moment of the death camp. The trauma may be conceived as a point in the patient's life when human time becomes defined by the narrowing of human space beat into him from the ashen welts experienced through repetitive trauma. The cumulative lumps of unreleased toxins bore witness to unspoken loss. It was perhaps Dr. Perls' attitude that did not recapitulate what this victim had experienced with others in clarifying and helping the patient gain the ability to express his considerable and cumulative loss. Because the therapist cared enough to help facilitate the loss being expressed, the transference was deliberate, passionate, nonjudgmental, and existential. His patient exchanged the map of hypervigilance (Gilmartin, 2002) for the vitality that hard work through direct expression of traumatic loss freed. Hiakawa offers linguistic perspective: "the map is not the territory, the self concept is not the self" (1963); to that I may add, the trauma symbols are not the loss in the trauma as each unique person experiences it, qua his individual style.

CLINICIANS CORNER—
PLACING THE WET ELECTRICITY OF THE
SIXTH SENSE IN FOCUS

The hyperintuitive officer's narration of trauma and loss may be viewed as a map, which may guide us into a clearer understanding of how he processes loss in trauma. It may also clarify what defenses have emerged, offering us clinical evidence for our hypotheses. For example, the officer-patient may express a hypersensitivity and vigilance against loss as feeling vibrations; having a sixth sense about people no longer present, but felt; or sensing an aura is present somewhere nearby. These few examples may suffice as an attempt to reach out to the therapist and to engage the therapist in facilitating expression of his loss. It seems labeling the patient as schizotypal offers little help, stigmatizes the patient, and may stultify your willingness to invest in the necessary grief work. In turn, cognitively disputing his metaphors as irrational or engaging in psychoanalytic confrontation of the officer-patient's experience may lead to premature termination.

Rather, I suggest understanding these symbolic representations as the officer-patient's own idiosyncratic meaning of constricted and indirectly expressed loss. This opens the door for using the Socratic and heuristic eco-ethological approach to help define, normalize, and more directly express the loss experienced in trauma. Normalization and expression are two important goals. Enabling the officer to become a participant and not remain a detached observer subject to superstitious forces (depersonalization) is another important goal as R. R. Ellis suggests (see chapter 4).

The payoff is that in many cases, the emergence of lucidity and creativity as the reality of repetitive trauma and loss is fleshed out. An officer who is healthily cautious may gradually replace a defensive constellation of hyperintuitive and overwhelming avoidant strategies. To illustrate how to begin to effect this change, let us refer back to the verbatim example given for the hyperintuitive officer-patient. Think how you might practically approach this public-safety professional. In the following case example (a snippet of our work), Sergeant U presents with a style of cryptic, illusive, and overvalued metaphors that indirectly invite me to explore his experience of loss in trauma. At this point, we have an alliance together and have clarified working on trauma and loss as an important aspect of the therapy. Our task is to facilitate a lucid and direct expression of the loss in the trauma while valuing this highly intelligent, intriguing, and pleasant Sergeant U.

Sgt. U: Doc, just tell me what to do. I'm tired, okay? I just can't figure out how an innocent girl can die like that. The pictures pop up again and again. The miasma of the Grim Reaper hovers around her face. I cannot feel anything. [Sgt U presents this trauma with minimal emotional expression, but in a deep and strongly pitched voice]. Well how do I get rid of this Grim Reaper?

Dr: U, once again, I have no magical technique or pill. In fact, it seems like you'd like me to give you the answers. I would like to understand what comes to mind with the image of the Grim Reaper coming up when you think of death? [I pause to allow a protest, in case a visual or auditory hallucination is present. Thankfully, this is disconfirmed by her silence.] It is no wonder, but understandable. If I am getting it right, and I may be far off, you are sick and tired of the physical arousal each time you see the face of the girl as the Grim Reaper hovers around her face. The Reaper's sword you've described may be the long knife that stabbed T, and the Grim Reaper's face replaces the girl's grim expression while dying and pleading as your eyes picked up and held her there for a long time. (silence) [I let my understanding of Sgt. U's genuine experiences underlying the metaphors lead me. They are quite rich, although seemingly awkward at first. I feel and think Sgt. U may be too scared to identify vulnerability, fear, and cry openly. I chose not to remain silent. I grab for the metaphors to clarify what I believe is blocking her expression of loss.]

Sgt. U: [Eyes becoming slightly teary with gaze aversion] You know, I've done all I could [Alluding to guilt, I make note to return at a later time]. Why did she have to die on the landing on the thirteenth stair of the seventh stairwell, upside down? She told me Ms. L. and her had disagreed about a boy. T gave me a dying declaration. T said, "Mrs. L told me that will teach me to be disrespectful. She pointed at her stomach. She said she was scared." [I saw a slice cut deep inside and the thick red blood.]

Dr: What are you experiencing right now as you are seeing her at this moment?

Sgt. U: Wet electricity jumping up and down my body, you know that sixth sense we discussed when she was dying. The EMT thought she may make it and told me so. The miasma was all around; I knew she was worse off than she made out. Then the fucking job and anyhow . . . (distracted to unrelated event)

Dr: (Interrupt). The wet electricity sounds like a very painful experience, while it is difficult, it is important to stay with it.

Sgt. U: It's the striding through circumstances, a jolt, a miasma is there, [directly looking at me intensely studying my responses] it's a real miasma when her face pops up. I feel the Grim Reaper is right there with us. It feels like wet electricity right now. [I don't attempt to get to the roots of these metaphors no matter how interesting, unless it offers an entire gestalt to the most pressing loss.]

Dr: It appears if we look at what's happening now, your experience of the Grim Reaper is not a ghost, or evil spirit, but the painful loss of seeing a grim face on T, a dying girl—flashing some real fears back into your mind's eye. The experience of striding through circumstances makes sense as a homicide seen again and again. The shock of the death and seeing such a young woman murdered by another older woman is jolting, shocking to your depth. I imagine for you, Sgt. U, it felt like wet electricity. Mrs. L stabbing T was your first homicide as a detective fifteen years ago if that's not a miasma, I don't know what is.

Sgt. U: [Silence and sadness in tone of voice, teary eyed, no expression for a few minutes, a deep sigh.] I remember the time I started to feel the miasma, and see the Grim Reaper in the shadows of her face like a dream or vision. I feel weird talking about it. It's chaos, like the feeling I told you about. You and I are Greek soldiers in ancient times, and you are my Centurion Doc, healing me from the bad stuff we saw.

Dr: (Silence) [I need to process where she is going. I get frustrated and think I may need a new hypothesis. I have not disconfirmed the original one yet. I know she is not psychotic, or paranoid. I choose to continue and keep to my stance. I go for putting the riddle she has presented to both of us as context for clarification.] It seems like the journey you are taking us on is one of finding clarity in a miasma, a miasma that makes a lot of sense in the context of ancient Greek times. [The patient had shared with me her readings about the oracle at Delphi where Socrates went on his quest to find order in chaos—reason and purpose behind the tragic comedy of murder.] The Grim Reaper moves in and out of the miasma of sorrow unexpressed. This miasma is where you courageously endured wet electricity as jolts to your soul, seeing her stab wound, red blood and the urine smells you described before as senseless offering to a false god of rage. It may be in part you wish to invite me, as your therapist, to find order with you in the senseless murder through your beautiful metaphors. As long as we remember they are metaphors, why not in the sacred relationship we are building? [This is a paradoxical intervention to help her realize what her metaphors mean through a dynamic interpretation, as well as to let her know on an existential level of experience I witness and value the pain and loss underlying her metaphors, and cognitively I support her expression of a more direct expression of her loss through modeling and positive reinforcement. My intervention tends to be helpful to the patient, Sgt U.]

Sgt. U: [Tears in eyes, crying, followed by a smile that is genuine] I mean it hurts to see this young girl's beautiful life wiped out by this self-righteous, mean-hearted bitch! Imagine, how evil is murder? Over what, Doc? Being dissed? Come on, that's madness, isn't it? It's not me that's mad, it's this chaotic situation and many more like it.

Dr: No, it not you! It's hard and difficult to express. As you're doing right now.

Our work continues; the paradoxical intervention worked well. Clarity and directness followed. By not relinquishing the quest to find sensibility and a rational creative approach to Sgt. U's overvalued use of metaphors, we have begun to establish a new and healthier way of expression, identification, validation, and exploration of losses in our therapeutic alliance.

THE CONTROLLED HYPERFOCUSED PUBLIC-SAFETY PERSONALITY STYLE

Intrapsychic Level of Defensiveness for Survival

How does an officer capable of intense concentration—attentive and pragmatic—deal with the quantum psychic moment of trauma? What happens to the rituals that served as predictable security against what is now shattered by the impact of original trauma? A search for structure and order intensifies with the aftershock of a crumbled facade of safety.

Practices that *should* have kept the officer safe invariably fail. Many times the symbolic and meaningful value of these rituals are not consciously recognized by the officer as selective affordances that signal a feeling of security. By hyperfocusing on a retreat of complex rituals heightened after a trauma, an attempt to undo loss is, of course, an even more intense defense against that very loss. The original symbolic value of the wish for rituals to ward off harm to the officer is not forgotten, but may be lost to repression.

Moving in for a more intimate view is helpful. Let us look at a case example, officer-patient TQ. Officer-patient TQ is in his mid-50s. He has made an active decision to retire after two-and-a-half decades of public-safety work. While he begins emptying out his locker, he finds an older radio holder and begins to cry profusely. Initially, many labels were used and affixed to officer-patient TQ: histrionic, possible borderline, intentional distortion, possibly decompensating. By using an eco-ethological approach, we discovered the radio holder had significance through every frayed line of leather that folded in on itself. It represented many positive, timeless moments shared with his partner of over a decade before he died in the line of duty. This was not absurd, not histrionic, or borderline pathology. The radio holder was a symbolic affordance for this FD officer. It anchored an existentially rich transitional object that held the moments that were meaningful and shared with his partner. In dynamic terms, it was a wish to be with the partner and all that evoked in psychological meaning. The defenses were opened and provoked genuine expression, which led to an insight that a dynamic exploration revealed. The death of his friend and partner invoked shared vulnerability, survival guilt, anger, anxiety, and buried loss that emerged upon his viewing and discomfort with the antiaffordance hidden in the radio holder. The telescope was a long one that burrowed down to a spiral of death, denied agape love, and a loss that remained buried and unheard.

Usually, the response to trauma is intense hyperfocus leading to a search. That search is to recover what was lost and what remains lost. Reciprocal to hyperfocus is an implosion, where aggression, excitement, and loss ever-present is masked in new and more involved rituals to defend against grieving. That implosion may be an attempt at compensation, when rules and rituals are no longer effective in keeping away the repressed loss. The invariant rituals no longer afford the ability to ward off danger. When a critical mass accumulates, exhaustion sets in, and an emotional implosion may occur; it is more of a recompensation then a decompensation. The officer healthily begins to express his loss emotionally through grieving that is largely unconscious at first.

Biophysical Level of Mood

What stands out is the constant overdrive of this patient. This nonstop energy includes anxiety and expressed agitation. A resistance against pleasure, relaxation, and genuine levity exists hand in hand with disavowed traumatic loss. The hyperfocus may be a way of communicating the biophysical aspects of mood. How? Ethological aggression communicated through a passive-aggressive behavioral pattern may signal to others agitation and pain in a way that is acceptable in public-safety culture. For example, mordant gallows humor, may not be real humor but avoidance of loss through distancing oneself. This avoidance and denial for the short term is adaptively functional, however, cumulatively toxic and maladaptive in the long term. When gallows humor is all too common and idealism is high, dissonance is not unusual. I have witnessed this a number of times in working with officers. *Peer pressure initially pushes an officer to exchange shock and grief for giggles. The pressure to not allow expression of grief is keen. This is particularly so when the victim is considered as not innocent or sacred as a victim.* In many cases, the officer experiences spiritual, religious, cultural, or philosophical existential angst silently. Apathy due to depletion of energy invested in these transient coping tactics may lead to chronic functional numbness. The therapeutic value of this so-called defense of humor is as effective as all paper tigers, when the real Bengal tiger of grief emerges in the living chamber of one's memories, with all its ferocity.

PHENOMENOLOGICAL LEVEL OF SELF-IMAGE, COGNITIVE STYLE, AND OBJECT REPRESENTATIONS

Internalized emotional constriction is forced into a Draconian self-discipline. The public-service officer with this personality style is prone to reducing his achievements as another phase of growth. The commitment to work is a straight-edged razor, no ridge of imperfection allowed. A unique clue is the procedural guide of the public-service agency/department, sometimes hundreds of pages of minutiae is committed to memory along with a rigid adherence. Asking for a procedure and witnessing the officer dictate encyclopedic knowledge is confirming. It is when vulnerability reaches its climax in defense as impenetrable as armor. It is functional and important as a defense that works in the context of the public-safety identity. However, no matter what is accomplished, one never lays down his chisel of symmetry for a wreath of calm achievement, not even for a blinking moment.

While most officers would feel a deep sense of accomplishment, efficacy, and pleasure when promoted to the rank of Captain (Executive level) and achieving an MA degree, many officer-patients with this personality style consider it just another goal/phase accomplished. What's next? This restless search for perfection is never satiated in the waters that flow through the straits of self-imposed exactitude. The wish underlying this armor in part is a desire for invulnerability and immortality. Reaching the accumulated mental and professional knowledge of one's profession means achieving a walking armor that renders him impervious to pain, loss, and ultimately death (Becker, 1967; Campbell, 1973).

The more this officer experiences traumatic loss, the more goals are established to detour the inevitable confrontation with PPS-PTSD. Drive is the key ethological emotion. Idealism and selflessness are both strength and weakness. Idealism is sparked in the young recruits and burns as a fire in senior and tenured commanders with this style. The self-image and cognitive style is cemented in a matter-of-fact attitude, imperious toward cumulative trauma. Truth be told, emotional repression may lead to a psychophysiological distraction that stalls genuine living. In its place is an automaton mentality that replaces spontaneity, flexibility, and pleasure.

A religiosity toward the work ethic is piqued. The wish to be a perfect soldier is enforced with Draconian masochism and alacrity. The perception that one has violated a standard is remonstrated through intense guilt, anxiety, and even more hyperfocus. This hyperfocus and functional numbing may carry into interpersonal object relationships. Tough presentations are put out by these officers when confronted by traumatic loss.

For example, it is typical to hear "Ahh, I let it roll, like a duck" or "I snap out of it." This veneer is sensible when put in developmental perspective. Many came from childhoods with role model(s) who evidenced a tough presentation and the ability to endure without flinching. The same public-service idealism is likely to be transmitted to loved family members and friends. Some of these expectations may be an altered form of action empathy, selected tactically to protect loved ones from vulnerability in a perceived dangerous world. This perception is not without evolutionary value and perceptual sensibility.

This phenomenon in holocaust survivor's children includes guardedness, hoarding, rituals to defend against vulnerability shaped by trauma. Assumptions of suspicion, agitation, and anxiety may be selectively transmitted to family members across generations and into careers (Benner, 1998; Bettelheim, 1979; Epstein, 1979; Gilmartin, 1986; Horowitz, 1999; Kelly, 1985; Silverstein, 1992).

It is far from accidental that this style was represented by veterans from the armed services, and extended police and public-safety families. *Rituals may be learned and shared defenses that help keep danger away from one's family. This can turn into situations that may provoke extreme overprotection. The term "control freak" is a pejorative taken out of developmental context and may contribute to simplistic notions of little value. Control may be parsimoniously understood in the eco-ethological perspective as a defense against perceived vulnerability to loss.*

An extension of this perspective is observed in adaptive functional disso-ciation where behavioral consequences become apparent. For example, an officer carries out everyday duties without missing a day of work while being severely depressed, that is, fighting to stay on duty rather than be relieved of full-duty status even when warranted medically, without penalty.

Adaptively, officers with this style epitomize the backbone of public service, the good soldier that goes on and on in spite of all adversities he faces. The problem is that eventually he collapses into an implosion of loss in trauma that erupts into the present.

DIFFERENTIAL DIAGNOSIS

The idiosyncratic patient uses the defense of withdrawal from vulnerability and hyperintuitive avoidance against loss in the shade of fantasy and abstraction; the hyperexcited become addicted to higher and higher thresholds of excitement and risk taking to ward off loss in trauma. The hyperfocused use control as a concrete, automated armor of defense to seal off the discharge of intense aggressive drive derivatives (Brenner, 1974, 1976) hostility, anxiety, shock, guilt, and energy. Under intense pressure of PPS-CPTSD, this armor splits. Approach strategies in relational terms are different across each personality style. How are these differences manifested? In part, the hyperaggressive officer displaces and projects rage at feeling any hurt or losses. The officer inflicts stinging sadism, pain, and control; he hurts others. The hyperexcited jumps into situations risking great damage and pain to self, undoing his vulnerability and sense of loss of an ideal self; the hyperintuitive shuns the traumatic loss through metaphors that fantasy veils in her shadow as intellectual and unreachable echoes of loss; the hyperfocused officer may develop a tolerance for more and more pain through masochism (Millon, 1996; Panken, 1973). This conditioning is self-directed, and hardly conscious.

Behavioral Level of Expressive Acts and Interpersonal Conduct

This professional is likely to present as Dapper Danielle: flawless, meticulous, fastidious, down to the pressed, button-down, starched, Oxford blouse. The shine on her shoe is spit polish. Another clue is Dapper Danielle's service record indicating hardly any absences, sickness, or rarely line-of-duty injuries. Although these events may have happened, unique for public safety is this officer's reluctance to report it, or if she does so, a tendency for extreme minimization becomes apparent.

Adaptively, the ability to think and act in critical moments is automatic. This officer is likely to excel climbing the rank order of strategic responsibility. I suggest adaptively because this style's strength is apparent in outstanding acts of courage, team, and role consistency necessary for public service. Survival is embedded in the ritual compulsions as a learned behavioral strategy for coping with the experience of trauma.

The Epitome of What Motivated These Officers to Join a Police Career

These officers joined a police career for "Job security. Being an officer felt natural to me. I wanted *to maintain peace and order* in peoples lives. As an EMT, I knew I could *accomplish* saving lives."

Verbatim Record of the Most Traumatic Event

Approximately 15 years ago, while working for EMS in Brooklyn, I responded to a call for a woman in labor. This would normally be a routine transport to the hospital, but it was not. We arrived on the scene and proceeded up to the apartment. The door was slightly opened. We knocked, but no one answered. We looked in, and we could see an elderly lady mopping the floor.

We called out to her that EMS was here, but she did not respond. We then saw a male walking in the apartment and called out to him, but he also did not respond. We then entered the apartment and asked the lady who was mopping up water if she called for an ambulance. She did not say anything, as if we were talking a different language. We proceeded as protocol, went further into the apartment: to our left in another room, we saw a female on the couch with blood dripping down from between her legs. We ran over to her and quickly thought she was the female in labor. However, we soon realized she had already given birth. We shouted, "Where is the baby?" Still nobody answered. After a short time, I pieced it all together and ran into the bathroom. It was there that I found the baby in the toilet with its head actually looking like it was stuck in the hole in the bottom of the bowl. I pulled the newborn infant out of the toilet. I had a job to do.

My partner called for the police as I was attempting mouth to mouth on the infant. The baby had a pulse of about 50, but for a newborn this is not enough to sustain life. The baby was also in respiratory arrest. I continued resuscitation efforts until the police arrived, and I immediately told the officer to take me to the hospital in the RMP. My partner stayed to care for the mother. The baby died a couple of days later. The mother was charged with murder. Sometime after the incident I ran into a police sergeant who became involved in that investigation that night. He told me that it was in the paper that the mother was acquitted in a jury trial. I do not understand how this could be. When I testified in front of the grand jury as a witness, they had tears in their eyes and were shaking their heads.

Her defense was that she did not know she was pregnant and the baby just fell into the bowl, a ridiculous story. Her past history involved prostitution arrests, and she had two other kids somewhere. This incident has stayed with me over the years. Thinking about it, talking about it, I am angry how someone can betray a beautiful little baby. Every once in a while, I relive this incident in a bad dream. I guess I have gone over this event for many years when I was remembering it. I have gone over my steps in responding, and I did everything proper. I studied hard and long as an EMT and was the third top graduate in my class. . . .

DISCUSSION OF PERSONALITY STYLE DEVELOPMENT

Strengths of officers with this personality type are likely to be seen through acts of courage, being a good team player, and consistency in the most optimal task completion. We have reviewed some dynamic aspects of this style. In turn, let us shift our focus to an integrative dynamic and cognitive-behavioral perspective. The motivation for survival appears to be expressed in the ritual compulsions (behavioral repetitions) that may be understood as a compromise formation (a defense against unconscious wishes for immortality, perfectionism, and merger with an idealized omnipotent ideal). Brenner sheds light on this process in which unconscious impulses from drive derivatives (sexual and aggressive) emerge during development. Inhibition of these very impulses creates conflict, which may evoke anxiety and depressive affect. In part, the anxiety and depressive affect may be appreciated as complex compromise formations, which are dynamic constellations responsive to the individual officer's conflict, where expression of drive derivatives conflicts with defense against expression. The moral defenses, the structure of ego reality, and libidinal and aggressive drives fuel the individual manifestations of dynamic and evolving aspects of the ubiquitous nature of these conflicts (Brenner, 1974, 1976, 1982, 2003; Richards & Willick, 1986).

The behavioral repetition cycles a pattern of familiarity while distancing the officer-patient from insight. The rote behavioral patterns motivated by deeply layered conflict with loss is defended against in a manner that prevents that very loss from being expressed. The repetition compulsion, as Freud viewed it, is put into clear perspective in the context of this officer-patient's presentation. The ideal incorporated is part of the training that is rewarded instrumentally, and failures to this ideal are experienced as narcissistic injuries in many officers with this tendency. Insight, whether through psychodynamic interpretations that are iterated or in direct cognitive clarifications and confrontations, are likely to be experienced by the officer-patient as a hostile attack. This perception of a hostile attack ripens the heightened resistance of the officer-patient.

The eco-ethological situation of peers and supervisors often instrumentally supports the recalcitrance of this resistance and repression toward change. The ethological survival value of behavioral repetitions is likely to be perceived accurately as beneficial to the officer-patient's peers in his ecological niche, the unit, and police service area. Remember, these officers are adept at making their ability known and to make themselves invaluable to others in the unit. They are without doubt the officers who do not embarrass the agency/department by stepping out of the role assigned and forged. Their rebellion is likely to be expressed in subtle passive-aggressive resistance. Doubt and uncertainty may arise when change, pleasure, or stepping out of his assigned role occurs. It also arises when trauma is experienced as a failure in one's roles and the ritualized compulsions fail to thwart the accumulated losses of repetitive trauma.

The content of trauma processing includes *objective fear* and *moral anxiety*. Objective fear is ethologically based and expressed through emotional fear, agitation, shock, approach avoidance, and freezing responses. Existentially, moral anxiety is processed through self-evaluation, guilt worthiness, and responsibility weighed by the scale of impossibly high, personally set standards, adequacy or inadequacy comparisons, and achieved or failed spiritual goals.

In this style, a tendency for redirecting objective fear and moral anxiety (objective/emotional and moral/cognitive) may be achieved through a higher level of behavioral overcompensation. The self-conditioning is compulsively ritualized through extreme discipline which may act as a buffer to vulnerability and expression of fear, shock, anger, anxiety, and guilt over traumatic loss. Perhaps the compulsive training of the body and mind may ward off disease through exercises of the brain and body. Agitation and high energy are diverted into behaviors that may help redirect the anger into professional activities. Sadly, this is not usually sublimation, it is repression wherein conflict abounds.

Ritualized activity may also be explained as a self-directed competency within one's niche offering the officer a sense of control by overcompensation against disenfranchised trauma and loss. The alexithymic/functional numbing of doing replaces cognition and emotion, splitting the emotional from the cognitive in the extreme service of the behavioral. This may explain in part why and how the officer continues enduring pain on the job with stoic perseverance. The officer is impervious to pain and imperious with equanimity in the storm of natural and unnatural trauma.

The extreme assumption of the world colored by danger and unpredictability hyperfocuses survival. Outside fortresses cannot protect you. Internal rituals and obsessive thoughts create a constant plan—A, B, C, D, E, F—the officer-patient becomes trapped in his own too-literal and inescapable alternatives, where decisive action is surfeited in uncertainty of choice. This is yet another clue to the ideal of superfitness and readiness. Genuine humor and relaxation are perceived in an extreme form as killing time, laziness, and harm. While the professional may attend parties, the other clue is "it is a thing to do"; "a function"; a "step ladder" in which little or no joy is embraced. The problem is all of life exists as a means to an end without the means being lived as part of genuine life being lived in the here and now fully and pleasurably. I am not suggesting this is an innate inability for joy and healthy living. It is conditioned largely by an unconscious process of selective shaping afforded through the eco-ethological niche and endogenous interaction and influences.

Vulnerability, risk of interdependency, and change in status or domestic situations hold the greatest opportunities for the officer-patient to visit for therapy. Specifically, physical injury, marriage, divorce, promotion, or change of status may be cause for initiating therapy.

INITIAL SUGGESTIONS FOR INROADS FOR THERAPY ALLIANCE MAINTENANCE

The novel event of trauma disrupts ethological invariants. Decompensation on many levels may occur: mental, physical, emotional, and perceptual. The focus on grievance and injustice collecting may become the focus of therapy, while the earthy pain and loss is not recognized. In many cases, a family history may suggest roots of intragenerational traditions of public safety as fecund soil for a belief in invulnerability (Kelly, 1985).

Another way of looking at the hyperfocus is as a legitimate rite of passage in openly expressing and sharing a survival value in active empathy. This is a redeeming quality when not extreme. Reality may also become a spiral of fear with an outward mask of indifference, a "who cares?" attitude. This bravado may distort reality in the service of saving lives and personal invulnerability. Anger is acceptable; sadness and crying is not. In one participant's words, "it is OK for a man to be pissed, but never a crybaby. After all, how long should I cry, day and night?

Why bother in the first place? It's an issue of snapping out of it; simple as that." This type of distortion, which says one must be an ideal police officer who can snap out and shake off trauma and loss, is hidden from others. As a matter of fact, even if it is hidden from one's self in repression it is not forgotten.

Behaviorally in this style, tasks started are completed from A to Z. This is a positive adaptation. Extant is a rejection of addictive outlets that are destructive.

High levels of frustration tolerance occur. There is an ability to fit into the rank structure of public-service agencies. The hyperfocus is extraordinary in staying with complex problems until their solutions arrive. A high-action empathy as a strength is exhibited.

Further, a stoicism dating from Epicetus and Marcus Aurelius as a living philosophy, not in place of religion or faith but in an attitude toward life, may be helpful. This philosophy is formulated by Dr. Ellis in his seminal contribution through Rational Emotive Behavioral Therapy (REBT) (Ellis, 1962, 1973). Stoicism suggests a style of responsibility, choice, and tolerance of frustration without naïveté and an ingratiating style toward others. Using stoicism may help this officer gradually enjoy more self-acceptance and pleasure. Self-direction and rational experiments to tolerate and express emotions and pleasure may gradually facilitate the ability to tolerate vulnerability and growth.

In public service, to vaunt a challenge is responded to with the officer offering himself as an oblation in the service of duty that can become all too real. Consequential thinking and boundary setting can enlist a healthy limitation to overly excessive commitment while enlarging the ability to balance duty and pleasure. This is no easy task. Supportive interpersonal as well as cognitive and emotional interventions may be optimized (Seligman & Garber, 1980).

Practically speaking, complexity that requires putting disorder into a doable routine is challenging and potentially a passionate channel for energy with this style. While many others find this irritating and annoying, this officer will likely find it gratifying. Accommodating for this style are certain readily available niches. For instance, administration, analysis, desk duties, operational duties, training and inspections sectors in which details can be organized and imple-mented. Learning the meaningfulness of actions taken and involvement in one's profession is encouraged and made an explicit goal through structured exercises (Selye, 1974).

The strategy of your approach is to gain a holistic, rational, and emotive, behavioral intervention from the right pole through the left pole. I suggest the following model I developed for expressing emotional empathy and wisdom is supported and structured from A to Z as followed by your skill as a therapist:

Idealism <_____> Pragmatism
Perfectionism <_____> Realistic allowance of fallibility
Selfless <_____> Self-interest
Indefatigability <_____> Limits of boundaries
Functional numbness <_____> Emotional empathy and action empathy
Anhedonia <_____> Responsible hedonism
Silent martyrdom for others <___> Team player with your own voice
Silent agreement: peer pressure<_> Experiment: your own example as unique
Self-image: must be perfect<____> Accept and value yourself as imperfect
Worthy of insults: self an others <__> Unconditional self-appreciation.

Avoid pleasure < _____ > Pleasure is positive and healthy experiences
Rationalization, intellectualism < __ > Experiencing life in all its hues
Impervious to pain < _____ > Learning to say I'm hurting and can use a hug

The idea that this officer is mean-hearted and cold is a therapeutic error. Identifying loneliness and expanding circles of friends and community involvement with non-public-service professionals helps expand to pleasure, involvement, and growth.

CLINICIAN'S CORNER— PRACTICAL APPROACH—PARADOXICAL INTENTION AND REDIRECTION

Lieutenant XP is a Hispanic American, patrol veteran, married with two children. He presented with feeling worn out and anxious, but could not understand why. He let me know right off the bat, "therapy is not really what I need, but I am here to get to know what a Cop Doc is all about. I don't mind as much now because, after all, you are a sergeant and retired uniform psychologist." I accepted his roundabout excuse for coming in. I began in earnest to develop a working relationship with him on his terms. Initial sarcasm filtered in to our sessions. I tolerated it, gently returning to identify his thoughts and feelings related to his current burnout. I did not confront his attempt to get me to repeat an attitude I suspected would confirm yet another hostile response. This was not easy. It was elusive and unproven. The alliance soon became successful by keeping my attitude consistent with a dynamic approach.

In our work together, a context emerged in which his family and his style were transmitted by intragenerational family members from military, police, and public-safety circles. My first hypothesis was that he was alexithymic and did not learn to identify his feelings; his polished surface and at times gruff attitude barked out resistance. The second hypothesis I had was the major trauma in Lt. XP's life was the catastrophe of 9/11/01. He was an active member in recovery efforts, and his loss remained unspoken. The first hypothesis of alexithymia was on the money, the second hypothesis regarding 9/11/01 was on my sleeve; I had to revise my second hypothesis after disconfirmation. Note his description:

> Going through the rubble, the dogs looking like they were battered. Seeing them, you look and say, what did I do? . . . Look at the heavy and real job . . . just to see we're on the outskirts of the morgue. They looked like zombies, the cops and EMTs, the walking dead on this job, *after you see bodies the first few times, you take your mind off of it*. Then it don't bother you no more, matter of fact. [He giggles with a fearful expression, not genuine.]

The first few sessions, I structured my approach (a bit autocratically) on the trauma of 9/11/01. I ignored my own advice to track the path of trauma and grief history to its core whereever the patient may lead us. I pick up my own "aha," hearing him repeat his phrase again, "after you see bodies the first few times you take your mind off of it." I pursue this offering as a path to possible disenfranchised loss and seek to find out what first few times he is referring to. My approach is Socratic, gentle, and heuristic.

Revising and moving with the natural unfolding account of original trauma as the patient presents it is the mainstay of the heuristic approach. The historical context of the segment I choose to present illustrates this point. Lt. XP was a former seminary student who became an all-but-ordained Roman Catholic priest. He aspired to be the only male to be a priest in his traditional Roman Catholic family. Instead, he exchanged his priest's frock and vows of celibacy for marriage to a lovely nurse practitioner with whom he fell in love and to the uniform and shield of the NYPD. He never grieved the loss his aspiration to be a priest. Compounding this loss was ambivalence in his drastic change from a priest to marriage and a war zone as a rookie street cop.

A tendency in many hyperfocused officers is to disavow feelings toward a loss and to move on in the cadence of whatever beat another drummer is playing. While he maintained being happy and content in his current position, he had adopted a strategy that was functional in performance goals, and intrapersonally supportive of an existential vacuum. This vacuum telescoped to traumatic loss, the earliest of original trauma, where two events merged. The first homicide and first dead person he experienced telescoped back from 9/11/01 to a decade ago. Being a rookie beat officer shocked at the indifference among his fellow officers was compared to sacred treatment he had used as a harsh moral standard to compare his own performance with. His cultural and religious training and his personal beliefs and assumptions colored his trauma and grief (Benner, 1991, 1998/1999, 1999/2001; Gilmartin, 2002; Silverstein, 1992).

A point not to be lost is if I viewed his loss as being a crybaby or whining, my stance would have helped silence his own voice and values. I could have also interpreted his traumatic loss as exaggerated hysteria, accepting gallows humor in its lighter shade, rather than the dark side from which he viewed it. Understanding his perspective is key. Helping him recover his lost voice was part of his self-healing. His making an active self-directive stance of redemption in an impoverished setting was his own value, long lost. You can do the same in your work. 9/11/01 was a historic turning point in masculinity, in which public expression of emotions, including grief, was made more acceptable. In Lt. XP's experience, 9/11/01 was a painful reminder of how different he experienced his response to death and loss over a decade ago.

On 9/11/01, Lt. XP observed officers and dogs hurting badly. As a lieutenant, he was a far cry from his life as a rookie, where he experienced overwhelming loss and its suppression. The shared expression of communal grief and trauma was not experienced as something normal. Instead, it was a rather painful event, which emerged when what he held sacred was first disenfranchised and experienced as shame, guilt, and cowardice in his conformity to gallows humor.

The image of police dogs in the craters of dirt and clay digging for any vestige of life was a sacred experience in which the rituals and public-service respect of the dead was equilateral across the board. This flew in the face of earlier repressed experiences in which his own expectations of how his ideal image of self and other officers were long discarded. How it *should have been* and how he *must have acted* was a harsh internalized taskmaster.

This cognitive distortion may have in part led to self-loathing with accusations against himself "for being a moral and spiritual lame duck." This type of self-denigration was a significant schema in underscoring a feverish pursuit of rituals and other activities without rest. Why? It turned out he could no longer bear the motif of what he perceived as the cross on his back in the face of a catastrophe. His harsh self-deprecation and castigation without respite may well have served a masochistic need. That masochism in part may have satiated his guilt and need for self punishment. Under the surface of his anxiety was a desire to express his loss so long and perpetually reexperienced through the rituals surrounding his life. Panic attacks signaled a desire to flee both his sorrow and the process of exposing his loss. It opened an avenue to explore his objective fear and moral anxiety.

I listened to the associations for their underlying dynamic that led to his original trauma. Looking at what happened from another dimension, we moved from a cognitive-behavioral level of exploration to a complementary dynamic exploration in which an overly harsh idealized view of performance standards were clarified. This led to a specific avenue of intervention wherein the Lt. XP's perceived failure to live up to ideals he wished to fulfill were disenfranchised with abrupt coercion to conform to the group norm. It led to an existential, dynamic and cognitive reassessment in response to his individual presentation of loss in his experience of PPS-CPTSD. With this brief context in mind, let us attend to a segment of my exploratory work with Lt. XP and how the shift from 9/11/01 moved in a facilitated telescope to original traumatic loss a decade earlier.

> **Dr:** Stop for a moment. Let's go back together to what you just expressed, *after you see bodies the first few times you take your mind off of it.* What comes to your mind?
>
> **Lt. XP:** We were going through the rubble . . . the dogs looked like they were battered, seeing them you look and say (in comparison), what did I do? The K-9 units did the heavy and real job. . . . What did I do?. . . Just to see them. We were in the outskirts of the morgue. They all looked like zombies. They looked like the walking dead. On this job, after you see bodies *the first few times you know and then you take your mind off of it. The first few times you see dead bodies you turn away you know* [looking up, as if asking himself, why this ordeal? Staring into space and saccadic movement from his eyes, are closed with a giggle as nervous laughter].

Dr: I would like to know where that giggle signals us to go. Where are you first seeing dead bodies?

Lt. XP: The first few times, you know, you're horrified. I mean, with my background, I see dead bodies as holy. No matter what. You know, guys are there taking pictures with Polaroids; they love it and get into it (nervous giggle spells anxiety and fear about even discussing it).

Dr: You said you learned to live with it, meaning you may have felt very different at first. Seeing the dead bodies and the pictures taken and placed in albums, what was that experience like for you?

Lt. XP: You don't like it, you know, sometimes you get where, someone died and you think it could be someone's father, husband, wife, or sister. Show some respect, you know! I realize the academy and puzzle palace is one thing—reality another. A lot of times I kept silent, but I was trying to figure out what was so funny. Someone died, you would sit on the body and wait until the ME (Medical Examiner) came, after the EMT (Emergency Medical Technician) confirmed it. With a body tag on the toe.

Dr: Tell me what body tag comes to mind right now. Tell me about the victim and where you are. My big ears are open. [I lean forward attentive and look in his eyes, undaunted in my message of accepting, not avoiding what he will say.]

Lt. XP: A lot of times in the back of my mind there was nothing I could do. It's part of life, but I thought, what if the guy's got no relatives? What's left when you're all alone without anyone to even ID him? I feel bad I keep everyone together, its part of life. It adds pressure. Sometimes when you think about it, *you almost feel like a robot.* You go through the motions. You feel awkward, you really don't know what to say, you got to keep everyone together in these situations.

Dr: It's very hard, I imagine, for you to be able to express that feeling of going through the motions and that experience of feeling like a robot in your mind's eye. What comes to mind right now?

Lt. XP: I remember my first homicide, December 30th, 1988. It's snowing on xx Street and yy Avenue. I am eating with my partner. Windows cracked. Midnight tour, about O430 hours, and it's starting to snow flurries outside. We go over to this job of "man down" with sirens blaring. It seemed like forever, after we arrived for night watch to come. Big xxx case, two years the wife set up her husband. I never forget his face, the guy lying there. I had a few months of nightmares afterwards. I first did the paperwork, then feeling bad for the guy. He was set up and murdered to collect on an insurance policy. She never got to it. The guys were giggling. I never forget how I kept it in. I was a rookie. One guy takes pictures and says this is a good killing, like as if it is an animal being displayed. I kept it in.

Dr: What did you keep in? [The nightmares will be addressed later. His major association in the therapeutic moment was the repetition of his expression "keeping it in." I choose to follow what meaning this phrase "keeping it in" held in Lt. XP's thoughts. I followed his lead in our exploration by attending to his own associations: His associations were not free and loaded with symbolic and psychological meaning.]

Lt. XP: I kept it in.

Dr: I would like to hear what you kept in. (Silence)

Lt. XP: I can't. (Silence, then expression moves to real anger; a smirk, then followed with a defensive grin, and then a vanishing giggle) They were acting like they just couldn't care less. One detective just lit up a smoke. Even my partner said, "well be happy, don't worry, it's all over, dude." This guy was barely dead, murdered without hope and he was so young; it was sick, depraved.

Dr: It appears you felt sick over the murder and seeing the victims on a street gutter. No one realized how nauseated and hurt you felt when you witnessed the murder and then what appeared to be a callous response by your fellow officers right in front of the body of the dead husband murdered for a few thousand dollars. That image would not go away, huh?

Lt. XP: It was sick and depraved. All I did was stay silent instead of saying what I felt. What did I do? I just giggled!

Dr: What did you want to express, if you felt you could?

Lt. XP then moves into expressing righteous anger and self-rebuke at what he believes was a betrayal of his values for the sake of conformity. The injustice and sordid cheapness of life coupled with the betrayal from the wife was a hard cross to bear for Lt. XP. He wished to continue in his role as the healing priest, with all the other wishes and expectations lost and unacknowledged until we began to explore these multiple losses. While we begin our work in earnest on his insight and active reassessment, he spontaneously describes shock at seeing a 60-year-old man at his first DOA. This man was dying on the bathroom floor of a heart attack.

The victim was in the process of defecating. The gallows humor of seeing the body, followed by picture taking of a few officer's is expressed this time openly: anger, shock, and disillusionment at the loss he experienced in witnessing this man who died so alone. Again, these situations are in part his depressed affect, infused with aggressive tension that remains unexpressed toward peers, while he absorbs all the blame. These cumulative disenfranchised losses remain largely unconscious.

It is through the eco-ethological approach that Lt. XP learns to use insight garnered from a dynamic exploration into the meaning of loss and how it impacted on him. The situation of 9/11/01 is connected through a telescope to what has emerged in a number of original trauma events. It is at this point that the grief and trauma work of Lt. XP begins. He gradually is helped to make sense of how he has replaced his genuine warm and empathic self with a hyperfocus in becoming a perfect soldier. By blocking loss, he stultified expression of disillusionment, shock, hatred, and disgust. This became his own issue with death as his personal onus. What was guilt around his imagined violations and self-punishment was exchanged through insight into an alteration in self-assertion and less harsh judgment of himself, others, and the world.

What was sacred was made profane. This was understood through a number of works that helped Lt. XP process the "numinous experience" of the holy through the work of Rudolph Otto (1982), trying to reclaim what is sacred for him and lost in his identity of the ideal cop, to the real cop. I suggested he write a log expressing his thoughts. We reassessed this together at his pace, including changing extreme idealism to a more genuine valuing of self and others. He was able to express loss without feeling compelled to conform to anything he did not want to. This was an existential success as well. While his conformity with regulations is crucial to survival of self and others, he found his self-growth by being able to offer a different perspective through self-example to his peers in place of conforming to a voice that was not his. The improvement in diminished emotional disturbance, lessened agitation, and ritualistic repetition of defenses intimated a growth in his ability to process trauma and loss in his life.

We slowly achieved initial growth by valuing his own beliefs as an ongoing choice, not a fixed appendage, and tolerance of others. *In vivo* rehearsals and role plays achieved getting Lt. XP to work on awakening and stirring his own style and thoughts, absent the bug of obsessive devaluing of his own voice and extreme demand on self and others. His growth advanced. We simultaneously worked on accepting the "profane" nature of some fellow officers as different styles he could not change. Lt. XP gradually achieved accepting his peers different coping strategies without internalizing hostility and exercising compassion for their different, not evil, means of dealing with loss.

In our trauma and loss work, I also offer a didactic explanation of the death albums without lecturing or devaluing this custom (see Epilogue). It helps him put this ritual in a more understanding perspective while valuing his own. The best way of change is through a model. His was one that other officers may embrace, absent the hostility. As a leader among his peers, he now flexibly models his reverence for the dead as a gift, unapologetically.

THE ADAPTIVEINTUITIVE STYLE

Intrapsychic Level of Defensiveness for Survival

What makes this officer's style resilient and socially intuitive when practical, emotional, and creative intelligence come together in a way that maximizes healthier adaptation? If a natural adaptation is active, what tendencies are present punctuating the landscape of repetitive trauma with an ability to thrive? Malleability, hardiness, and curiosity toward novel situations are a key to understanding officers with this style, regardless of other tendencies, traits, and features. It seems they take responsibility for their own actions in the agency they work for, yet, they remain somewhat aloof to maintain integrity and autonomy in decision making—a practical wisdom.

They are not paragons of justice, strength, or courage. They're with it by being able to communicate without giving into apathy or overt hostility. This is not without work. I suggest this style emerges within the crucible of loss in trauma. It is the upheaval that comes with trauma on an emotional level of experience that may pique the ability to embrace the opportunity for development. The selective value of this adaptation requires an exquisite emotional intelligence and the ability to use it and learn from it. The ability to confront the meaningfulness of life is not without a price. Here the lessons are not fleeting but are learned and are in part stable. Rather than become bitter from the hard luck handed them, they have a tendency to establish alternatives and optional paths where some don't exist. When given crap, they heap it together into fertile hills and till the seeds of their own insight until fruit grows. There is a strong sense of commitment to actualization that is not pursued but lived. This style has a range from positive adaptation to being highly actualized.

Biophysical Level of Mood

One aspect of mood appears to be a self-regulation that is expressive and on an even keel. Absent is an exaggerated masochism or sadism; but there is an ever-present assertiveness. The mood reported and the emotional regulation observed is generally on that even keel. This is not to say this officer has no issues with anger, anxiety, relationships, or PPS-CPTSD. I am suggesting he has learned to balance the extremes with moderation of mood and affect. He does this not with serendipity, but with hard work, which entails motivation and resilience. Spontaneity rather than extreme impulsiveness, avoidance, or procrastination is apparent.

Behavioral Level of Expressive Acts and Interpersonal Conduct

Activities include being involved in the community and being culturally aware and service oriented (Gilmartin, 2002; Wilson, 1968). Many bring spiritual/existential beliefs and meaningful activities and hobbies outside of public-service culture. They actively seek the gaining of unique skills for establishing themselves in their area of interest and responsibility. Pursuits include art work, sports, and martial arts. Many have varied interests and even dual professional or vocational certifications ranging from attorney, teacher, architect, to funeral director, nurse, engineer, auto mechanic and chef. Equally, many had obtained rank at one level, or appointment, represented in greater numbers than the other styles.

Expressively and interpersonally, a willingness to tolerate the discomfort, pain, fear, and anguish of working through the material of traumatic- and loss-filled experiences makes this officer resilient, unique, and able to thrive.

For example, one patient, a corrections officer who had a serious trauma in which she was injured in the line of duty, used her time off to enjoy quality time with family and friends. She did not blame herself and appreciated the good work she had done. At the time, she was pursuing a BA in engineering, wherein she did not demand straight As, but attempted just that nonetheless. In considering becoming a Captain, she carefully weighed her choices. She realized it would be worth it, set out a realistic strategy, and pursued it. She succeeded.

The Epitome of What Motivated These Officers to Join a Police Career

"To help people, to learn, and try to do the best job I can while making a secure living for myself and family. To have a respectable profession and to make an honest living."

DIFFERENTIAL DIAGNOSIS

This personality style epitomizes sublimation of the tendencies that become exaggerated in the other styles presented. For instance, while excitement, aggression, vigilance creativity, and ideals are present, none are dominant, none neglected. They are channeled productively in a mature social altruism, which includes self-interest and the interest of others—interest, not the idealism of the hyperfocus, or a need for excitement to feel good, or a vigilance hidden in abstraction as main conduits of maladaptation. Sadism, masochism, and overt aggression was absent. Compassion and emotional empathy were more freely expressed.

PHENOMENOLOGICAL LEVEL OF SELF-IMAGE, COGNITIVE STYLE, AND OBJECT REPRESENTATIONS

Self-image here is one of a professional and private person who is confident and relaxed about life and its challenges. Yet, this officer is not blind to the very real dangers inherent in public service, including personal vulnerability and psychological burnout. Believing, rather than knowing one has a personal, sacrosanct right to peace of mind.

Cognitively, an internal locus of control embraces the here and now of living. Tolerance of ambiguity is infused with cautious optimism. This is neither without hard work, nor innate as much as a desire to learn and use what is learned. This is adaptation. Consequential thinking, including planning for the present and future, were delivered with passion and with alternatives in mind. Rigidity and impulsivity were not in the forefront. Letting go and relaxing was balanced with hard work toward long-term goals. Notably absent was short-term hedonism. Existential meaning and choice certainly was a pivotal factor in the protean effort of these participants to confront their problems, styles, and disorders respectively. In most cases, they were motivated to vertical (promotional advancement) or horizontal mobility (appointment or assignment to positions of better opportunities). Healthy competition was not a dirty phrase; neither was single-mindedness when it came prospectively to important values.

Maintaining friendships with public-service peers as well as civilians outside of the job are strengths of this style. A refusal to buy into the tendency of being a stuffed shirt in which the hub of ones identity—being a public-service officer—is left on the hook of one's locker. This officer is likely to be open to assignments that offer enjoyment outside of duties as a public-safety officer. Quite pertinent to the therapist is an attitude for this officer-patient to embrace therapy, as well as a desire for growth and creative expression. These patients were active in taking responsibility for their own direction. Significant involvement was with people, not objects and routines. They earned the respect of their peers and subordinates by supporting both with empathy and humility, not with a controlling, sadistic, or avoidant style. The ability to trust or learn to trust even after experiencing severe trauma and loss was coupled with optimism toward life and their fellow human beings. Supervisors usually accorded them the respect to follow their own initiative. A key element in this trust was a willingness to accept change and actively to seek novel learning experiences. Self-interest was openly avowed without self-effacing apologetics. Supervisors knew they could count on this officer not hiding his genuine thoughts, including suggestions, and critiques without hostility.

Verbatim Record of the Most Traumatic Event

> The most traumatic police experience was being part of a volunteer search-and-recovery team with the U.S. Coast Guard for the TWA Flight 800 recovery effort. As a ranking member of the department, I spent many days and nights recovering, searching, and photographing bodies and body parts. The tension physically grew once we were notified a boat was coming in with bodies. As we suited up, I knew each group would be in worse shape than the one before. I didn't know what to expect. *Those sights and smells will never leave my memory.* I was truly saddened and upset for a while after the loss of so many lives and imagined how they felt at impact. Their family members' tragic loss and anger at the senselessness of it all, with the possibility, it could have been prevented.

DISCUSSION OF PERSONALITY-STYLE DEVELOPMENT

Protean is not to be mistaken for a chameleonic (Lifton, 1993). Flexibility is the core in this personality style, along with stability and consistency. Moral anxiety, objective fear, and existential angst commingle in an officer who sublimates this energy in a willingness to speak her humanity, voice, sensitivity, and empathy with action.

It is not easy to maintain an even keel in a profession replete with multiple detours to dissociation, complicated grief, delayed/chronic trauma, and addictive disorders—PPS-Complex PTSD. This style does not exude invulnerability. Not only are the heels of the feet vulnerable, but so are everything along the path leading to the parietal orb: They were not dipped into the River Styx as with the heels of Achilles.

The key is rather an openness to change, risking vulnerability and listening to other perspectives without relinquishing one's own moral compass. This is complemented by self-disclosure active in expressing one's vulnerabilities. For example, an officer who came in for a few sessions told me directly she was feeling troubled about retirement, "and wanted to explore options for insight with me." Money issues and choices related to practical aspects of retirement were expressed along with her feelings, including loss of a meaningful profession and career. Since she was young, in her mid 40s, enjoying the prospect of a new challenge and career "seemed logical to me, and why not," she asserted. She was fully aware it would be difficult, a novel experience, and one at which some peers jibed. After working on an existential calculus, in which she weighed the pros and cons as a valence of experience and emotion with the practical benefits, she choose to retire. She set time for relaxation and set about doing it. She was stimulated and interested and pursued her new career. The likelihood is our job as therapist is made stimulating by a public-safety officer with natural felicity as pilot in response to our navigational skills.

Another level of differentiation was the use of two defenses. One was the mature defense of sublimation, a successful and gratifying channeling of loss in trauma to resolution in spite of the odds against her. The ability to channel her neurotic conflicts into productive and rewarding substitutions ranged from creative work to ingenious adaptation.

The mature defense of altruism drove achievement of a professional standard combining equity and empathy toward peers, subordinates, and supervisors, which was realistic, not idealistic. She earned the respect of her peers, and she was liked by most of her fellows. She established a place for herself in the ecological niche she experienced, even when there was none, out of ingenuity and tenacity, willing to take the risk and accept her own vulnerability.

The altruism and sublimation were bolstered without exception by a remarkable level of resilience to hardships with genuine high frustration tolerance without avoiding responsibility or compartmentalization. Loss and trauma were confronted, not avoided, repressed, or diverted. A high level of motivation toward genuine well-being and self-insight was established. This makes our work no less stimulating or challenging.

Initial Suggestions for Inroads for Therapy Alliance and Maintenance

The officer is likely to be a participant with the ability to engage in the full encounter of a therapeutic relationship. Bibliotherapy, including films, are excellent tools of entry into insight and renarration, depending on the dynamic nourished. Active behavioral interventions work well. A seriousness alongside commitment provokes new developmental experiences for the patient. Cognitive interventions easily lead into narrative and insightful discovery for therapists by plumbing depths hardly reached with other patients. An inside caveat is to respect a person who has not achieved their gains easily. Usually the most hardy are those who have put in hard work before ever seeing us. *Hidden resilience may belie the initial presentation.* That is why I suggest the heuristic approach in practice, regardless of therapy. *Emotional intelligence and the resilient officer is a discovery in the therapeutic encounter that is priceless. It is a combination of adaptation not as centered on mental, cognitive, and behavioral goals as much as existential and philosophical.*

Staying positive in the fulfillment of your calling is key in the work you do with officers, which is more difficult than I can possibly say. What helps is the results you will see. I choose to illustrate this with one case example of some essentials with one special patient, eloquent in heart and soul. *The end of our work, truth be told, was a loss for me, as for him.*

> I remember when I sought help from you, Doc Dan. Finally, I refuse to blame myself. I remember contemplating how easy to put myself in the dust with one shot or booze my way to extinction. I became friends with some of the other workers who experienced trauma with me and continue to share peer support informally to this day. I read your recommended book, *Man's Search For Meaning* by Dr. Frankl (1959), this is my fourth reading since we began. I am not ashamed. I will read it many more times. I accept my own story as unique; I own up to it. I can't attain perfection, I'm only a human who wants to be only human. Only God can be perfect. I learned that the rough way, but I learned this lesson for life. I just want to live well and be socially productive. I understand each man must find his own meaning of life. We have a choice and at times and in different situations of our life, meaning may change. We are different at a younger age versus an older age, but we make the choice to choose not caring, to overcome rage or avoid everyone. I made a choice from within to live fully. I agree man must have hope, love is his basic meaning of life, and he need not be ashamed of that. *Through my traumatic experiences, I now realize I have become closer to*

God, I have a spiritual freedom; I talk out my problems through prayer and not condemnation. I pray for strength and like Frankl, I pray I can come out of it more of a man and not get down on myself for tragedies I know I didn't cause. I know my responsibility to my wife who is very ill, my children, and I know she needs me very much. So I stand by her suffering meaningfully. I endure for me as much as for her. As Frankl says, "Happiness will eventually ensue, when you know, and have a how and why God is God for all people." I have faith in the same God he did. No need to say more here.

Suffice to say the rewards are worth every bit of effort and resilience you will need, to cherish qualities in yourself that this line of our professional work will bring out. It is not politically clever, but wise to say that with each patient we see, we either grow or allow ourselves to diminish if we do not learn as well, professionally and personally.

CLINICIANS CORNER— SHARDS OF GLASS AND STEEL

At this point, we have done serious work on trauma, reassessment of moral anxiety, survivor guilt, inadequacy, shame, self-blame, objective fear as psychophysiological inevitability, and renarration of experience. Yet the existential angst and ontological anxiety (ultimate meaning in question) is gnawing at the patient's core. The following example illustrates a fragment of my existential work together with an officer-patient.

Capt. A: I have been working hard at not avoiding the death and bodies at Flight 800 [1996 TWA plane crash]. I've come to realize the recovery effort is in part successful from my corner of the universe. I can own up to that fact now. I still feel an ache when I see the victims: the brains are all over, the carnage in the sea. I try to see the meaning of it all. Don't get me wrong, Doc. [Capt. A delivers a stare that means no punches pulled. I accept with a reciprocal look back, "I hear you loud and clear" in my silent nod.] I mean, I stopped second-guessing myself. I accept I did what I had to. I dispute this as irrational. I do believe I did what I had to do, it is good enough. But then what about my faith, why is it so damn hard to accept? (Silence looking up and down, teary eyed) How can . . . ? (sobbing).

Dr: [Silence, allowing expression of grief] It's very hard to express how it's so damn hard to accept. As you were going to say, how can . . . ? (I let him fill in the blank and lead us).

Capt. A: How can a higher being allow this to happen? How can innocent people be killed like this, and their families shattered. What is there afterwards? I know I have faith, but I feel my faith in God is pretty weak right now. I feel like I have let go of the strength of faith in a higher being. I feel I am weak in what has been my strength through faith. To tell you the truth, at times now I have my moments where I have little confidence after Flight 800. [Pause] But I still believe I think it's my own weakness.

[In many public-service families a refreshing belief in a higher power shines through. I will address what he considers to be weakness, which in his case means he feels inadequate to his real faith. To slip this under the table is to ignore a genuine experience of his life. Not I.]

> **Dr:** Is it weakness, or are you and I, and every thinking human being, trying to seek definitive answers we just can't fathom. Asking the questions means you feel it deeper and care deeply. Is it enough to ponder the questions, rather than pound yourself for having healthy moments of skepticism?

> **Capt. A:** I do ponder, and I guess pound myself at times more than I like. I find it hard to think life goes on when it ended for them. Whole lives ended that day on a flight that ended in the sea. Maybe life is purgatory, a truth that lies under all the coincidences or destiny of our lives.

> **Dr:** Maybe it is purgatory; but it seems maybe that truth as you put it under co-incidents may help us witness the dark moments to remember our life right here and now is precious. Maybe not heaven, nor hell, nor purgatory, nor paradise, but precious is the mystery and hard truth of death and tragedy.

[The tragedy of flight 800 is very difficult to process; putting it together in Capt. A's way of looking at life through faith is a strength he has shared with me. It is fair material to work on and to balance in coping with the trauma and guilt. Again, the vast majority of officers believe in God, whatever religion or creed.]

> **Capt. A:** You know, I jump to magical thoughts at times. I even think I was meant to experience this event and the trauma. I feel like Frankl, that Doc who was in the death camp and came out with faith in God more intact. I mean, that is silly, and my ego gets high falutin, I mean comparing myself to his ordeal, right Doc?

> **Dr:** Why ask me? You know yourself; I trust your truth, do you? Lets look at it together. What do you experience when you go back to Flight 800 as part of your history?

> **Capt. A:** It sucks in part; I hate the death, the bodies, the blood, the violence. Maybe shoot down or accidental, it hurt the innocent. Being a Police Captain, African American family man in a second marriage, with an estranged son from a first marriage, I know how it feels to hurt. Suffering is history seared into my blood. But I have not let it make me bitter and hate others. Like Frankl, I know it's not easy; you just keep going. But I let out the tears, and I don't blame myself like I did years ago.

> **Dr:** You bet. Like you're doing now, and the hard work you do each day of your life. No retreat from reality. How have you convinced yourself not to let your history, police experience, and beautiful cultural tradition not

make you bitter and biased even though you've dealt with racism from all angles and hatred?

Capt. A: I realize rather, I trust our work. I am not responsible for what I learned is tragic. I did the best I could, and my prayers count. The silence of God does not mean he is not listening. My blue color does not run, our police culture has a tradition and pride too. I have a why, a how; I have faith in a creator who has no race and loves us all. I have confidence in myself and others like you, Doc. I choose to believe in good and evil; I need not apologize for my race, my faith of Judaism, nor my shield by hiding any of it.

Dr.: Bravo, well said Captain A. Doesn't sound like you are weak in faith, but expressing some doubts firms up what you know and believe in your heart of hearts. That's what counts.

Our work continues traversing the trauma in specific ways as depicted in chapter 4. An existential need seeks to quench a parched inner thirst. A thirst calling for sensibility and kindness in a world shattered by trauma and grief. Without a deep sense of calling, a courage to embrace a vocation in which life is imperiled, most folks would not join up as public-service professionals, uniform and civilian alike. A dry, pedantic style that denies "the unheard cry from meaning" (Frankl, 1988) is bound for an excursion that docks one's real humanity and leaves the port vacant of his essence, no matter how efficacious the technique: Louis Armstrong called it soul.

The difference is your level of compassion, empathy, and persistence, which goes a long way with your unique use of technique. Pure objectivity is a tombstone. I, for one, cannot deny the expression of humanity of self as well as my patient.

CONCLUSION FOR PUBLIC SAFETY STYLES

This chapter in its entirety may be viewed as a guide, a path, a bridge into the styles that public-safety officers are likely to present. My hope is that it is not used as some modern day guide to disorders and styles of personality in a prescriptive way. That use may erroneously achieve a delineation reifying a humane being into a diagnostic category (Ryan, 1972). I also hope it is not used as an overly optimistic formula, implying this work is easy. It is not.

The offering here is some insight, awareness of possible oversight or nearsight of quick interpretation, and far-off sight that attempts to fit any officer into a snug quadrant. When this is done, the officer becomes an imperative through categorization. Pure objectivity is found in granite tombstones and porcelain dolls. The real, warm human being may be lost through compartmentalizing patients unless we are careful to avoid taking labels too seriously, including my use of police-personality styles. The caveat is that the language of science is qualitatively and historically limited. It is relative. The human being who is your patient is not—ever. It is all about semantics, is it not? Including ones we can be tempted to guide us, as our own ideals. What we do best in our resilience as clinicians is complemented by the resilience in each of the public-safety styles presented. In writing this book, I have come to the realization, public and private, that if we go out of the shadows of our private sense, we all have a common sense waiting to be discovered! As long as I live, I suggest you may follow your adaptive, intuitive senses as well as your scientific senses.

To legislate what is right and wrong can only be a disaster. The key is to remind ourselves almost always that we are mere mortals and that our active listening means self confrontation and growth, not miraculous interventions with strict and impervious boundaries. When as clinicians we take up the line of a single therapeutic approach with public-service people, we can only fall into a unidimensional perspective. Integration is a wonderful idea, an even better blueprint, because the vast array of vectors, complexities, and prisms afford many different views.

The one minority that generality has not achieved real understanding and empathy is the police and public-safety officer. To serve is a profile in courage! Therapists serve too. The deeper the excavation, the more resplendent the transubstantiation of darkness collapses into the fulgent light of hope.

REFERENCES

Baumrind, D. (1978). Parental disciplinary patterns and social competence in children. *Youth and Society, 9,* 239-276.

Baumrind, D. (1980). New directions in socialization research. *American Psychologist, 35,* 639-652.

Becker, E. (1967). *The denial of death.* New York: Free Press.

Benner, A. (1991). *The changing cop: A longitudinal study of psychological testing within law enforcement.* California: Saybrook Institute Publication.

Benner, A. (1998/1999). Personal correspondence: The practice of necessary separation of peer support officer as independent from an Employee Assistance Program structure.

Benner, A. (1999/2001). Personal correspondence: Cop Doc and the forging of a new role for the Uniformed Psychologist.

Bettelheim, B. (1979). *Surviving and other essays.* New York: First Vintage Books.

Bishop, M. (2001). *Managing addictions: Cognitive, emotive and behavioral techniques.* New Jersey: Jason Aronson, Inc.

Black, D., & Larson, C. L. (1999). *Bad boys, bad men.* New York: Oxford University Press.

Brenner, C. (1974). *An elementary textbook of psychoanalysis.* New York: Doubleday/ Dell Publishing Group.

Brenner, C. (1976). *Psychoanalytic technique and psychic conflict.* New Haven, CT: International University Press.

Brenner, C. (1982). *The mind in conflict.* New Haven, CT: International University Press.

Brenner, C. (2003). Personal correspondence about trauma at New York Psychoanalytic Society.

Brent, A. D. (2001). Is impulsive aggression the critical ingredient? *Cerebrum Journal the Dana Forum of Brain Science, 3,* 43-54.

Buscaglia, L. (1978). *Personhood: The art of being fully human.* New York: Fawcett Columbine.

Campbell, J. (1973). *The hero with a thousand faces.* New Jersey: Princeton University Press.

Chamberlin, J. (2000). Cops trust cops, even one with a Ph.D: Psychologist and police officer Alan Benner helps San Francisco police cope with stress on the job. *American Psychological Association: Monitor on Psychology, 31*(1), 74-76.

Cleckley, H. (1976). *The mask of sanity: An attempt to clarify some issues about the so-called psychopathic personality.* St. Louis: C. V. Mosby.

Dekovic, M., & Gerris, J. (1992). Parental reasoning complexity, social class, and child rearing behaviors. *Journal of Marriage and the Family, 54,* 675-685.

Dekovic, M., & Gerris, J. (1994). Developmental analysis of social cognitive and behavioral differences between popular and rejected children. *Journal of Applied Developmental Psychology, 15,* 367-386.

Ellis, A. (1962). *Reason and emotion in psychotherapy.* New York: Lyle Stuart.

Ellis, A. (1973). *Humanistic psychotherapy.* New York: McGraw-Hill.

Ellis, R. R. (1999). Personal correspondence: Individual differences in officer responses to loss.

Epstein, H. (1979). *Children of the holocaust. Conversations with sons and daughters of survivors.* New York: G. P. Putnam's Sons.

Erikson, M., & Rossi, E. (1989). *The February man.* New York: Brunner/Mazel.

Ferenczi, S. (1933). *The clinical diary of sandor ferenczi.* J. Dupont (Ed.). Cambridge, MA: Harvard University Press.

Figley, C. (1985). *Trauma and its wake. The study and treatment of post traumatic stress disorder and its treatment.* New York: Brunner/Mazel.

Frankl, V. (1959). *Mans search for meaning.* Boston: Beacon Press, Inc.

Frankl, V. (1988). *The will to meaning: Foundations and applications of logotherapy.* New York: Penguin Books.

Freud, S. (1894/1963). *Therapy and technique.* New York: Macmillan.

Freud, S. (1922). Beyond the pleasure principle. In J. Strachey (Ed.) in collaboration with Anna Freud, *The standard edition of the complete psychological works of Sigmund Freud* (Standard ed., Vol. 18). London: Hogarth Press.

Freud, S. (1926). Inhibition, symptoms, and anxiety. In J. Strachey (Ed.) in collaboration with Anna Freud, *The standard edition of the complete psychological works of Sigmund Freud* (Vol. 20, pp. 77-174). London: Hogarth Press.

Fromm, E. (1951) .*The forgotten language.* New York: Grove Press.

Goffman, E. (1961). *Stigma.* New York: Simon and Schuster.

Gilmartin, K. (2002). *Emotional survival for law enforcement: A guide for officers and their families.* Tucson, AZ: ES Press, Inc.

Hare, R. (1993). *Without conscience: The disturbing world of the psychopaths among us.* New York: Pocket Books.

Hatfield, E., Caccioppo, J., & Rapson, R. (1994). *Emotional contagion.* New York: Cambridge University.

Heidel, A. W. (1941). *Hippocratic medicine: Its spirit and method.* New York: Columbia University Press.

Hiakawa, S. I. (1963). *Symbol, status and personality.* New York: Harcourt Brace World, Inc.

Horowitz, M. (1999). *Essential papers on post traumatic stress disorder.* New York & London: New York University Press.

Kassinove, H. (1995). *Anger disorders: Definitions, diagnosis and treatment.* New York: Taylor and Francis.

Kelly, W. (1985). *Post traumatic stress disorder and the war veteran patient.* New York: Brunner/Mazel.

Laing, R. (1965). *The divided self.* New York: Penguin Publishers.

Laing, R. (1971). *Self and others.* New York: Penguin Publishers.

Laing, R. (1985). *Wisdom madness and folly.* London: Macmillan.

Levant, R. (1997). *Men and emotions: A psychoeducational approach.* New York: Newbridge Communications, Inc.

Levant, R., & Pollack, W. S. (1995). *A new psychology of men.* New York: Basic Books.

Lifton, J. R. (1993). *The protean self. Human resilience in an age of fragmentation.* New York: Basic Books.

Lorenz, K. (1962). *King Solomon's ring.* New York: Time Incorporated.

May, R. (1983). *Discovery of being.* New York: W. W. Norton & Company.

McCord, W., & McCord, J. (1956). *Psychopathy and delinquency.* New York: Grune & Stratton.

Millon, T. (1990). *Toward a new personology.* New York: John Wiley and Sons.

Millon, T. (1996). *Disorders of personality: DSMIV and beyond.* New York: John Wiley and Sons.

Otto, R. (1982). *The idea of the holy.* New York & London: Oxford University Press.

Panken, S. (1973). *The joy of suffering: Psychoanalytic theory and therapy of masochism.* New York: Jason Aronson, Inc.

Perls, M. F. (1978). *The gestalt approach and eye witness to therapy.* Toronto: Bantam Book.

Perls, M. F. (1979). *In and out of the garbage pail.* Toronto: Bantam Book.

Reese, J. (1987). *Behavioral science in law enforcement.* Washington, DC: U.S. Department of Justice, Federal Bureau of Investigation.

Reich, W. (1970). *The mass psychology of fascism.* New York: Farrar, Straus & Giroux.

Reich, W. (1991). *Character analysis.* New York: Farrar, Straus & Giroux.

Reik, T. (1948). *Listening with the third ear.* New York: Grove Press, Inc.

Ryan, W. (1972). *Blaming the victim.* New York: Vintage Books.

Richards, A., & Willick, M. (1986). *Psychoanalysis: The science of mental conflict.* New Jersey: The Analytic Press.

Rudofossi, D. (2007). *Working with traumatized police officer-patients: A clinician's guide to Complex PTSD syndromes in public safety professionals.* Amityville, NY: Baywood.

Ryan, W. (1972). *Blaming the victim.* New York: Vintage Books.

Samenow, S. (1984). *Inside the criminal mind.* New York: New York Times Books.

Sass, L. (1994). *The paradoxes of delusion: Wittgenstein Schreiber and madness.* New York: Cornell University Press.

Scharf, R. (2003). *Organizational structure of character, defenses, and psychoanalytic formulations.* Lectures given at New York Psychoanalytic Institute.

Schlossberg, H., & Freeman, L. (1974). *Psychologist with a gun.* New York: Coward, McCann & Geoghegan, Inc.

Seligman, M. E., & Garber, J. (1980). *Human helplessness.* New York: Academic Press.

Selye, H. (1974). *Stress without distress.* New York: The New American Library.

Siegal, B. (1990). *Love medicine and miracles.* New York: HarperCollins Publishers.

Silverstein, R. (1992). *The correlation between combat related trauma processing and male development.* Doctoral dissertation. Michigan: Bell and Howell UMI Publications.

Toch, H. (2002). *Stress in policing.* Washington, DC: American Psychological Association.

Wambaugh, J. (1975). *The choir boys.* New York: Delcorte Press.

Williams, M. B., Zinner, E. S., & Ellis, R. R. (1999). The connection between grief and trauma: An overview. In E. S. Zinner & M. B. Williams (Eds.), *When a community weeps: Case studies in group survivorship.* (pp. 3-17). Philadelphia: Brunner/Mazel.

Wilson, Q. J. (1968). *Varieties of police behavior.* New York: Harvard University Press.

Wilson, J. P., & Zigelbaum, S. D. (1983). The Vietnam veteran on trial: The relation of post traumatic stress disorder to criminal behavior. *Behavioral Sciences and the Law, 1,* 69-83.

Winnicott, D. W. (1984). *Deprivation and delinquency.* London: Tavistock Publications, Ltd.

Yalom, I. (1983). *Existential psychotherapy.* New York: Basic Books.

Yalom, I. (1985). *The theory and practice of group psychotherapy.* New York: Basic Books.

Yalom, I. (1989). *Loves executioner.* New York: Basic Books.

Yalom, I. (1996). *Lying on the couch.* New York: Basic Books.

PART III

Eco-Ethological Existential Analytic Therapy on the Front Line

CHAPTER 4

Provoking Motivation through the Field of Despair in the Multiangular Polychromatic Lens of Dissociation via Eight Officer-Patients Odysseys

Tis true my form is something odd,
But blaming me is blaming God.
Could I create myself anew,
I would not fail in pleasing you . . .
If I could reach from pole to pole,
Or grasp the ocean with a span,
I would be measured by the soul;
The minds the standard of the man.
Attributed to Sir John Merrick (Survivor of Complex Losses and Trauma)
(Howell & Ford, 1981, p. 189)

Digging our heels into the ground of loss in trauma includes dealing with sensitive and particularly difficult problems the officer-patient presents to the therapist. Achieving a successful intervention leads to a more effective navigational chart for the therapist treating PPS-CPTSD. Tapping out a heuristic cadence orchestrates the impact of loss in each trauma regardless of therapy.

What is presented in the current moments of therapy are existential opportunities to redress distortions, lesser than effective compromise formations, and to correct self-destructive cognitive, emotional, and behavioral patterns. Emerging existential opportunities unfurl in the context of all therapy hours. However, hearing them and acting in the moment on these opportunities requires a therapist who has gained the skill to listen to what is being said on a number of levels. What I offer here is a focus on listening to the moments that are deeply influenced by the eco-ethological niches that support the psychological context of each officer's daily life. Whether you are a psychoanalytic, cognitive-behavioral, logo-existential, or a gestalt psychotherapist, enhancing meaning within the nondescript poverty of death, violence, and cruelty of the officer-patient's experience is the core of my suggested approach to PPS-CPTSD. Finding motivation within the existential meaning of each officer's pain and suffering is not a byproduct of therapy, it is an explicit and potent core of the therapist's intervention. My supervisor in the NYPD, Chief Surgeon Dr. Martin Symond, left a strong prescription for me. He said, "If you can figure out how to motivate an officer-patient to keep up his/her resilience, then you have the key to healing." While I suspect that key may have rough edges and be fragile, in part I suggest his wish and dream is closer to fulfillment. The cases I present highlight how that may be done one officer-patient at a time.

In part, achieving motivation means understanding why the officer-patient's guilt, rage, depression, and anxiety is not only overwhelming but a self-imposed prison. Without a clear understanding on the therapists part, the officer-patient may remain lost in an existential prison. Gaining a different perspective of the same situations in which he has persecuted himself, the same officer-patient may redeem his own strength, resilience, and courage through insight. Losses accumulated over time and left disenfranchised and ungrieved are toxic to healthful living: losses are poison in trauma. Left untouched, they remain preserved in timeless tumors in the body of the officer-patient's life. Gaining insight for the officer-patient is facilitated via healing toxic loss—human freedom to choose another path that ought not be passed over. Putting a time frame on the process of grieving is like putting a time frame on any fluid process: it is illusory at best, a shared delusion at worst.

By returning to the pain, suffering, and human anguish of trauma, there is much that goes unheard regarding what may have been passed over of what was done right with courage and humanity in the face of very harsh losses. That task of discovering the courage, humanity, and resilience for motivation and creativity is in the real and personal level of encounter. The task of therapist and officer-patient becomes visible through identifying and validating the courage, resilience, and ultimate humanity of each officer's experience with his own trauma. This process of therapy is what I offer and suggest as the core of meaningful intervention and effective therapy in the case examples that follow. What may be most helpful in an age of terrorism is an existential attitude to grab logos that humanizes the officer-patient, the therapist, and the therapy process. It is so basic to all therapy that it may go unacknowledged as one of the most important and neglected of all tasks to achieve.

The most difficult of tasks for the therapist is helping the officer-patient confront very human disappointments, suffering, and anguish at intimate moments experienced in blinking terror, shame, and anguish. Facilitating the mourning of these losses can be fully achieved only by understanding the individual manifestation of such losses. Some are personal redemption of the officer-patient's will to live without slow suicide; addiction, depression, and nihilism of sorts is replaced with a desire to live more healthier life styles. Social contributions and the impact officer-patients have had on other lives is redeemed from the ugly trauma they have endured in silence. That trauma is ugly in very real terms and experience, as I have illustrated throughout this work. Frankl was a master teacher who suggested how important redemption is for human beings. He quotes Einstein, who summed it up well: "The man who regards his life as meaningless is not merely unhappy but hardly fit for life" (Einstein, 1954).

Dr. Frankl elaborates on Einstein's point:

> This is not only a matter of success and happiness but also of survival in the terminology of modern psychology. The will to meaning has survival value. This was the lesson I had to learn in three years spent in Auschwitz and Dachau . . . it is true that if there was anything to uphold man in such an extreme situation as Auschwitz it was the awareness that life has a meaning to be fulfilled . . . uncounted examples of such heroism and martyrdom bear witness to the uniquely human potential to find and fulfill meaning even in extremis . . . we must never forget that we may also find meaning in life when confronted with a hopeless situation as its helpless victim when facing fate that cannot be changed. For what then counts and matters is to bear witness to the unique human potential at its best which is to transform a tragedy into a personal triumph, to turn one's predicament into a human achievement. (Frankl, 1978, p. 37)

Nothing is static and complete in any psychological manifestation, whether it be trauma, loss, mental health, psychological growth, or resilience. I suggest rather than this being a dreaded problem for the therapist and for the officer-patient, this is an opportunity in which the process of genuine growth in therapy is forged. Extending Frankl's suggestions into a core approach to dealing with loss in trauma, I use the term "redemption" as in correction of misconceptions—conscious and unconscious—in the officer-patient's maladaptation to the events in the past. The event of the past, whether the recent past or the distant echoes of the past, is what needs to be worked through to get to the opportunity awaiting the officer-patient in the here and now of human time and space, as I have suggested explicitly in chapters 1 and 3. Hence, listening and achieving insight into the context of loss in trauma the officer-patient presents is key to intervention. That loss in trauma always is an issue of individual responses and different manifestations on an unconscious and conscious level. Encounter is the ongoing process that is ever-changing in the dialogue of loss and redemption. Encounter is fostered in the major core of the eco-ethological approach to trauma and loss by using the insight of psychoanalytic ego-psychologist's understanding of conflict and compromise formations.

Establishing your encounter with the officer-patient means that you understand his impulses; satisfaction of those impulses as wishes may be at the level of an unconscious wish influenced by tendencies of an aggressive and at times sexual nature (drive derivatives). Yet, *conflicts emerge over the fulfillment of that officer-patient's wishes and the defenses against fulfillment of those wishes*. The result of these wishes and the defenses is what Brenner originally supported and established as compromise formations (Brenner, 1974, 1976, 1982; Richards & Willick, 1986).

Compromise formations are fluid and dynamic and open to change. They are ubiquitous. What Brenner suggests is original and relevant to the therapist seeking to effect change with an officer-patient who is traumatized. This is evidenced when the officer-patient presents his own unique compromise formations that are ever-changing in the face of conflict. Brenner's science of conflict suggests the therapist's attitude and stance toward conflict is critical in effecting change in the patient. Brenner suggests an effective therapist's attitude includes consistency of stance through empathically listening, clarifying, elaborating, and confronting the officer-patient's conflicts, of which his defenses are an important component. The defense against losses in trauma is highlighted in the eco-ethological perspective where the therapist identifies, clarifies, elaborates, and interprets losses through many iterations.

Brenner's science of conflict (Brenner, 1974, 1976, 1982, 2003; Richards & Willick, 1986) complements my suggested approach to therapists intervening with officer-patients suffering from PPS-CPTSD by the therapist being clear in his understanding that officer-patients make compromise formations to ongoing conflict in their daily and cumulative experiences with trauma. The immediate benefit is that the therapist's illusions of a quick cure for the officer-patient is less likely. The consequence of this is that the patient is gradually familiarized with the toxic and cumulative layers of loss in trauma—premature termination is countered by a more effective integration that now becomes possible. The alliance as enduring and evolving complements the approach suggested in a consistent and reliable means through the therapist's stance toward PPS-CPTSD.

For our purpose, ethology and ecology, compromise formations make superb yet parsimonious sense in approaching loss in trauma. A point that may be missed as long as rigidity in any therapist's approach does not blind him is that the insight gained from approaches that differ from a psychoanalytic perspective with benefit for the officer-patient may be used. This point becomes evident as we realize compromise formations are not only fluid in the patient's development but may be changed in response to and effected by insight and associational growth through the process of therapy (Brenner, 1974, 1976, 1982, 2003; Richards & Willick, 1986; Scharf, 2004).

To effect such a stance, the therapist would be well advised to learn about each officer-patient's unique and evolving constellation of compromise formations within his ecological niche. Therapist's understanding includes specifically learning what meaning a traumatic event has in that officer's life. That understanding is still insufficient until the therapist learns how the officer-patient unconsciously and consciously uses his/her own ethological strategies for preserving motivation in defending against cumulative losses. Therapist's understanding of the specific strategy and motivation underlying each officer-patient's defenses includes the specific understanding of what challenges, impulses, and defenses will emerge in each officer-patient's uniquely individual response to intrapsychic conflict.

The compromise formations of conflict that the officer-patient presents initially holds promise in durable change effected over time and with a consistent approach. Through the therapists intervention, the individual officer-patient may achieve compromise formations that are healthier as a result of achieved insight.

When insight is reached, it is almost never complete, yet the severity of symptoms is likely to be reduced. Helping the officer-patient reach a level of insight takes time, effort, and an attitude that demands repeated attention to what is ethological, ecological, and largely unconscious and conscious, real and fantasized in each officer-patient's individual response to trauma. That insight in the eco-ethological approach includes the third core for building a psychological context: identity modes and multiple losses in the officer-patient's handling of past cumulative and daily trauma (see Rudofossi, 2007). Rather than engaging in a passive, descriptive accounting of trauma and loss, the eco-ethological therapist actively seeks to understand the unconscious and conscious impact of loss in all trauma. The direction of evolution is hardly conscious in any of the world's species, including homo sapiens. Yet the unconscious pursuit of sexualized aggressive satisfaction, however hidden, can hardly be denied. Psycho-analytic insight in a classical sense may shed light on this process, regardless of treatment modality.

As Frankl put it, "Destiny is not fate" (2000). Drive derivatives may be the rake of destiny until the field is exposed and tilled a different way. The harvest from exposed loss in trauma takes time to ripen from the initial sprout of its promise in change and development along new furrows for each officer-patient in his unique compromise formations and existentially meaningful path.

This harvest cannot be achieved with a cookie-cutter approach, according to this author and others, who include private and police practitioners (Balter, 2004; Barnes, 2005; Benner, 1974, 1976, 1982, 1999, 2003, 2004; Gilmartin, 2002; Mansfield, 2004a, 2004b; Myers, 1940; Reese, 1991, 1996; Rudofossi & Ellis, 1999; Scharf, 2004; Southwick, 2005; Thorp, 2005). Gain may be achieved by taking the humble goal of improvement, rather than attempting to extinguish trauma and loss by instituting treatment plans forced upon officer-patients. What is economical is based on sound theory—economical in terms of psychological, mental, and existentially sound cost-effective efforts. Simplicity is slicing away with Occam's razor the idealism in mass producing a linear, all-encompassing treatment plan. Improvement is a substantive gain and demands an approach that deals with realistic differences, one case at a time. When disenfranchised losses are made tangible and concrete, the grief may be then expressed.

I suggest the witnessing of one's own trauma may eventually be shifted from an external source (the therapist) to an internalized witnessing in each officer-patient's own conscience. This internalization is not a simple externalized witnessing by others via the therapist as yet another cliché and proscribed strategy. I suggest, in a sense, we can anticipate with confidence that internalized witnessing occurs as the officer-patient *achieves a worthwhile and meaningful change in other people's lives* through his own police actions.

How important internalized witnessing may be, in a case-by-case approach with police and public-safety patients, is suggested by the accumulated wisdom and the historical context of clinicians dealing with war trauma. The therapist's goal in combat-trauma therapy was to help each soldier-patient reenfranchise what was horrific and traumatic by not watering down or insulting his sensibilities by grouping together his unique experiences.

No hell is as vivid as war, with its dehumanization, death, and losses that are heaped upon a never ending pyre—no matter how legitimate, the combatants never remain unscathed—except for war fought in one's own backyard, which is the additional shock, disgust, guilt, anxiety, and depressive affect that officer-patients deal with. Clarifying that truth is therapeutic. Clinicians who worked with the combat veterans of both World Wars shed light into the darkness with clearly calling horror what it was, horror! The treatment approach was to identify what was called the "culminating event" (Rado, 1939, 1956) in the soldier-patient's experience, which is similar although expanded in what I have called "an original traumatic event" (see chapter 4) in the officer-patient's experience of trauma (Freud, Ferenczi, Abraham, Simmel, & Jones, 1921; Myers, 1940; Rado, 1939, 1956; Solomon & Yakovlev, 1945).

The second stage was helping the soldier-patient work gradually through that original trauma with all its "agitation and terror" with the task of helping the patient as an individual gain mastery and reposition that culminating original traumatic event in his life (Freud et al., 1921; Myers, 1940; Rado, 1939, 1956; Solomon & Yakovlev, 1945).

While many differences can be garnered to challenge the combat experiences of the soldier-patient during both World Wars, enough similarities exist in the disruption of intrapsychic development for the officer-patient, which is relevant to the attitude gained within the eco-ethological approach to PPS-CPTSD throughout this book. What is timeless is Rado's advice to the clinician on how to deal with combat trauma's immediate systemic effect on terrorizing and agitating the solider-patient, which is as informative and relevant today as it was to his contemporaries more than half a century ago:

> In my opinion the decisive factor to be introduced into the therapeutic procedure is de-sensitization of the patient to all memories of the war, whether repressed or not. In other words: His war memories must be stripped of their power to perturb him again and again and be turned into a source of repeated pride and satisfaction. (Rado, 1956, p. 162)

This means the officer-patient is guided through clarification and elaboration to take an active and introspective look at his trauma and reprocessing through his own initiative. That may be achieved in the transference during the therapy situation if handled with support, clarification, elaboration, and confrontation while helping the patient gain insight to the successes that remain hidden and disenfranchised in the losses unveiled. Facilitating an internalized witnessing of one's personal achievement as a police and public-safety officer may help create a meaningful bridge on which the officer may move toward, asking for social support and love of family members and friends. An internalized witnessing of one's resilience and redemption may facilitate a self-initiated renewed commitment to public service. That renewed commitment can enhance an ability to tolerate tragedy and maintain one's own sacred optimism, triggering other areas of growth and healing.

Expanding your unconscious and emotional wisdom as a therapist seeking to do work or to enhance your work with police and public-safety officer-patients cannot be offered in cookbook fashion. What I hope to relate are ways to facilitate initial interventions likely to work with officer-patients. I present real composite case examples of trauma and loss to guide your odyssey. The inherent challenge in this process may be a motivation for you, as it was for me, each session being an evolving renewal of moments of opportunity for encounter. That sensibility is bidirectional and an exquisite hidden pleasure of therapy; it is unique in potential for each therapist.

Case 1: Vicarious trauma through media trials of sacred victims—What if it's me?

Biography

Officer B is a 14-year veteran of the Police Department and has worked for four years in what is typically called a war zone. He is a proud "blue knight," as he calls himself, after Joseph Wambaugh's character (1972) of a beat cop who pounds the mean streets of San Francisco. Officer B is of Scottish-German ancestry and was appointed a Patrolman Benevolent Association delegate in his current precinct, (substantially slower than his former command). He is well liked by his peers and is proud of his feisty attitude. At 44-years-old, he started a second marriage to a wife who is an African American beautician. After a period of cultural adjustment, they have maintained a balance between both professions while raising a beautiful baby girl. Officer B presents as overworked and fatigued. He has not lost his sharp wit and a survivor's spirit. He is estranged from his ex-wife and their son. While he had a drinking problem in the past, Officer B has remained sober through his own initiative and with the help of Alcoholics Anonymous. This sobriety has continued for over a decade.

Officer B has a cumulative experience of around 300 traumatic events; that may be a very conservative estimate. The most significant reported traumatic event for Officer B was witnessing the incarceration of a fellow officer. Officer B worked with this other officer on patrol. He felt that fellow officer "was a time-tested, reliable stand-up cop in his unit; not a shaky cop." Officer B witnessed his fellow officer being indicted, arrested, and now serving time. Incarceration of Officer B's fellow officer was for what was deemed to be excessive force in an arrest that arrest led to the death of the perpetrator and a manslaughter conviction for that officer.

Hostility and anxiety emerged in Officer B's presentation, frequently expressed in a particularly vehement manner. It should be noted that an officer who is convicted of a serious crime loses benefits and is often disowned by the police department and unions alike. Truth be told, wrongdoing has little to do with the loss and anticipatory anxiety of seeing a fellow officer being imprisoned. This loss is one of the most typically disenfranchised. It was exacerbated for Officer B because he was also one of the delegates involved in representation of this accused and later indicted and prosecuted fellow officer. Officer B expressed how he considered the past police experiences they shared and how life-threatening events had created the bond with this fellow officer.

As a therapist, my goal was helping Officer B in his less articulated goal, which was to come to terms with what he considered to be injustice and depravity in a system gone bad. While in this case example, my approach is cognitive-behavioral and existential, it does not neglect the psychodynamic underpinnings of his disenfranchised losses in the trauma.

An Eco-Ethological Existential Analysis with Officer B

Officer B's presentation was a very difficult case—my emotional reaction of extreme empathy had to be tempered with the clarity of a strategic approach and framing the problem without being overladen with my own sense of abstract justice. I had to keep my own responses in check, which was difficult in this specific case.

Officer B was relating to me through transference. I used my unconscious experience of how I was experiencing Officer B's transference itself to gain insight into his rage, his feelings of helplessness, and his sense of loss. Achieving this objective was assisted by allowing myself to gain insight by processing the emotional intensity of hostility initially displaced at me by Officer B. His attitude toward incarceration was made clear along with the feeling by holding back my own responses of over-identification with Officer B. Whether your philosophy veers right, left, or center of the spectrum, by allowing your own unconscious feelings and ideas to silently guide your pick-up, by not reacting judgmentally whether you'd like to be supportive or rebuke by remaining neutral, you can gauge the direction and intensity of the patient's directed aggression, which will likely be displaced on you through the transference.

Being aware means seeking the advice of a peer who is an expert, going for supervisory consultation, or at minimum, acknowledging your own biases that may emerge. Personally, in part I felt revulsion for the actions of the officer in custody, but I equally felt compassion for his plight. I felt he was likely a highly traumatized officer, based on his command experience, and likely acted in a state of extreme dissociation, with tragic consequences for all involved. While my insight was helpful, I took the following three steps: I sought consultation to deal with my reactions, I disputed my *demand* for saving anyone and changed it into a *wish;* and I used my empathy as an active strategy, which helped Officer B to process the rage, the helplessness, his guilt, and losses associated with his fellow officer, now incarcerated.

Eco-Ethological Existential Analytic Focus

The cultural influences that shape becoming a delegate leader include identifying a number of maladaptive beliefs that can develop when ideals become extreme. Often the role of delegate is that of advocate, especially for officers in a bad spot. Many delegates I have met are extraordinary in their outreach and maintain intact boundaries. Some become overly identified with the plight of a fellow officer when self-preservation and interest become a hazy shadow. This is not unusual and not unreasonable—it happens. Why? The trauma to a delegate is intensified when he has to deal with frivolous, unwarranted vendetta allegations against officers by criminals, which are prolific and wearisome. The appraisal of Officer B's experience of a fellow officer's incarceration frames three cognitive interventions. The first is the triad of self-blame, other blame, and societal blame: "If I only observed and acted on Officer X's behalf"; "If only the cops and superior officers did"; "If only society cared and there were no vicious perpetrators and repetitive events this would not have happened." This is clarified in the following brief segment:

> **Delegate Officer B:** Officer X was a decent guy who was at the wrong place at the wrong time. He was building up a lot of anger and did not deal with it. He lost his cool and hurt a perp in explosive rage. You've been there, Doc. You know exactly what I am talking about. When an officer loses it. . . . Why didn't I do anything about it? Why didn't the Department or anyone else, before it exploded in our face. I mean, it sucks, it blows. I did squat, I feel I should have known.

> **Dr:** It seems like you have every right to wish you could have known and helped more. Still, it was impossible to really know what Officer X was going to do. After all, he had built up of a lot of rage and he let loose explosively. How could you have predicted this unless you had a crystal ball?

> **Delegate Officer B:** Yeah, it blows badly, it does. All the crap on the job and I mean he just couldn't handle it.

> **Dr:** Let me ask you B, what did you do when you felt you were at your wits end and last straw? [I also address the vicarious fear that Delegate Officer B one day may be in the same situation, act out, and then be targeted for prosecution.]

Delegate Officer B: I came to see you. So?

Dr: Well, that option of seeking help and expressing that one is at their wits end is available. Yet, many officers do not use it. They still do not act out, committing manslaughter. You had the good sense to seek help. Why?

Delegate Officer B: Because I got the damn good sense to seek help when I know I am ready to blow.

Dr: Right on. That is why extreme ultimate force is almost always a choice, and that is the officer's responsibility. Not everyone has that good sense. But you do. That's evidence you can choose to use among many other alternatives as we agreed if you have a crisis. When someone acts impulsively, is that your fault or anyone else's?

Delegate Officer B: No, its not, but it's upsetting.

Dr: So, if I got it right, it's sad, very sad, even more so it's tragic. In Officer X's case, didn't he too act without thinking? Is that not tragic and you wish it was different as I do too? It appears in his case from what we know, it was his choice. A tragic one, not one forced upon him.

Delegate Officer B: I hate when you do that Doc, you twist it around so it's not that bad.

Dr: Meaning?

Delegate Officer B: I am tired of the liberal left-wing politics and cops being scapegoats.

Dr: I'm with you. But how does that translate into putting yourself down and blaming yourself for the tragedy of Officer X?

Delegate Officer B: I don't know, doc.

Dr: It appears it's hard to acknowledge, but you do. What do you imagine you're telling yourself about Officer X?

Delegate Officer B: I guess I'm blaming myself, but I am upset.

Dr: I suspect when you say upset you mean, you're feeling sad and hurt he is in jail.

Eco-Ethological Existential Analytic Integration

[From here, I continue to identify the sadness and feelings of loss about the incarceration of Officer X. I confront his exaggeration of self and others' guilt for the tragedy of Officer X. A reappraisal gets B to realize he, not fellow cops and supervisors, nor the community is responsible for Officer X's actions.] Evidence used for an empirical challenge is that while risk assessment may have spotted potential for abuse of authority, any prediction that actual abuse would occur was simply not present. It would be a wrong and arrogant accusation to say

Officer B should have been able to predict any aggressive outburst and prevent it. To expect *anyone* to have done that would be wishful thinking. The explosive episode was hardly predictable in reality. [The irrational belief that one is omnipotent and must be able to see the future correctly is unreasonable at best. That wishful fixation is also Officer B's intrapsychic reality. By gaining insight into the distortions of his wishes and the defenses against his awareness of those wishes as a compromise formation, he learns how to better negotiate this conflict. Holding these wishes as unexamined truth obfuscates self-sabotage, leading to self and other blame, guilt, and hopelessness over the loss of his fellow officer and friend being incarcerated. I will relate that to Officer B while respecting the values of his role as delegate and investment in doing his best. I genuinely clarify how initially sensible his advocacy on the officer's behalf was. Insight is used as an intervention in changing the way Officer B views his plight.]

From an REBT perspective, his wish was transformed into an absolute demand, a behavioral withdrawal in which he is ready to resign from being a delegate—which he loved in the past—and even resigning as an officer has emerged. Cynicism and pessimism about peers, the department, and union leaders who appear indifferent has been a core defense (compromise formation), displacing the insult to his sensibilities from his niche as a delegate in his command onto others as guilty saboteurs. While there are elements of truth in his accusations, the exaggeration and persistence of blame and aggression suggest destructive sabotage. Secondary consequences include emergent distancing in his relationship with his wife, who is not privy to what is going on.

Finally, a somatic presentation of pains, aches, elevated blood pressure, and cholesterol level spiral into further declining health. [I identify actions to be taken to ensure fairer treatment is accorded, and the incarcerated officer is given special consideration due to the complications surrounding his imprisonment.] My clarification is dynamic while employing at this point a functional, empirical, philosophical, and existential challenge to his self-guilt, blame, and recriminations for what is beyond his control. I target Delegate B's fear of being arrested for doing his job by getting him to clearly discriminate between use of force that is justified (a reality), and total loss of control leading to manslaughter. This is framed with genuine empathy and acknowledgment of the fact that the Officer is not a villain, need not be related to in that way, and the fact is his options include a strategy to be proactive in educating fellow officers. I will return to an insight-oriented approach as we move in addressing his multiple losses in trauma.

A practice segment follows:

> **Delegate Officer B:** Doc, what if a perp comes out and tries to shoot me. I had garbage hit me from housing projects. While we are talking, his life goes right by. He's rotting in jail. You know this cop went through hell with you and now he's rotting in jail. It could be me on the hot seat and burning for just trying to do my job. He's left holding the bag. I remember picking up the garbage bag and saying to myself, "If that hit me I'd be

gone." The images are all in my head, and I can't make anyone believe the cause we are fighting for now is worth it, getting him out of prison.

Dr: It seems like the experiences you have been through together make it all that more painful to see Officer X put away. So being the advocate and realizing change is not taking place really hurts bad, huh?

Delegate Officer B: It's really hard! It's extremely hard because nobody really gives a fuck. You are just a number on a shield. You don't mean anything. You make a little mistake and they want to grill you and fire you. Nobody is really going to care for us except for us.

Dr: The realistic insight is it's not a benevolent bureaucracy. That's true enough. What about the stand you're making. What is the cost to you in self-blame, making yourself helpless, and the situation hopeless?

Delegate Officer B: I feel I'm making a stand right now. I'm demanding that he gets out of that pit of hell. [Red in face and really agitated.]

Dr: When you demand he MUST get out, I MUST be the one to save him, and you blame you, the union, and the job (PD) like right now, how do you feel in the pit of your tummy when you let it hang out and get out your righteous anger? On a scale of one to ten, one being slightly irritated and ten being aware of sharp pain, dullness, and dizziness, and your pulse starting accelerating to a racing pace?

Delegate Officer B: Ten, I mean, it gets up there. But it works. I get it out and feel better.

Dr: So when you let it out and you get real angry, it's worth having the pain physically, perhaps getting dizzy, thinking in a fuzzy hazy way, its worth it because it works with the guys in the precinct?

Delegate Officer B: Well, they did get worked up and excited.

Dr: I'm with you then. Even though you get physically sick, getting the guys stirred up is the goal. Did you meet your objectives for the cause you believe in?

Delegate Officer B: No. They get upset and it becomes a griping session. I join louder than all of them and then we go at it with each other.

Dr: So if I got it right, you feel physically sick, and you don't get your point across and your goal suffers?

Officer Delegate B: Yeah. Okay, but what should I do—nothing?

Dr: Well, what about your strategy. Are you thinking clearly, advocating on target, and getting what you set out to do?

Delegate Officer B: No. I get it, Doc. But I'm working too hard and, I mean, doing all the right stuff and getting a stiff break instead. Why even bother?

Dr: Good question, if you only really believed that. I think its clear, you do care. In fact, you care so much, you tear yourself up inside by demanding things go your way in place of wishing that. When you demand, you must get your way hollering till it does, and if it doesn't, you get even angrier and more disturbed when you've drawn yourself into a circle. Yet, if you don't, you feel you're giving in and not doing enough.

Delegate Officer B: Doc, did you read my mind? Okay, that's what happens in my mind.

Dr: No, I didn't read your mind. But, it follows that when you make your preferences into demands, the evidence is, it stops you from meeting your goals. So let's work toward a solution together?

[As a delegate, B has many unique solutions, some more ideal and some grounded and realistic. We come up with ideas that turn into behavioral goals, as tactics. A heuristic approach elicits his solutions and is more likely that he will invest in them on an existential level. Some solutions are internal tactics, for example, political raising of funds and working on alternative healthy outlets for officers who are stressed out.] We go on to explore Officer B's sense of hopelessness and loss in regard to Officer X. As in other cases, we set up a journal and activities to mourn the loss, advocating for active engagement and communication with his former colleague. As we progress in our sessions by grieving the losses, energy and optimism returns. Officer B moves to being more objective and passionate. He remains a delegate who serves as a model for his peers, an extraordinary, fully fallible delegate.

Case 2: Stuck in the double bind of Catch 22: Lashing one's way out of grief.

Biography

Fire Officer Emergency Medical Technician (EMT) Y is a Hispanic American public-service veteran with eight years of public-safety service. EMT Y is married to a teacher who is supportive. He experienced approximately 230 traumatic events. The one presented here was initially disenfranchised but was evoked in the spontaneity of our therapy.

The presenting problem was anxiety, confusion, and feeling as if he was sometimes outside looking in (depersonalization). At the time we began therapy, Officer Y was reticent about presenting to me how seriously anxious he was and how scared he was about going crazy.

Officer Y's presentation of a nonverbal genuine distress was matched by a silent resilience and an equally amiable personal style. As our alliance grows, an obsessive fear that Officer Y may lash out and hit someone he loves emerges. As we work on his compulsion, it is associated with his perception of feeling helpless and being stuck in the same situation. That situation is gradually fleshed out to a specific trauma. Denial of suppressed guilt, anxiety, and rage at his performance during a rescue of a mortally wounded aided case was brought to awareness. [(I have avoided elaboration on the medication issues and the psychopharmacologic interventions along with the physicians involved). Please refer to chapter 2. To reiterate, I strongly advocate a team approach and having at minimum a physical examination and a psychopharmacological evaluation from the onset].

Eco-Ethologic Existential Analysis

My pick-up of extreme anxiety, fear, and agitation was largely by being aware of my own responses to his presentation that was largely nonverbal. A need to flee was expressed through the gestalt of his posture, as clear as the fear expressed through his facial expressions and his attentiveness to any noise with perking up his nose and eyes with dilated pupils, tracking the suspiciousness and magnified distraction. My need was to model equanimity and empathy, not patronizing sympathy, not neutrality.

Focusing on not getting distracted is key to modeling calm while using the Socratic method of getting at Officer Y's cognitions underlying his disturbance. I do not hesitate to interrupt his incessant flow to clarify, confirm, and confront the terror of his trauma and self-recriminations and existential lacunae. My approach here may be conceptualized as crisis intervention. I suggest it can also be conceptualized as ambulatory intervention by initiating significant change in provoking the patient's realization of his avoidance of the lack of meaning in his life work. The achievement of that goal includes lessening secondary depression, anxiety and helplessness that result in a loop of behavioral malaise and burnout existentially.

I focus on understanding how an original traumatic loss may be involved. While not first discussing the childhood causes or roots implicated, I work on the trauma he presents first. Why? The immediacy of his fear of going crazy and striking out at loved ones is the immediate problem and the most intense. At present, it is entirely rooted in fantasy. The classic model of psychoanalysis cannot be avoided. However, the modification of impulses and defenses against those impulses are represented by the fantasy that emerges in the context of original trauma in its eco-ethological presentation.

I use Freud's cornerstone of life and love to deal with my curiosity and desire to delve deeper first. How? Putting it in perspective in the context of love and his desire to destroy that love (striking at loved ones) and work (his life passion) as more fundamental. As Freud himself said, love and work (*lieber* and *macht*) are the two strongest human desires and the stuff that helps make life meaningful. It is clear that in Officer Y's case, this emerges as well.

An Eco-Ethological Existential Analysis with Officer EMT Y

Traditional methods for treating Obsessive Compulsive Disorder (OCD) vary with systematic desensitization, implosive therapy, and flooding, to name a few. The loss initially is a quantum antiaffordance. For EMT Y, it was the first time in the field that he became aware of his hesitation and was conscious of his emotional reaction when an aided case suffering from a cardiac arrest brought up an image of his old girlfriend (transference), whom he loved. In addition, stab wounds were not noticed as the immediate rescue was responding to a young person in cardiac arrest. These two incidental aspects of momentary lapses in his rescue efforts in reality were negligible to the actual rescue. This fact was pragmatically and heuristically drawn out and became evidence that he did not have any complicity in the tragic death.

Fact does not always influence one's personal truth until it is processed and accepted in one's own narrative. By structuring a heuristic approach incorporating an eco-ethological reconstruction, it became clear to us that the anxiety and hostility were related to his experience of an abrupt break in his sense of invulnerabilty and perfection. His idealized expectations were disenfranchised. Our work was to pull together a sensibility that what appeared as an urge to strike out was not being crazy. In the eco-ethological perspective of his unit's affordance, he could not express hurt, guilt, or anger openly. The belief that he failed was interpreted through internalized anger and recrimination. His loved ones became the target of his hostility as they were the ones he paradoxically cared most about.

Eco-Ethological Existential Analytic Intervention

The following is an example of the way Officer Y processed his aggression:

> **EMT Y:** I feel guilty. I have constant thoughts about it. I feel embarrassed and would rather not talk about it, Doc.
>
> **Dr:** I hear you. You trusted me with talking about it in some detail—that was courage as well. I am interested in knowing why you feel embarrassed? (Silence)
>
> **EMT Y:** What if I lash out? I mean, what kind of a person have I become to think of striking my partner, my wife, and to just start to scream?
>
> **Dr:** Have you ever done anything like that in reality?
>
> **EMT Y:** I was worried you would send me to the state hospital and EDP me as a threat to myself and others.
>
> **Dr:** For what, a fleeting fantasy? I guess then I may be sent away with you, too, as a quack—hmm?

EMT Y: (Nervous laughter turns into a genuine smile.) Well, you know, like I said, something stopped me from doing my job (exterior locus of control is noted). I love my job, but now I just don't want to be there (conflict). I'm not me anymore (depersonalization). I no longer want to do my job (avoidance). [That classic stare into the wall and eye movement (dissociation).]

Dr: Tell me, what did you just see when you stared so deeply into your minds eye?

EMT Y: [Without hesitation] The ACR in my jacket with patient K. (Ha, ha literally strong and nervous laughter, which signals to me he is feeling intense anxiety and avoidance. Nonverbally, through my silence and focus on what he is saying and listening, I encourage him to continue and trust me.) I mean, it was weird, real weird (meaning we may be onto the event triggering his interpretation of his irrational belief of going crazy). We were hanging out and it was, you know, real nice and quiet that night. We got the call a woman was in cardiac arrest. The other team of medics was first on the scene, and we came on the scene where resuscitation efforts were underway. I like the medics, I know them well and always liked them. They are really good (when a phrase is repeated a number of times, it alerts me to ambivalence that may be related to an event or avoidance of people associated with the experience). Now, I'm standoffish. I don't why (this ambivalence will be approached, but not now). I know my job and my task well (justification of competence). At the time, I felt like time stopped literally.

Dr: When did time stop for you?

EMT Y: It stopped for a long time when I saw her eyes, the brown eyes and her tears—it is too much (Fighting back the tears is followed by sobbing and letting it out. Y's face slumps downward, there is a dead silence. Long pause is followed by the default disclaimer:) It's fine Doc. I am better, really! That's my problem I am becoming too soft. It's life. Period. You know let it roll off like a duck. Honest . . .

Dr: (Interrupt) Stay with it, Y. You and I are no ducks, we are human beings. I'm with you, Y. This is painful, it takes courage, don't let it go. You saw her eyes and tears, then . . . (Silence)

EMT Y: (Crying) I thought she looked like an angel and I felt attracted to her. I wanted so much for her not to be hurt, to wake up. I had my gear and then I began to finally get into it and did my part. If only I had not stopped and looked like a gawking civilian Joe. I think it was a long, a long time (he is attempting to get me to collude with him in self-denigration: masochism, guilt, and confirmation from an authority like me when he is more than adequate to come to his own choices).

Dr: It seems like you were changing gears from anticipation to your rescue identity mode, to your comforter identity mode by easing her passage into death, all the while your fellow medics were working on the patient.

EMT Y: I was doing what I have to do. It was a minute.

Dr: How long did it feel like you were stuck?

EMT Y: Honestly, I feel like I am still stuck there. It's real weird shit. It's me not doing what I have to do, looking at her even now, she appears frozen.

Dr: What are you thinking as your mind's eye visualizes, her frozen right now?

EMT Y: She's young and beautiful, and I cannot do anything to help her. She shouldn't be suffering and dying. She is too young. I touched her. That is when I felt we ought to turn her over and then we found a wound and scars all over her body. (He turned pale and I felt a jolt in my face and back.) I still feel the sweat on my back—it was dripping.

Dr: How long did it stop you in real time, even though in emotional time it feels as if you are still there?

EMT Y: About as long as I told you my thoughts now.

Dr: That's around 40 seconds, yes?

EMT Y: Yeah, about 7 seconds. It feels like much longer, hours and hours.

Dr: This makes a lot of sense that you are trying to sort through the very real tragedy for hours on end by reliving it in your mind again and again. Holding it keeps the toxic stuff in and just builds up. Allowing release by crying is part of the process, talking about it another, and then exploring your association and thoughts about this trauma, yet another. Your experience of compassion and even attraction to this young beautiful woman of 25 years of age who was mortally wounded makes superb sense. [Normalizing, refocus and assess with empirical evidence for him to use in his own renarration. It also helps him appreciate his own humanity and compassion without self-recrimination.]

EMT Y: You know, if I think back now, it wasn't really that long in reality; it was only a few seconds.

Dr: So you did exactly what you had to do, you were cautious and hesitant before engaging in rescue work for a few seconds. Hardly an eternity, even if it felt that way.

EMT Y: Hmm, I didn't realize it was that short time. I thought it was much longer than that. I didn't realize it, but I started acting strange since this happened. I would be joking and laughing and being easygoing. My partner and other people told me I'm not driving like I usually do. I'm not my usual self. Seeing her lying down with colored bruises all over her body. It was a homicide and a cardiac arrest. Who knows what happened to her murderer and even if they sort it through? (Another very real loss—not knowing what happens after his investment as an EMT ends the imagined guilt, and failure begins to mushroom from his multiple and complex identity modes.)

Dr: How did you feel not knowing what happened?

EMT Y: You learn to just forget it . . . put it aside let it go. period.

Dr: If it is only that easy. Does it work?

EMT Y: I realize more and more now it doesn't work. I got upset, I felt really upset, and I wanted to let it out really bad and I couldn't let it out. I felt like just yelling and getting it out.

Dr: Say that again. Did you hear what you just said?

EMT Y: (Y nods and says with real sadness and expression.) I was unable to express my fears, guilt, attraction, and being really peeved at the injustice and then not even knowing what happened to her. What could I do?

Dr: I imagine you know, that one is to go back and honestly see what you did do. It seems you are so conscientious at times, you give yourself little of the credit you truly deserve. While you were sad and at a loss, that did not block your ability to do your share in the rescue on the scene.

An Eco-Ethological Existential Analytic Intervention with Officer EMT Y

Here, paradoxical intention was refined and impactful through three conduits. One was a behavioral assignment of reading *Catch 22* by Joseph Heller (1961). Another paradoxical intervention to address his fear of losing control and striking those he loves most was to place a hammer in his hand and ask him to do with it as he will. Third was to go out and to focus on his fantasy of striking those he loves and to write out all his thoughts and fantasies in explicit detail. It worked exquisitely. In a series of role plays in which I was the patient, an EMT blaming myself without surcease, he took the role of doctor. I persisted until he gave me some concrete evidence and means to challenge my thoughts. He was superb.

In addition, allowance of his loss and the hurt heart he felt was complemented by an active *in vivo* exercise of asserting his feelings and stance in the field. In one exercise, he dealt with inebriated aided cases to openly express compassion when he felt it, rather than keeping it in regardless of approval or not by his peers. To his surprise, nobody ridiculed him, although they ribbed a little. Some came around to his viewpoint, enabling him to be competent and assertive and not to hold in his genuine expression of compassion, loss, and mercy when he experienced these feelings. Perhaps my bias, but he agreed that although we cannot change a culture, it is absurd not to change one's perspective and expression while one is alive. Finally, mourning the loss of this beautiful young woman's soul was not left unattended but memorialized in our work of candles and renarration for him to take as motivation.

EMT Y: (Laughing nervously) I feel guilty fleeting thoughts. I feel embarrassed to talk about my possibly lashing out and hurting someone. I was thinking about it; it must be stupid. I had to do a protocol update. I know I don't want to hurt myself, but I feel stuck.

Dr: Stuck where?

EMT Y: I was worried that I'll be sent to the state hospital. The scene comes into my head and I got drunk with my friends that night.

Dr: (Interrupt). Let's go there. Tell me what happened that day.

EMT Y: I was thinking a lot about what had happened. I couldn't get it off my mind. I felt really bad.

Dr: So far you're not crazy. Highly anxious, but not crazy. But go on and construct some challenges to the maladaptive belief that you're crazy for embracing the tragic comedy of public service work.

HW: Read *Catch 22* by Joseph Heller (1961). See what insights you can glean.

This is an excerpt of my putting a reclaiming of his sanity in an ecology of trauma into practice with EMT Y:

EMT Y: I got the book and the video. I mean what really struck me was they think they're crazy and really not. Yossarian was sane. The whole idea was to get out; figure out how and get out of a nutty situation. The scene where the plane blew up made me feel I know exactly what Heller was getting at—the numbness or pretending of indifference. It was absurd, not of the situation's tragedy, but the mad ignoring of the tragic as if it was a comedy. I got the bulb. It was a tragic comedy of life you were relating to me, Doc. Is that what you wanted me to get?

Dr: I didn't ask for you to get anything from it but your own insight. That is exactly the interpretation you brought to the table, as evidence—Bravo! Hence, evidence you are not crazy but really sane for knowing a tragic comedy we are all part of in public service.

EMT Y: It really makes sense now. I really am not crazy. It is the every-day situations that are like a MASH unit you can get so used to it. You can numb yourself by drinking it away or hiding from it, pretending to be indifferent. It's not a good thing or something to brush off. It is sad and frustrating and tragic to see life and death unfold. It's not routine for the normal Joe in the street, but it is not for me also. I can say it's shitty and express my sadness and frustration. But I didn't cause it and can't change it—only respond the best I can. It's like I was told if you can't take it, get out of the kitchen when I was a rookie and expressed feeling sorry for a drunk. After realizing it is part of being a man to express myself and mercy or compassion, I can say out loud I feel sorry for the guy. I don't hold it in.

Eco-Ethological Existential Analytic Intervention

This is the paradoxical *in vivo* assignment with FD EMT Y:

> **Dr:** What you are doing now is getting it out without covering over what you feel because you do trust our relationship. Then going a step further by realizing that the tragedy is real; your loss and grief is important to express, and rethinking your experience and challenging your maladaptive beliefs is where it's at. You hid it in and it felt like being trapped. You are an avid naturalist. What happens when an animal feels trapped?

> **EMT Y:** It wants to run or bite.

> **Dr:** Isn't that in a way what you naturally and more cleverly hid from yourself? (Y nods assertively) Does it make sense that is why you had such a strong fantasy to strike out, perhaps even at me?

> **EMT Y:** Doc, I was so worked up, I had that fantasy for a moment.

> **Dr:** Let's do an experiment. I trust your sanity 97% that you would not act on it then and now about 99.97%. Here is a hammer. Do with it as you will. (I hand him an office hammer for picture frames. I look relaxed and in fact shuffle a few papers. He holds it while getting a little sweaty and then gives it back.)

> **EMT Y:** Wow, Doc. Have you lost it giving it to me and knowing my fantasy.

> **Dr:** Let me ask you, is a fantasy reality?

> **EMT Y:** Of course not.

> **Dr:** No, you bet you're right. I know and trust in your sanity. Here's evidence for you to use when you challenge those maladaptive beliefs with the evidence. Nothing will make you act on fantasy except you. You clearly know the difference between reality and fantasy. If every guy or gal who ever fantasized about the sordid things we all do at times actually acted on them, we would all be put away. [I go on to assign a homework to fantasize as much as he can to actively "whack this one and that one" for every reason under the sun. He leaves with a sense of humor seen for the first time in many weeks. EMT Y reports back he has been able to resume sexual relations and really enjoy himself with his wife and try as he did to fantasize about hitting someone, he couldn't. He initiated visiting some museums and getting to attend some events he put off for a while.

[As in the other case examples, we set up a living goal to memorialize the dead starting with his role as part of the witnessing, memory, and active work. He agrees this is meaningful and will include losses he is not responsible for predicting and causing.]

Case 3: Internal Affairs: Don't trouble your own house or you will inherit the wind.

Biography

Detective Sergeant G is a single female college student—educated career investigator, groomed for a key position through increasingly complex cases. She had aspirations to go to law school and become an attorney. Most recently, her position has presented challenges within the Internal Affairs Division. Det. Sgt. G presents as an intense person with a highly verbal style of expression. She is focused and has a strong core of high values associated with her position. While she has had an ambivalence about being an Internal Affairs Investigative Supervisor, she has been fair, yet tough-minded in her no-nonsense approach.

She denies being bothered by politics, yet she describes in detail what she says is "Internal Peyton Place Puzzle Palace Politics." This denial appears superficial; we will explore emotional upset together. She remains inordinately enamored with an "ideal performance" that barely covers over perfectionism in her standards and a harsh standard toward other investigators. She maintains that being a totally serious investigator helps her root out misconduct by officers. Recently she has been feeling burnout after a series of trauma experienced vicariously with officers involved in off-duty incidents, ranging from minor violations to serious crimes. She believes that she is not able to deal with the loneliness of isolation after joining Internal Affairs and not being able to mingle with the general police population.

Unidentified traumatic loss emerged in an operation wherein she supervised a sting in which an officer was indicted for a serious corruption charge of drug dealing. She was treated by a cold wall of indifference by former professional colleagues after this sting went down. One of the officers involved seriously hurt himself and she felt enormous guilt. Being called a rat and given the cold shoulder has exacerbated her isolation. While her unit members were supportive, she felt they were disingenuous. She believed they were not to be trusted; "One can never know who is watching her," this disturbed her sense of whom to trust, which no doubt included me.

Eco-Ethological Existential Analytic Perspective

My countertransference was frustration at being a recipient of desperation, agitation, and burnout. A hatred of many of the injustices she had witnessed put me as a Cop Doc squarely in the middle of her displaced anger. Because I am a Cop Doc, she felt she was able to relate to my "essence as a fellow sergeant, and investigator of the mind."

A deeper feeling of desperation to connect with me was countered by fear and distrust at being vulnerable, misunderstood, and hated because she was an

Internal Affairs investigator. This came up each time we got close to the heart of her discontent. Her anger was surfeited by a plastic smile: disingenuous, and plastered on. I dealt with my frustration by considering the objective reality of her position before clinical judgment was exacted (i.e., paranoia and border-line tendencies).

My approach was to acknowledge to Det. Sgt. G that as a psychologist I was interested in understanding her—not ever to betray her trust—tolerating her hostility. I silently took the attitude of any professional therapist, maintaining my optimism and perseverance that she could learn to trust again through the consistent attitude I would take to her ongoing transference. That transference of course includes negative as well as positive processes, and as Brenner reminds us, is ubiquitous (Brenner, 1974, 1976). However, for me being a container for Det. Sgt. G's hostility was frustrating. I kept my tolerance high by focusing in on the underlying emotional interpretation that her demand for me to validate her right-wrong, black-white, whore-madonna judgments were tests of my trust. I stayed firm on why she needed my approval, working through inference, chaining to the root of her core maladaptive belief in perfectionism overly harsh damnation of her own actions and others in her unit. Her attitude was too serious and hyperfocused. Behind this was an attempt to squelch real and disenfranchised human emotions related to traumatic loss. That loss was associated with her ideal demands for her own performance as a ranking supervisor investigator.

Eco-Ethological Existential Analytic Perspective

One objective was to get Det. Sgt. G to realize that her position is not "being a rat" as she half-jokingly derided her own detail, but rather one of critical importance. Her performance was ethical, not overly zealous, and with the internalized goal of being fair, which she had successfully achieved quite well. In fact, some criticisms of Internal Affairs are appropriate. It is an operation that allows a breadth of venue, but is subject to great abuse of power (revenge) and privilege (to ignore certain people's misdeeds). Like most investigators (not all), she did a remarkable job of not falling prey to either temptations. This is not different from most public-official appointments in which public safety is at a premium and loyalty to ideals are important and need be balanced by one's own tendencies. I ensured she would recognize this fact via the Socratic method, leading her to identify maladaptive beliefs about herself, others, and the importance of her work as a nonzealous investigator doing unpopular but nevertheless important service. On the other hand, I told her that her integrity would for the most part go unnoticed by the department brass, and in fact, would be a form of derision in certain commands. This is not different from many of the covert operations of investigators who are members of national and international security agencies, largely unrecognized for the extreme sacrifice expected by personal mental, physical, and existential demands.

In gaining cultural competence, being a fair-minded investigator is difficult, especially when fellow officers are subjects of investigations, which is tragic not only to witness, but to be involved in as an arresting officer. It is a disenfranchised traumatic loss when an officer arrested or charged inflicts self-harm or harms others. It is unacknowledged usually within the unit because the officer is dehumanized as a rogue. As in Detective Sgt. G's case, she cannot get solace from peers in the unit when she feels responsible for the officer who commits criminal activities and is dehumanized or viewed as being framed. Support is highly unlikely because of the sensitive nature of her work. Even officers outside of the Internal Affairs are unlikely to be trusted as witnesses of her distress. The loss of other uniform friends when an officer joins Internal Affairs is also a very hard loss for her to accept as reality. Yet her identity modes are replete with all these conflicts.

I do not suggest she change her detail; rather I get her to explore her attitude toward it. Included is one goal to continue on with her ideal in mind, but with less harshness and zeal in her self-condemnation. I relate to her fervor as supervisor and investigator, getting her to identify and mobilize her high frustration tolerance and tendency to hyperfocus on a resilient attitude toward the jibes sent her way.

Eco-Ethological Existential Analytic Intervention with Det. Sgt. G

The following is a brief example of such an intervention:

Dr: It seems like this case really bothered you a lot.

Dr: What comes to mind now?

Det. Sgt. G: Well, I feel like he took an oath and betrayed it completely. He's no better than a perp. Then I just cannot believe he tried to hurt himself; that's the way of a cop turned bad, *as simple as that.* I don't really care, not an iota. I'm not guilty, not one ounce! Not even a kernel of truth, he can accuse me of that, but he is a rat. He caused his own downfall. (I respond to her guilt feelings by clarifying her truth, that the officer did act criminally, and acknowledging her difficult position, while getting her to own up to and express guilt to simultaneously disabuse herself of it.)

Dr: It is interesting that you're say your not guilty, you really don't care not even an iota. It seems like you very understandably feel incensed that he betrayed his oath. He put you in a position you hate to be in. Then he accuses you of being a rat. That's grating on you, huh? I can imagine it's painful.

Det. Sgt. G: It was not. I felt good that he got what he deserved. (Her denial is strong, and passively accepting what she has presented as guilt is almost an invitation to clarify her guilt and help her to express it.)

Dr: Yet you needed to prove with evidence to me, and perhaps yourself, that he deserved what he got. If you felt he was so deserving, why repeat what he said unless it bothered you? [I repeat the dynamic and cognitive intervention to get her to focus on her denial.]

Det. Sgt. G: Do you think I overdid it, Doc? Do you think I was overzealous?

Dr: You tell me. Did you overdo it in being overly zealous by discarding the fact he may have been totally innocent? [This is risky, considering our relationship is somewhat ambivalent. I, however, test her ability to see the point that she did try to disconfirm his guilt, which was blatant in his behaviors and which included collaboration with drug dealers.]

Det. Sgt. G: I know many times officers are unjustly accused by drug dealers and civilians with a gripe: a vendetta by others for whatever reason. I am never overzealous.

Dr: So, if I got it right from your history, you personally have been involved in thwarting those who would tarnish a good officer's name?

Det. Sgt. G: Yeah, you don't know how many times, and no one seems to sing my tune.

Dr. Ahh, so why do you react so harshly on yourself for doing your job, clearly you know you are not overly zealous. Yet, you remain so unsure and so harsh on yourself. I am turning my large ear right in your direction to listen. I am listening intently, if you care to share with me what comes to your mind. She smiles begrudgingly.

[We go over a few times the actual case and other associations emerge where she witnessed drug transactions, sordid deals, and disregard of colleagues, civilians and others.]

Eco-Ethological Existential Analytic Perspective

It appears that Det. Sgt. G suffered from a great deal of pain in her position as investigator, often not realizing that her assignment was meaningful in finding officers who are in fact innocent of charges that were directed by vengeful criminal organizations. Det. Sgt. G achieved getting innocent officers by the scores exonerated and free of unsubstantiated accusations when they were proven false. This is inestimable in reducing the harm inflicted by her peers. This achievement was also disenfranchised when we began our work and yet was redeemable to her own edification and to counter her disenfranchised losses. The point here, as in many cases I have presented, is that in the eco-ethological approach to loss in trauma, the disenfranchised courage and resilience is redeemed and made conscious. One growth in our work is Sgt. Det G's choice to present to her superiors the suggestion that exacting equal prosecution of those individuals who have targeted public servants by creating false allegations is a stance she can present internally with more credibility than if she chose to leave and be part of a different command. Her keen debating and polemical views are repositioned from sour grapes to humble raisins: choice morsels that are shaped by her existential struggles with justice, not in the abstract, but in the complex crucible of field experience. A potent result that emerged in our work was her choice to pursue what started off as a scoffing of her disowned dream to be an attorney. In the course of our work, she achieved her existential reward, realizing the only obstacle to becoming a law-school candidate was her own self-imposed limitations to her considerable ability.

When she gave up some of the dichotomous ways of thinking she found she could reappraise her identity mode as one clear and united entity as an investigator. That identity mode was a necessary check and balance approach to allow those officers who, in the vast majority, are honest and putting their lives on the line, to be free of those who would undermine this goal. While the option of leaving exists, there is a great deal of negative mythmaking about Internal Affairs. She does not have to buy into that negative labeling. I mobilize a series of rational coping statements, coupled with analytic explorations to earlier losses and trauma. We work on expanding her circle of boyfriend candidates outside of exclusive law-enforcement officers. The trauma of witnessing the self-harm inflicted and the disenfranchised pain of seeing the officer arrested, crying and in anguish, was elicited in the following abridged piece. [While reviewing her thoughts, her expression turned ashen and sullen, tears started to well in her bloodshot eyes as she fought letting them out. My tears were less noticeable.]

> **Dr:** It seems like you are holding back what you are really wanting to let out. [Silent and waiting till she is ready to express what is on her mind.]

> **Det. Sgt. G:** I felt terrible that I had to lock him up. He was young, and I felt this was serious. He was going to do time. The other cases were minor in comparison: DWI first offense and other minor offenses. The officer usually had a loss of days, mandatory counseling, referred to early intervention unit, or alcohol detoxification through the counseling unit (these units are manned by outstanding mental health professionals who are usually uniformed members, Certified Alcohol Counselors, and Certified Social Workers). I supervised the sting operation. I mean, I shouldn't be feeling sad—he is a perp, right? I mean, you were a cop too, you know the deal. Of course, you probably think I am a rat too?

> **Dr:** [I do not respond to enlisting me for confirmation, but rather I normalize her feelings of distress.] Why shouldn't you feel as you feel, including sadness?

> **Det. Sgt. G:** (Teary eyed and crying.) I can't think of him that way because he is a rogue cop, a degenerate, he went to the other side, including drugs. I mean the way he looked at me…

> **Dr:** Does that make him a totally evil person, although his actions we can agree on were evil by supporting the drug dealers who are involved in hurting brother and sister officers?

Det. Sgt. G: I can't think of him that way because then I can botch the investigation. It's weakness, Doc. You have a notorious reputation to put almost any member of the service on the couch.

Dr: Is that so that you can't feel the way you do? Tell me that again.

Det. Sgt. G: Oh, I really hate you. [If I only had a dollar for each time I heard that.]

Dr: I'll take that risk. It seems he made a bad mistake that will cost him his career, his freedom for a while, and yet he still is a fellow human being. You feel sorrow. Is that a crime?

Det. Sgt. G: I guess not, but it's hard to keep on thinking of him as a human being even though he acted that way. It's easy for you, like I said, you put everyone on the couch.

Dr: [I do not negate her statement because it has some truth in it. I use it to bring some humor into our dialogue and, more importantly to encourage her to think of me in human terms in our relationship (typical REBT/existential style). I then reassess her thoughts.] It seems like the only difference is while I may find some peoples' behaviors patently absurd at times to downright obnoxious, I work hard at not damning anyone as a whole person. Why? Because I will invariably lose the fact of my own humanity the moment I start to consume myself in the hateful actions I witness and encounter at times.

Det. Sgt. G: You're a shrink. It's easy for you with all that training you've had and your experiences.

Dr: Not easy at all. It seems like life as a cop and sergeant for me involved real losses, some I can never replace. The challenge with my losses, although different, is parallel to yours. The challenge is our personal attitude, choice, and responsibility toward the tragedy our lives traverse. I have become more of an enlarger than a shrink, by choice. My choice is different from your exact choices, but I agree they have similar components. I have a choice of my attitudes, responsibility, and what to take on and what to let go.

[While I do not disclose the specific losses in my personal life, I equally let her know I, too, had to work hard at dealing with my experiences of trauma and loss, and I am no different as a fully human and alive person than is she. This is not without obvious problems. It is a choice I make, and it works in helping Det. Sgt. G put her situation and her existential freedom in perspective.]

This type of confrontation, while not typical, is necessary considering her command and the style she brings to the table. Sometimes being a therapist with police and public-safety officer-patients demands command decisions, no apology given nor demanded. Keeping that in mind in your approach may be helpful at times as it was in mine.

Case 4: PPS-CPTSD: Experimental Traumatic Neurosis—Excited Type

Biography

Sgt. Z is a German American First Rescue Responder. His significant other is an Emergency Room physician. Although an intimation of folie a deux related to a craving for excitement, and hyperstimulation may exist, intimacy and love in this couple has sustained the relationship. Another dynamic here is that both are highly committed, no-nonsense professionals, who share a goal of work as an essential to meaning in their life. Both have a *hyperfocus* toward achieving those goals. Predictably, both also help the other when there is a crisis.

Sgt. Z expressed one problem he had in his mid-40s. He believed "life is too unpredictable after so much crap on the street, I cannot commit to marriage." This fear of commitment is related to intense worry about loss. That fear of loss through violence and death has kept him from expressing the love he feels. In place of the love he feels he exhibits an overprotectiveness for those he considers significant in his life: his significant other, family, friends, and the officers in his elite unit.

Sgt. Z's major complaint was sleep disturbance. He wrote down his dreams in a log as per our behavioral plan. He reported, "feeling bored, unappreciated, and upset about a lot of things on the job. Recently it's caught up with me."

Paradoxically, Sgt. Z focused on doing a great job, "I will be one of the best bosses in the department. I loved being a cop. I will be a great boss as a sergeant too." Over seven years, Sgt. Z responded to an estimated 300 emergency situations involving officers and civilians in dire straits. This is likely an underestimate. He presented me with multiple letters indicating personal extreme risk and bravery. He was not foolhardy, running in without caution.

He is a highly trained and skillful police supervisor, who expressed "loving the mean streets and rescue-call excitement." Yet, he is exasperated with these same jobs. He "demands perfectionism or nothing," and is hyperfocused in his approach to public service. He presented with many achievements, commendations, training certifications all of which requires a great deal of savvy and increasing sophistication. He is very involved with officers who work for him on and off duty. While I was taking his trauma history, he described what was one of the worst events in his career.

Sgt. Z's Account of his Most Traumatic Event

About seven years ago I responded to an Emotionally Disturbed Person (EDP) job in the confines of Pct. X. Upon arrival, we were informed by the sectors on the scene that there was an EDP in the house, possibly with a gun. The male involved was at the window shouting at the police. I made contact with him by telling him my name was EZ and I was here to help him.

I do not remember exactly how he responded. But I do remember it was with viciousness. For about 130 minutes I tried to talk with this male and establish some kind of (rapport) mutual trust. No matter what I said, he would not respond directly to me. He responded only with hate toward police, including me.

Because the radio run said he was armed, I came in armed with an automatic weapon. This made him more mad. I tried to explain why I was armed; he didn't want to hear it. *No matter how I tried, and I really tried* to give him a pitch, it failed.

He would not have dialogue with me. During my attempts to talk with him, he would leave the window, come back a short time later, and then back and forth. It was wait and try to talk, and he would get that *look of hate, then pain in his face*, then hate. The last time, he came back with a gun in his hand. Before I could say anything, *I saw his face and eyes filled with such hate. And he looked straight at me and said, "Let my blood be on your hands."* He then put the gun into his mouth and blew his brains out. I remembered a short time later him lying on the floor with brain matter all over. *I wondered why he did this. I did not understand. I still don't understand.* I remember we were all getting our gear together. We were then called to another EDP job. *I didn't have any time to talk about this. I do remember going home and wondering all night, "Why did he do this?" I had a lot of dreams. Why couldn't I reach him? I didn't ever discuss this, until now with you.* This was one of the *worst things that happened to me in my life. I just feel this can never go away.*

Heuristic Reconstruction of PPS-CPTSD with Sgt. Z

Sgt. Z's dominant sensory mode and memory appears to be primarily eidetic in both visual and auditory modalities. It is likely that Sgt. Z has a more than average awareness of emotional expression in others (i.e., hate, viciousness, and fear). The keen perceptual skill is likely endogenous and, in strong measure, exogenous. My use of the term exogenous is nested in the ecological with ethological shaping of behavioral and cognitive patterns. In Sgt. Z's case, his behavioral and cognitive appraisals are influenced by evolutionary demands. After all, Sgt. Z's survival value depends on being correctly attuned to severely disturbed and violent offenders.

What distinguishes Sgt. Z's processing of this dimension of trauma we are analyzing from the prior one presented, Officer T's case (see p. 217), is in part style, rank, and unit responsibility, as well as the identity mode and situational demands both experience. In Officer T's case, his roles were clearly delineated with five distinct situational demands. This is not the case in Sgt. Z's experience, whose roles and situational demands remain indeterminate, volatile, and uncertain. In Sgt. Z, the roles are not as sharply delineated in comparison to Officer T's experience. The mental state and intention of both disturbed men are very different, as is the conclusion of Sgt. Z's event that ends with the death of the emotionally disturbed person. However, there are similarities that exist between Officer T's and Sgt. Z's experience of trauma as substantive and core dimensions of PPS they share—Police Experimental Traumatic Neurosis.

To review, these substantive dimensions include a minimum of intense situational demands that rapidly change; are simultaneously experienced; or are so vague as to be indeterminate to the participant. To these ecological demands is added the ethological motivation of extreme role conflicts. Let us review why this is so.

In Sgt. Z's own words, the existential conflict is intolerable and is evidenced by the symptoms ripe for development of a trauma syndrome. Sgt. Z is forced to become active, and hold himself back simultaneously. He is unsure of what will come next for 130 minutes. Yes, 130 minutes! The stimulation is as intense as it gets. A psychotic man is threatening to kill himself and possibly Sgt. Z and anyone who gets in his way. This person is attempting to place the full responsibility for his destined outcome on Sgt. Z through unrelenting and extremely unstable behavior.

The situation is not simple. The possibilities make it a complex situation that demands the utmost of emotional intelligence and strategic cognitive intelligence. The strain on Sgt. Z's ability to inhibit his own arousal toward self-defense, and the increasing provocation toward confrontation, is exhausting. The memory is absorbing these toxic elements into his neurological encoding tracks, both limbic and frontal executive structure and function. This memory may become part of his "ethological memory," triggered whenever cues and stimulus are evoked during similar trauma he is likely to experience.

What is evoked with certainty is a simultaneous collision between two opposing forces—inhibition/excitation. Here is a reconstruction of that collision into four parts:

1. The inhibition of the use of ultimate physical force is effected in the context of the pursuit/attack and confrontation role evoked by the armed, barricaded EDP.
2. The EDP is exhibiting "a cry for help" through his erratic actions of hate and extremely aggressive gestures and behaviors. The words spoken by the barricaded EDP betray a possibility that communication may be bridged. Sgt. Z is attuned to his own voice of conscience to effect his custodial and rescue identity mode.
3. That psychophysiological conflict is complicated by yet another conflict in the existential realm. That conflict revolves around whether or not action that triggers the pursuit and confrontation role is to be unshackled or, at tremendous risk to Sgt. Z, embrace the risk of inhibition.
4. The existential dimension of Sgt. Z's compassion and mercy toward this disturbed person is intense. His investment in success as rescuer, and the investment in his idealistic goal, is enhanced by the highest standards he has

learned as a member of his elite unit. While the result of his intention could very well end his own life, he is not naïve, not ignorant of this choice. He chooses to place himself in the front line and to resolve this event.

What remains unclear is how much neurological, ethological, emotional, cognitive, and behavioral aftershocks will reverberate in the trauma syndrome that follows Sgt. Z's traumatic experience. What we are certain of at this point are Sgt. Z's supervisory responsibility and indeterminate identity modes relating to the extremely inchoate field demands of a barricaded and volatile psychotic person who is armed, suicidal, and homicidal.

To begin to appreciate Sgt. Z's experience, an individual perspective enhances our understanding. Our approach to Sgt. Z targets maximizing specificity in treatment plans, facilitating his healing process, and redeeming the positive outcomes equally disenfranchised from his own interpretation of trauma.

First he seeks out excitement and the challenge of his detail. However, unlike the officer who has a hyperexcited style and may be addicted to trauma (we will observe later), he appears to get, "little pleasure in being the first in the line of fire." Rather, we will now touch on his style of being hyperfocused on achieving ideals of perfection in his work. Specifically, in this trauma, Sgt. Z's hyperfocus includes success as he sees it unfold through his anticipatory schemas of trajectories—involving the identity modes of pursuit, confrontation, arrest, custody and rescue.

Elaborating on what we do know: Sgt. Z still is a sergeant and evaluates his sense of self and identity through his successes on the job. This original trauma was experienced seven years ago. Remember Sgt. Z called this event, "one of the worst things to happen to me, and what I did not discuss, until now." The hyperfocus afforded by his elite unit's survival value complements his perfectionism. His eco-ethological niche afforded the specific evocation of his development of PPS-CPTSD. While the psychotic man did not succeed in getting Sgt. Z to shoot him, unconsciously he used a form of projective identification to hook Sgt. Z into absorbing the hate, torment, and anguish from the initiation of the first event until his suicide. The suicide triggered the emotions of guilt, uncertainty and doubt. The personality style of Sgt. Z suggests vulnerability toward hyperfocus.

Thus, the various roles anticipated in the ecology of conditional situational demands could unfold at any time. Sgt. Z was keenly aware and hyperfocused for 130 minutes. The investment he chose was preventing death to himself, other sacred victims, and the person barricading himself. We know Sgt. Z had no chance to debrief, moving on to the next job. A critical factor of the shock and loss after intense investment is that his experience was disenfranchised. Seven years later, his impressions have gone through many permutations through a series of subsequent traumas. Strong evidence suggests an Experimental Police Traumatic Neurosis-Excited Type for Sgt. Z.

His extraordinary courage was not acknowledged in the least. The reality was that his bravery was considered a failure by performance standards. He did not prevent the suicide. While no one berated him, no one acknowledged the magnitude of this trauma, thereby adding another to the many losses for Sgt. Z.

Finally, in our initial heuristic construction, the stimulation that comes with highly exciting and dangerous events for ego enhancement or for thrills is not congruent with Sgt. Z's style. That raises a question about why motivation and desire to continue in his special line of work continues. It is here that ethological motivation can explain this desire to reenact the original trauma successfully. This type of trauma may offer an ecological reexperiencing of the psychophysical threshold of the original experimental traumatic neurosis. It makes exceptional sense that the repetition compulsion to search for this type of situation in part is a result of conditioning and reinforcement.

As a sergeant, his existential angst motivates schemas for anger, hopelessness, guilt, and self-recriminations in what he appraises as an unsuccessful conclusion—suicide. Every time he is successful in a barricaded situation, proof is confirmed by gathering what he considers self-deficiencies. Behaviorally, this self-reinforcement becomes psychologically toxic. The invariable success and failure stimulates variable conditioning schedules in the ecology of his world of trauma, which paradoxically reinforces the persistence of his search.

The personal toll emotionally, cognitively, behaviorally, and existentially is excessive. This type of trauma is what officers deal with repetitively as chronic, overwhelming, and extreme strain. It is overly complex and intense emotional shock that is inescapable. Pavlov predicted, "the excitatory type loses almost completely, (his) ability for inhibition, and seeks unusual arousal to repeat the excessive stimulation" (1941). Our work suggests clinically in the eco-ethological approach that this trajectory can be reversed through our persistent interventions.

Eco-Ethological Existential Analytic Intervention with Sgt. Z

Let's review the anticipatory and trajectory schema in Sgt. Z's executive strategy. His goal is establishing a relationship and reaching this psychotic fellow emotionally. His attitude is to stave off a confrontation. Sgt. Z established a high level of expectation, and anticipation of disarming, taking custody, and rescuing. At the same time, his role as a supervisor demands personal safety that weighs heavily on his tactical approach. His ethological motivation is to defend himself and others with the full weight of personal survival.

Existentially, an intense desire for rescue and connecting through his exquisite empathy is countered by the situational demands of confrontation with an armed and seriously disturbed man. This is a severe conflict including unconscious and conscious conflicts (too elaborate to present here). Tactically, Sgt. Z has assessed three possible and radically different outcomes:

1. Arrest and custodial identity mode with all the tactics in anticipation of a nonarmed struggle ensuing
2. Custodial and rescue identity mode if the person surrenders to assistance (this man's injuries are undetermined)
3. The ultimate confrontation identity mode if the EDP moves into an assault mode, entailing a full-blown firearm life/death struggle

These outcomes are dependent on the situational demands that unfold in relation to the EDP behavior, the ecology, and Sgt. Z's response. Each outcome demands radically different approaches, safety, action, or inhibition of action. The investment and response to any outcome involves risk to life for all involved. Sgt. Z has not dehumanized the EDP, and chooses, as far as he can, to desperately attempt, at extreme risk, an encounter. He has the following identity modes actively and simultaneously stimulated:

Sgt. Z has activated the identity mode of *strategic pursuit*: following every move, tactic, and point-by-point intention that the aggressor makes (there is an attunement and identification with the aggressor). This carries unconscious and conscious awareness of hate, rage, despair, excessive anxiety, sadism, masochism, and chaotic impressions.

Sgt. Z has activated the identity mode of *arrest and custody*: following every opportunity to capture this highly volatile emotionally disturbed person without effecting harm and using the necessary force to accomplish this goal. What this entails is uncertain throughout.

Sgt. Z has activated the identity mode of *confrontation* the moment he tried to encounter the emotionally disturbed man with a possible deadly weapon. He has anticipated whether and how he will use deadly physical force if necessary to stop him. He has also no doubt anticipated his own death if he is shot point blank. Sgt. Z reported he went over multiple times the alternative tactics to stop this person. This has been ethologically motivated and practiced many times. It is likely that vicarious trauma and anticipatory schemas complicate the experience. Sgt. Z is constantly monitoring the ecological opportunity to end the barricaded situation with the least harm to all participants.

Sgt. Z has activated his *rescue* identity mode as the most desirable. It is the most difficult in the face of all the other contradictory and oppositional roles. He anticipates gaining an inroad to lessen the strain and stress of the emotionally distraught and psychotic person, who thwarts each attempt with extreme rejection. Sgt. Z is painfully aware of the desire of the psychotic man either to commit suicide or attempt to kill Sgt. Z.

Factually, these identity modes are all activated, the potential outcomes are all lived through as trajectories with different intensities. Our specific understanding is clarified through the following facts as we re-construct the trauma with Sgt. Z.

Sgt. Z led the work of his unit with this barricaded EDP, who threatened suicide in an escalating ultimate confrontation through potential suicide/homicide.

Hateful emotions and vicious expressions were picked up as invariants that Sgt. Z learned to recognize accurately as affordances in his ecological niche as an Emergency First Responder.

There is communication for 130 minutes. High ranking officers are controlling the outer scene, yet another factor of escalation and performance anxiety. Perimeters of safety are set, established preparation is forged for contingencies where he is at the heart of the negotiations.

The ambient internal perimeter is highly charged. At extreme levels of sustained attention for Sgt. Z, the emotional intensity and mental exhaustion are neurologically overwhelming. Sgt. Z's communication with his unit, his bosses (superior officers), the sounds and cues of his ambient environment, and general communications are all in addition to his communication with the EDP.

Keep in mind, action and outcome are unknown. Indeterminate stress has been conclusively associated with high levels of cortisol and strain. The extreme affordances for all-out combat is established tactically. Sgt. Z adapts by what I have already proposed as adaptive-dissociation and adaptive-depersonalization due to the sustained attention the situation affords. The splits that are sustained by Sgt. Z may support crystallized splits of consciousness. He is running the equivalent of an emotional marathon.

The EDP's pattern of leaving the window and coming back and forth heightens intermittent stimulation and inhibition, episodic moments of uncertainty with peaks of aggressive readiness and anxious inhibition. Escalating rage by the EDP is in striking opposition to Officer B's strategic counterinvestment in establishing nonviolent rescue. Keep in mind that suggests his adaptation level is one of confidence in the success of his approach. Sgt. Z is left with the imprinting of traumatic shock and loss when the involved victim commits suicide, setting the fertile ground for delayed PPS Experimental Traumatic Neurosis—Excitatory Type, and Disenfranchised Complicated Grief within Complex PTSD.

With the clear understanding of how significant this trauma is, our approach to the PPS-CPTSD is not to force change for Sgt. Z. That choice is ultimately Sgt. Z's. Our choice is first to understand the toxicity. I structure understanding within the patient's style and the specific event in mind.

Structuring your initial intervention with Sgt. Z may be achieved with the following in mind:

First, I support and validate the patient's free association to the trauma in his own good time with my tool of active listening.

Second, I heuristically clarify all points of trauma and loss embedded in anticipatory schemas; trajectories of those schemas; the roles, conflicts, and situational demands and investments as delineated in my heuristic reconstruction. We will go back in Sgt. Z's good time.

Third, I will explicitly validate the impact of the multiple events separately. We clarify how these events can yield a quantum psychic moment with many antiaffordances for a new sergeant assigned to an elite unit responsible for rescue work.

Fourth, I clarify how stressful the simultaneous potential and actual unidentified expectations of model performance clash with reality, including behaviors and emotional responses in terms of stimulation and inhibition. The simultaneous stimulation of arrest and custody identity mode with compassionate-healer identity mode and executioner identity mode are highly charged and contradictory with inhibitory turn on and off switching. In clarifying the intense strain, Sgt. Z was forced into and helping him identify each contradictory identity-mode and conflict the existential dilemma is fleshed out in an eco-ethological map that makes superb sense out of chaos. This, of course, is done in language that the Sergeant can understand and relate to.

Fifth, our attempt is to bring Sgt. Z to verbally express his angst with his identity modes, behavioral repertoire, and emotional distress. He now begins to express the unacceptable.

Sixth, Sgt. Z's narration of each potential outcome is highlighted with his enhanced understanding of why each role emerged. I lay out the framework for later clarification and confrontation by beginning to destigmatize aggressive, depressive, and guilty self-recriminations in thoughts, behavior, and emotion as affordances shaped by field trauma.

Seventh, shifts in his awareness call for cognitive, behavioral, affective, and emotional states in which altered consciousness may be allowed expression under the safe haven of the therapeutic encounter. The defined, highly chaotic situation as a whole event produces extreme emotional arousal and inhibition, and a maladaptive pattern takes shape. This perspective helps bring the motivational change necessary by my facilitating Sgt. Z's emotional drainage of what had been compartmentalized through counterphobic defenses. Those defenses are given substance and understanding as evolutionary mechanisms. This understanding, while fundamental, begins to allow expression and reenfranchising what has been disenfranchised so long.

Eighth, Sgt. Z's courage, compassion, and wisdom, which has gone unheard, is gradually given expression. That positive aspect of his existential sensibility had been disenfranchised up to this point in our work.

We will now move on to disenfranchised loss in trauma that may be decades old but remains as preserved as frozen meat left in the frost of a tundra of emotional numbness. That telescopes and leads back to decades of accumulated grief in some officer-patients. We will review this in our next case example.

Case 5: PPS-CPTSD: Telescoping Original Traumatic Loss Background

Inspector C is an Italian American Patrol Commander in his early 60s with a diverse portfolio: commanding specialized units, detective-bureau assignments, and tracking down offenders who target uniformed police and public-safety officers. Inspector C remains married to his first wife. They have three children and many more grandchildren. Inspector C suffered a minor heart attack recently which may be related to his stress experiences. He affirms that his Lutheran religious faith is an important and meaningful commitment in his life. Inspector C has above-average intelligence; his organizational and analytic abilities, culled from years of experience, are adroit. He recalled his pride at being appointed detective 30 years ago, "an achievement I will never forget." In his long career, he investigated many high-profile homicides. What initially emerged in our interviews was an extraordinary resilience in this highly successful man. His background would rival that of Frank McCourt, with an equally warm amiability under a pugnacious exterior veneer. Inspector C's adaptive, resilient personality style shines in his ability to take the suffering he endured and sublimate it into productive and willful achievements. Yet, in part, he could not move beyond his trauma and loss over meaningfulness shattered by the legacy of death and brutal murder. Together we estimated he experienced 2000 traumatic events over almost four decades. The most recent was prominent in his choice to retire from public service after 37 years of duty. That most recent trauma also was the one that was quite difficult for Inspector C to describe. Yet, in his lucid style, he shared his thoughts with me.

"I just don't feel right (after a recent investigation of a sensational homicide), especially after this homicide. I am not feeling like myself. I figured I'd give this therapy thing a chance. I've decided it's time." How telling—his choice of words—how sincere.

Inspector C's Account of His Most Traumatic Event

It's not a good atmosphere. I felt I was in something tragic. I tried to do the right thing with my cops (who mistook an object for a weapon). The victim was shot multiple times. It was the end of my career. I realized I just did not need this crap anymore. I felt sick, real sick. My chest bothered me and I felt queasy. I just didn't want to go to trial and see this accidental shooting become a circus for my officers and detectives. There's blood all over. Cops in deep shit. I was not even there. Man, the trial brought back . . . naw forget it (looks away, stares, and pauses). Anyhow I just had enough of this. (He paused)

(I interrupted with, "That was something or someplace you remember that brought you back. Don't leave it, tell me where.")

Bad emotions. It brought back bad emotions. Real bad. I got sick. I had it. I got myself into two binds. I was involved in a shooting, we got the perpetrator later. Then the second one was . . . (I again interrupted him with, Let's go there. What's happening right now? What is it that your seeing in that shooting?) Oh, yeah. I was drifting into those bad emotions. You know, this shooting was that same sick feeling. It was all police orientated. (When is this happening, C?) Cop YY was shot on December 26th 197X (Note: this interview was December 1997). I was working my vacation week. Radio transmission, "shots fired at XXX YYY Blvd." Big gigantic building complex. HS was right around there. I knew exactly where, I knew that address well. His partner came over the radio screaming. We got there as the first car. We walked over to the alcove in Building A, in a row with Building's B and C. The grass is all around and he, Officer XX, was lying in the grass. His partner is in the alley taking cover from fire, shooting back, screaming back to us. We asked, "Where's the guy?" The perp answered by shooting two rounds at us. It hit the grass. XX was still lying there on the grass, staring alive at us."

The perp did a robbery and rape with a .44 magnum. XX and his partner had information he was at XXX YYY Blvd. They spotted him, he booked, they chased him. They told him, "Stop, police!" He turned around, as soon as XX was at the door. He fired three shots at XX.

All three shots hit him, (teary eyed) . . . My GOD, all 3 shots hit him. I had to go down next morning to the morgue. It was like cigarette burns. One was right between his breast plate, the second here, third over here (showing stomach area). He was almost like, almost like you know, he fell between the hallway and pulled himself to the window. He opened it up for air. His partner came to him and chased the perp up the stairs. His partner was yelling on the fifth floor stairwell. There was shells. He was firing down at us with a 44 magnum. I can hear pow, pow, pow, pow, pow. We got him [XX] into the radio car. I had his head on my lap. He was looking at me saying, "Mommy, mommy . . ." I told him, "Hold on hold on X." His family met us at Lincoln Hospital. I had blood on my dungarees. He didn't make it through. It was devastating. I couldn't believe this was a cop. I knew him. He was very active in the station house. Earlier that week, we made a collar together, we chewed the fat. I just can't believe it, it feels like I just went through it again.

Heuristic Reconstruction of PPS-CPTSD with Inspector C

Telescoping trauma to an original loss is a process in which complicated trauma and loss emerge after having remained unconscious for years. I suggest the dormant-grief behavior needs to gain an outlet, to gain expression in each officer-patient's unique voice. For the officer-patient, we may be reasonably certain loss involves the absence of eco-ethological and existential security in his world. Nowhere is this likelihood more evident than the murder of a sacred victim. Such an event is what Inspector C experienced over two decades ago.

Inspector C's current trauma spontaneously emerges first through an emotional uneasiness, fleshes out in a telescopic view leading to an original trauma. That original trauma reemerges, and he reexperiences it as we are working on the present trauma. The cognitions, behaviors, emotions, and feelings are eidetic and visceral. This may occur because a barrier of repression may have been breached. He expresses anxiety through verbal cues that signal its emergence. His anxiety gives way to avoidance of my suggestion to explore that past trauma. This is not a clear transition. It is not definitive. But it is one necessitating my heuristic approach to follow the cues he presents as original trauma.

While recounting the recent trauma, Inspector C expresses feeling victimized *again,* the feeling of being helpless activates once *again.* He tells us, "This shooting *was that same sick feeling, it was all police orientated.*" The clue is a presentation of something from the distant past, presented in the context of the present. That gives me a moment of pause, suggesting ambiguity that something from the past is emerging. That "same sick feeling" at this point may be the emotional track to invariants between what was to provide the clues leading to the ambient environment of Officer XX's murder and one he experienced recently. Both were "police orientated."

Officers are participants in both: in the first shooting, an officer from the same unit as Inspector C is the victim. An emotionally intense pursuit ends with a bloody crime scene. In the original event, there is a vicarious victimization as Inspector C is at that time a patrol officer. He experiences loss at the murder of his peer. Inspector C's perceptual process suggests the older trauma as an original quantum psychic moment with the full antiaffordance of imprinting and eidetic memory. I do not solicit detail. It is made sensible when eco-ethological motivation suggests the invariants of the ecological setting are presented: address, street location, weather, day, and time. We are made aware of this motivation through Inspector C's process of disclosure by acute detail to ecological invariants. Those details provide clues for us to employ in our reconstruction of the event. The why of this presentation of detail may be a way of provoking our empathic response to pursue the multiple losses, how intense they are, and which are more pressing to initiate grief work. The perceptual imprint of original trauma suggests you will be made privy to as veridical an account as you can get. The point is trauma-grief work is respectful, gentle, and requires patience; it also requires a degree of persistence in pursuing a hunch fully to disconfirmation, before letting it go too quickly as insubstantial.

As I Socratically explore Inspector C's original trauma of his genuine thoughts, beliefs, and feelings (disgust, hate, fear, revulsion, pain) all speak of existential despair over his conflicted identity modes during this experience. These related cognitions, emotions, and beliefs are disenfranchised and repressed in loss. For many officer-patients, loss unexpressed does not heal itself with time, but will seek its level of filling the gap that very loss created. I do not mean that as an analogy, but as another avenue to explore. The very fact that one observes what is seemingly an exemplary way of overcoming an original trauma does not mean the officer-patient has successfully mourned his losses. That remains to be seen.

Let us observe this easily overlooked clinical issue of major importance in our therapeutic approach. Specifically, the multiple losses young Inspector C experienced occurred when he was a patrolman. He was not capable of expressing them at that time. His choice of filling the voids his losses created was most economically served by enlarging his scope of mastery. That mastery included solving cop killings and other homicides in which sacred victims would not go unheard without justice. This achievement serves as a very ingenious defense and outlet that hides the anguish of grief. How so?

In part, he accomplished an unconscious fulfillment of a wish. He gained status in his unit and within his culture. His mastery ethologically was successful. Let's examine his words carefully within the context in which they emerged; as a bridge from the present trauma to the original trauma: "you see this accidental shooting become a circus for *my officers and detectives.*" [Yes, I see, I choose to not ignore what he wants me to see, a circus for his officers and detectives; as a commander, it is his responsibility and solidified in the context of the defenses he has built up over years to protect his officers from being exhibited in a media circus]. He goes on, "There's blood all over. Cops in deep shit. I was not even there. Man, the trial brought back. . . . [The trial was a trajectory meaning a linear anticipatory schema of what would unfold; it was a future forecast when he was experiencing the current trauma. But a trajectory based on what? The past is necessary for any trajectory, whether in fantasy or reality.]

Inspector C's trajectory is "survivor guilt" on a surface level. From our eco-ethological approach, we find a sensible answer in part. The future trajectory of a circus is based upon guilt over his perceived failure (idealized omnipotence as an alpha leader)—once failing to protect XX from death. Of course I am not suggesting a direct guilt that remained unchanged over two decades, but guilt and the defenses he nourished in an ecology of trauma, unspoken and with all the fantastic distortions on a cognitive and dynamic level.

His failure to stop the recent homicide and protect "his officers" from their own tragic error in self defense is part of his idealized demand for vicariously protecting his officers from any harm. Harm in an ethological sense is distorted, it is triggered by an equally harsh vicarious liability for their suffering, the quorum of judgment, and their punishment, linked to his ethological belief that he is their boss (alpha leader of his officers and detectives in his niche). To this was added his shame and humiliation, unexpressed, when he encountered his feelings of vulnerability and deflation as a patrol officer in the most toxic of disenfranchised loss—guilt over a peer's death.

But the difficulty of our approach is staying on track with the ethological position. Why is this so difficult to do? In reality, Inspector C did such a splendid professional job of tracking down killers that the suggestion that he is suffering disenfranchised loss would appear without substance. Is it not obvious he has mastered his trauma being the great sleuth he no doubt became? He did, in reality, become a most adept, adroit, and efficient sleuth, and a leader of sleuths. What is difficult for the therapist on a personal level is not to be seduced into being awestricken and losing clarity in the glow, but to help facilitate Inspector C's expression of loss.

We gain insight into reconstruction of the process that involved the stepwise genesis of Inspector C's processing and condensing of the original trauma as follows:

First, the loss of his ethological goal is made visceral, emotional, and somatic to us.

Second, as he recounts his eidetic memory of the original trauma, he presents the invariants in veridical order to give us the layout for vicariously experiencing with him.

Third, he presents his cognitions and emotions about the invariants of the homicide. Specifically, his cognitive appraisal of trauma included many branches of consequent self-recrimination about his own performance, other officer's performance, public apathy, and his helplessness about the unfolding of the murder of a sacred victim. We discover his guilt about his fantasy role in the homicide. Did he meet his own super-standard of being an ideal officer? That ideal standard was running to and saving the mortally wounded peer (member of his eco-ethological unit). Inspector C's fantasy was, "If somehow I was there as the patrol officer that day, I could have saved Officer XX from his fate. I would have directed the pursuit of the perpetrator successfully."

Fourth, as he starts verbalizing his grief about the original traumatic event, the event begins to emerge into more conscious awareness. We identify multiple levels of loss at this stage: shock (loss of stability and predictability), helplessness (loss of control and mastery), fear (loss of invulnerability), shame (self-ideal performance standard shattered), failure of fellow officers to hear pain and anguish (loss by alienation and aloneness).

The unconscious ethological goal for Inspector C is being an alpha officer among other officers. This goal requires an intransigent belief in his own invulnerability as well as evoking that same belief from his subordinates through a mirroring process. His perceived failure can occur only if his idealized goal included his vicarious responsibility for the errors of officers subordinate to him. In his reconstruction of the events, we have gathered evidence for our hypothesis.

This sequence suggests the order of his presentation, which I facilitate, not design. He presents his sequence naturally and then I, by attentiveness and intention, flesh out and detach heuristically and reconstruct the embedded events. It is our skill in listening and attention to the invariants (ecological and ethological importance) in the officer-patient that yields insight into our reconstruction of Inspector C's trauma etiology. That sequence suggests a reverse sequence from its actual occurrence. Reversing the presentation in telescoped trauma gives us an enlarged view of how the (mal) adaptation to trauma was processed as a defense against overwhelming ethological loss and existential despair. We are consciously seeking to disconfirm our hypothesis. That is done by our clinical sense to actively listen for emphasis, avoidance, attention, and excitement in Inspector C's responses to our Socratic approach. We have enough evidence that our hypothesis of telescoped trauma was not disconfirmed. We have achieved a partial reconstruction of PPS-CPTSD in Inspector C's trauma and grief reconstruction.

Eco-Ethological Existential Analytic Intervention for Inspector C

The emergence of original trauma that telescopes from the present to the past is challenging to both patient and therapist. It puts a tangible perspective on the range and life of traumatic loss. This past event may be more complicated than one presented as the immediate clinical problem. This angst can fuel real existential change if handled properly. A timed moment that taps into direct empathy for emotional expression of original trauma leads to insight, sensibility, clarity—not understood, even less expressed. Keep in mind that anniversaries of retirement and change in assignments may mask this trauma. Being aware suggests direct questions to guide understanding. Loss that is unidentified is not supported and becomes invisible to efforts to make it tangible. This can lead to distortions that severely subject the officer to self-guilt, depression, and learned distrust. Telescoped trauma, when uncovered, offers a center for ongoing trauma work. Making sensible what appears exaggerated or disjointed for our immediate initial task.

Now look at the specifics of telescoped trauma in Inspector C's case with the objective of intervention. It is important to realize that in our eco-ethological approach, we seek to consistently reconstruct existential meaning through Inspector C's retelling of his trauma, as he sees it. Primary losses and the defenses that thwart expression of fear, anxiety, and questions are respected and valued with him in his identity as a police/public-safety officer; in his case, that covers the spatial range of police patrol officer to the rank of police Inspector. His multiple identity modes evoked through conflicts that emerge in the situational demands of his experience need to be addressed in this developmental context.

Inspector C's original trauma is 24 years old. His inhibition at expressing loss is disarmed, allowing functional dissociation in the context of a very stressful trauma in the present, to be repeated in your presence. Why this happened is likely, although not definitively, due to his trust, commitment, and positive transference, which has successfully developed in our relationship. His spontaneous emotional abreaction is elicited with a few connections that open to the Socratic approach in the context of the positive relationship we have established. My approach is to facilitate the connections, and is achieved as follows:

I listen for the window of disclosure in Inspector C's account to tilt enough in his functional dissociation without provoking withdrawal or inhibition. I will attempt to gently but consistently gain a hold on whether or not he is experiencing some event that overshadows the current trauma. Let's probe deeper into the account of trauma in Inspector C's words. I Interrupt, "C, (pause) that was something, or someplace, you remember, that brought you back. Don't leave it, tell me where." [I was attuned to the possibility that an original trauma may have been ready to emerge.]

"Bad emotions, it brought back bad emotions, real bad. I got sick. . . ."

At this point, it is more likely that there is something painful being hidden and something very much in the past. You don't bring something back that is not distant and in the past. You are not likely to repeat words unless there is something intense. Listen to his words, "like *bad* emotions, real *bad*." [Bad enough, that is, to make one sick.] Inspector C says, "Anyhow, I just had enough of this." [By "this" he means whatever bad emotions and event behind those emotions were associated with getting sick. It was so sickening that Inspector C had enough of what he is seeing and I am blind about. That pattern of presentation is a *sine qua non* for motivating our therapeutic antenna toward confirming past trauma.]

What the past trauma hinted at may be primary rather than secondary. The context for this decision was observing a glaze in his eyes, followed by the rapid eyelid fluttering, the body movement away, the head down as the other event was abruptly mentioned. Through my own countertransference, I felt strong revulsion and nausea, and dissociation came to mind. The cognitive attribution "emotions are bad," and the somatic presentation, "these bad emotions are making him sick" all added evidence, supporting my hypothesis. Included in this evidence are visceral defensiveness and global judgments, (i.e., I'm out: not good; tragic; I tried; the end of my career; I felt sick, real sick; my chest bothered me; I felt queasy; I didn't want to go to trial; blood all over; deep shit; I was not even there; man, the trial brought back; naw, looks away and stares, pauses). Still, hypotheses are tentative predictions. Disconfirmation would direct our path to other possibilities. But direct empathy motivated my enquiry and persistence.

By direct empathy, I mean not letting the moment blink into active ambivalence that serves as a defensive resistance to disclosure. This was the cue for me to time my disruption and test my hypothesis. My heuristic approach is built around the patient's lead. What followed was confirmation of my hypothesis. The empirical evidence of eidetic memory emerged in emotional abreaction. I facilitated this process with minimal disruption.

1. [Interrupting, "C, (pause) that was something, or someplace you remember, that brought you back. Don't leave it, tell me where."] "Bad emotions, it brought back bad emotions, real bad. I got sick, sick, real sick. My chest bothered me and I felt queasy." [We have confirmation that what he is seeing is

something that suggests an original trauma that is emerging from his past into the here and now. We are now at a confirmation of our hypothesis, rather than a disconfirmation.]

2. Having confirmed that the older trauma exists, I attempt to allow the focus on it to gauge the emotional, cognitive, and existential meaningfulness in comparison to the more recent trauma. I attend to Inspector C's responses of sequences of presentation as highlighted in the prior section (reconstruction of the trauma).

3. Inspector C as well as his elicited state of mind as a patrolman 24 years ago requires my responsive support of facilitating disenfranchised loss in the original trauma he experienced. Why do I use the term disenfranchised? If trauma had been successfully resolved, it would not be emerging in the here and now emotionally, cognitively, and existentially in a spontaneous upheaval. The timing for my elicitation of this dimension of trauma is critical, as is my empathic attunement—I suggest, more so than any specific technique.

4. The evidence in our eco-ethological reconstruction is that this original trauma emerged in the face of invariants in the current trauma that telescope back to the original trauma. It is in this context of reconstruction that original trauma and loss make superb sense as a telescope back to the hyperattention for direct pick-up of information as affordances.

5. His experience of "bad emotions" and emotional upheaval was compounded by years of suppression. What was bad then has become even worse now. The original trauma emerged significantly when he was discussing retiring. Not an accidental choice and far from conscious awareness, retirement is stepping out of an identity with four decades of experience. That is an enormous loss hardly mourned, but chosen in the context of the original trauma and telescoped to the current trauma.

6. I then move on with tying the compartments together in the pressing gestalt, based upon Inspector C's presentation of the trauma. I consider the gestalt to be the bridge between the past and present made evident in the telescope. The understanding of this telescope is made clear to Inspector C. My explicit approach is to ensure him that this bridge between the original trauma and the present one is sensible in his eco-ethological understanding. His realization that his adaptation to loss helps diminish some of his distress about fears of being crazy, deficient, cowardly, stupid, and for not having worked through this trauma on his lonesome. I use humor to help him see the absurdity of thinking he can magically work through his trauma. I suggest, "You can don your Superman cape and work through your own trauma by osmosis, if you'd like." We establish a clear reconstruction by interpretation that he is led to by my use of the Socratic method. The sensibility and the eco-ethological mechanism worked well for him. Adaptation is valued and understood as well as the hard work ahead. That is an honest approach that helps him understand the investment and my confidence in him that he can

achieve this difficult goal we have embarked on. I ensure he is with me, and that helps us move on together.

7. I move on toward clarification of an intense ambivalence by Inspector C's choice of retirement as a high-ranking executive, young enough and near enough to promotion to Chief. The attainment of Chief is an explicit goal he alludes to. The status and social power of being an inspector is explicit, and I make it clear I appreciate that fact as a long-invested struggle. The rank that protected his vulnerability to direct pain and loss has lost its ethological function and motivation after two-and-a-half decades in this defensive bulwark. His loss is intense, hardly in conscious awareness, and painfully overwhelming. His paternal style as a commander with his troops, male or female alike, is a protective core. It also allowed his warmth and empathy to be expressed in a culturally acceptable style while protecting his own personal vulnerability to any feelings of dependency. He once again could not stop the harm of a spontaneous shooting. He tells us he was not there, but he has vicariously and personally absorbed the responsibility "as if he was responsible." The protective and paternal function is clearly without mercy as a superego function and as an ethological motivation. He believed he failed in the first shooting by not preventing it and not running in to save his fallen peer, although he would surely die. In the present, he wished that he would have prevented his officer's tragic error. Once again, he bore the responsibility and guilt for both. When we clarified this, the release for him was enormous.

His loss of status is heightened by his hints that, "He was on vacation when the original trauma occurred." In the here and now he tells us, "It was the end of my career" [another vacation of sorts, a wake-up call from numbness followed] "I realized I just did not need this crap anymore. I was working my vacation week." [The retirement choice was made in part by the realization that he could not "deal with the crap anymore." That crap was his disenfranchised loss, including feeling his investment was for naught. The loss of his ability to control the unpredictability of the shootings.]

In Inspector C's case, we realize the parallel and simultaneous conflicts also bridge the gap of space in physics within the dimension of "human time," which Gibson and Schiff reminds us are not equivalent (Gibson, 1966, 1986; Gibson & Gibson, 1955; Schiff, 1979, 1994). Minutes, hours, days, months, and years are counted as *quanta*. That is, events are imprinted, remembered, and at times recalled consciously or unconsciously, based on their meaning and our motivation in remembering or repressing them. In a world shaped by trauma, human time ultimately is linked to memories of loss—the search to find Inspector C's place depends on it. That is integral to placing the loss in its appropriate place and, as Worden suggests, is one task of grief work (Worden, 2001). *For Inspector C, it apparently was human time, not physical, that mattered most.*

Finally, somatic presentation masks grief, and the illness may serve as the consequence of years of suppression conditioned by eco-ethological demands for being the alpha officer. Inspector C's unspoken and cumulative losses may have culminated in part with an undiagnosed minor heart attack he sustained. That minor heart attack may in part be the cost of disenfranchised loss and unconscious existential guilt, owned in silent tragic ownership by Inspector C. The eco-ethological vicarious responsibility intensified with cumulative executive responsibility and exponential complexity in decision making. Helping Inspector C realize the genuine courage he has exemplified in the face of extreme threat offers comfort that can be easily forgotten and never recovered if you do not help him see that truth. Advocating and relieving this guilt and shame undeserved is our goal. In telescoping loss in trauma, we observe how trauma unresolved is crystallized and remains unhealed with of a festering toxicity lurking beneath the surface of a functional dissociation.

Case 6: PPS-CPTSD: Dissociation through Quantum Psychic Moments

Background

Officer R is a single Transit Bureau police officer, with eight years of patrol experience. He is of Jewish American background, not orthodox, and with a firm religious faith. Officer R's faith in God, he tells me, "helps me deal with the trial's of the job." He has confronted many violent criminals in difficult situations underground. Radio contact has been lost at critical times. It is not uncommon in his experience to be doing solo patrol in the subway. While the New York Police Department consists of three bureaus—City, Housing, and Transit—the Transit Bureau is often called the Marine Corps of the Police Department. A majority of officers hold that evaluation. Patrol is often solo for the transit police officer. He is still likely to encounter the most dangerous of situations alone. That terrain includes caverns and subcultures only these officers are privy to. The existential conflicts of not having a steady partner can be daunting. Escalating fear and vigilance are the norm when faced with overwhelming danger. Consider smaller departments and solo patrol is the rule, and factually most departments are small.

Officer R shares with me nearly 100 traumatic events he remembers as a patrol officer. These traumas include stabbings, shootings, and homicides, usually involving robberies. While he presents as somewhat jaded, in truth he is a nice, creative, and witty officer. His extemporaneous lines epitomize what Ker Muir described as a "street corner politician"—extraordinaire (Ker Muir, 1977).

> Officer R presented his trouble as, "feeling upset, snappy, and very anxious at times. I feel tired a lot. I feel like just staying out and not coming into work to deal with the crap I may encounter on the steel horse (subways)."

He presents as anxious and having panic attacks; he describes the most difficult trauma to process as being: surreal situations."

Officer R's Account of his Most Traumatic Event

The worst event is when I was called to a space case. (A space case involves a passenger caught between the platform and the train itself.) The aided, rushing for the train, fell in and got stuck between the broadside of the train and platform." (An "aided" in police terminology describes any person who is the subject of a medical emergency.)

The screeching train spun this aided around, severing the bottom half of his body. The train sealed his midsection allowing him to live until air bags lifted the train. You could smell the cauterized body. As cops, we have to hold the bags underneath the aided, because death is certain and the body falls into the bag.

In the meantime, before the train is lifted, I was the one who had to stand there and have a conversation with this person. The worst is that a cellular phone is there. I remember that cellular, and the person saying goodbye to the family. I listened as the wife and child began to cry. I was trying to make him feel better and be as comfortable as possible. *I cannot figure out how he really felt. I don't know.* We are not taught what to do, not trained to know how to make death notifications when the aided is still alive.

It is *very weird, surreal,* just do what we have to do. I offered food and drinks and was given the order and the train moves on. It makes you feel things that cannot be explained, only felt. It is hard to hold back the tears. *He is dead and alive.* What do you do but take the cellular back, and ship the body parts to the morgue. I cannot forget his smell.

Heuristic Reconstruction of PPS-CPTSD with Officer R

Officer R is up close and intimately involved with the victim who is alive, speaking coherently, and initially hopeful of being rescued. We are made aware of the conflict in modes and the disparate ethological demands of each mode as follows.

Officer R is hurled into this situation involuntarily, without preparation, *his immediate rescue mode is activated.* Seeing Officer R, the victim is likely to believe he is going to be rescued, especially being unaware of the massive internal damage. The cauterization of the body in the midsection is soon realized by Officer R, but not the victim. That hope is immediately conveyed to Officer R. That hope gets more desperate. His plea for reassurance from Officer R increases as he realizes he is not able to move.

The victim is unsure of what happened, but he is conscious and in a suspended state of dying, teetering on life. Officer R must tell the victim that the situation is dire, and attempt to achieve landline communication to the victim's family, letting them know he is mortally injured. At the same time this communication is heard by the victim, informing him he will die even though at this moment he is fully alive and ever-present as a human being. In addition, Officer R is establishing communication with his central command, these goals in preparation for activating what we will call *the death notification identity mode*.

The intimate bonding evoked by the aided person's distress and by Officer R's human compassion is intense. It is also infused with anxious uncertainty. The relatedness and vicarious experience for Officer R is unconscious, visceral, and nonverbal. In part, it is also conscious, verbal, and emotional. His overriding preoccupation and dominant role is infused with his wish to comfort the victim. We call this Officer R's *comforter* identity mode, which is now active.

These roles of death notification and comforter are replete with conflict. They are simultaneously active. Social distance is impossible to maintain, yet equally heartbreaking to let go. The situational demands of the psychic quantum moment for social distance is learned in part through impersonal descriptions and dehumanization by using such terms as "space case," and "body parts" transmitted by intragenerational meaning from senior officer to rookie officer in the transit bureau. The person to whom Officer R is responding is imploring with his eyes. The fact is the situation is beyond the control of Officer R to correct. A human bond is forged existentially in the life-and-death encounter with the innocent victim. This bond is ethological in terms of the functional value of Officer R's rescue role and the interpersonal relationship and existential encounter in the comforter identity mode.

This bonding is not afforded in Officer R's ecological niche. He and the victim become intimately bonded in their shared knowledge of life being literally held together by a thread. That thread is under the control of the officer's direct command through telecommunication. Although he will let central command know when to move the train, he is helpless against that imperative decision. The moment the train moves on, death occurs. It is Officer R as a police officer who will say move on to police communications. He has no choice. The existential burden now places Officer R *squarely into the executioner identity mode*.

In understanding the impact for Officer R, the surreal is the antiaffordance impacted by the death through the train being activated and the body organs being emptied into a body bag. *Officer R must safeguard all possessions and the body parts for collection by the city morgue in his custodial identity mode*, and then write up the professional report in the dry, vacant words of an incident report.

Officer R explains the space case to me methodically. His sensory modalities here are predominately olfactory and visual. The smell and visual memory is more than likely encoded in his brain for life. Emotional distance from the event suggests an active ambivalence and functional dissociation that is activated in the here and now. The perception in Officer R's description supports a gauging of the impact, "very weird . . . surreal . . . I cannot figure out how he really feels . . . I don't know . . . I cannot forget his smell . . . smell the cauterized body" [olfactory dominance].

Hints include a social distance of the victim being classified as an "aided" and in concrete terms of "body parts." This distance is usual when public-safety professionals discuss death. Social distance is afforded and learned as a functional adaptation to death, especially gruesome death. Emotional, existential, and cognitive impact is not adaptive by this defense. Answers are hardly afforded by a social distance placed between the officer who has shared the quantum impact of a developing relationship with a fully living human being in the most tragic of moments. While the event could be measured in physical minutes, the human time for functional dissociation is resonate with loss: trauma, guilt, anxiety, rage, fantasy, distortion, helplessness, and horror. That loss when complex, disenfranchised, and masked is indeterminate.

This type of trauma has all the aspects of an ethological antiaffordance; it is surreal, not afforded ethologically in his experiential repertoire. His own mortality is at stake too. This is unmentioned (not as bravado) as much as it is a denial of personal vulnerability. Factually, one jerky movement of the train could crush him too. Through training and experience in his eco-ethological niche, he is aware of this outcome. The affordance of the cellular phone is now an altered object. In terms of eco-ethology, it affords a radically changed symbol of an antiaffordance. Fear and anxiety related to the event is inhibited. His cellular phone is symbolically transformed as an antiaffordance. This serves a therapeutic usefulness as a symbol that is more likely to be accepted in helping the therapist ease communication associated with the violent accidental death. The cellular phone is confirmed as an invariant symbol of the trauma by Officer R avoiding any type of cellular phone off duty as a painful antiaffordance.

Eco-Ethological Existential Analytic Intervention with Officer R

Clarifying Officer R's trauma includes understanding his experience of personal vulnerability, mortality, and meaning in light of the train accident and the multiple conflicts in his emergent identity modes.

When the modes are examined more thoroughly, as we will reconstruct them, there is denial, depersonalization, derealization, and inhibition of loss. The demands on this officer are multiple, contradictory, and once again he is disenfranchised. This type of accident is not rare in the public-service officer's eco-ethological niche. There are many similar cases of accident events in which the service professional has multiple and conflicting roles without a prior adaptation. The eco-ethological perspective I present is psycho-educational, insight oriented, and existentially meaningful to Officer R. It is the first time a heuristic perspective is offered, where Officer R learns how to make sense of what he perceived as surreal and made acceptable in our reconstruction and confrontation of the loss in the trauma. This approach is highly effective in relieving stress.

Multiple conflicts emerge in the situational demands of the five identity modes experienced. Let's clarify the conflict within each mode and between each with the other. That clarity of role conflict will help us in our strategic interventions as follows:

1. *The rescue identity mode:* Officer R's objective here is to save the injured person. The effort, training, and all energy is to render medical first aid and get the victim to a medical facility. The rescue identity mode is complementary with the comforter identity mode, and oppositional with the identity modes of executioner, death notifier, and custodian. The rescue identity mode values the victim as a fully human being. The reality is due to the severe injuries, there is no way for Officer R to effect his goal.

2. *The custodial identity mode:* The objective here is identification and removal of body parts and an accurate collection of information and witness testimony, including the officer who reports his account in the third person— the reality is identifying a human being as body parts. The interviewing of the victim to gain information, before death, while actively coordinating the other identity modes, is dissonant in cognitive, existential, and emotional goals of rescue and comfort to the victim. The dehumanization helps in the moment to distance the officer from the reality of the tragic medical emergency the victim is experiencing. The "as if" schema in which a human being is reduced to body parts is part of the functional dissociation necessitated by Officer R's custodial identity modes.

3. *The death-notification identity mode:* The objective here is informing the family of what is happening, while the victim is witnessing the entire communication as it is unfolding. The reality is that the victim is alive as Officer R is explaining his imminent death to his family. Officer R is there not as witness but as a participant in the man's death. Death is made morbid by the situational demands that are contradictory and functionally dissociated, meaning the victim is proclaimed dead before he is dead. This reality is made explicit without resolution in existential terms for Officer R.

4. *The comforter identity mode:* Officer R's objective is to engage in a genuine relationship with another human. His forging an encounter with the victim is achieved with intimacy, fear, and hope that few people may encounter in an entire lifetime. R activates his rescue identity mode, leading up to the tragic moment when life ends abruptly—he invests his energy into saving life. At the same time, he reduces the reality of an encounter with a human being into a dehumanized dead human being.

5. *The executioner identity mode:* Officer R's objective here is compliance with the situational demand to make a police command decision for the train to move on. In making his choice, the simultaneous release of the train will sever the body parts into a body bag, effecting death. When Officer R decides to move the

train, the dismemberment begins. Putting it in the perspective of conflict, a functional dissociation is forced when the comforter identity mode is followed by the executioner and custodial identity mode in one "blinking moment" to another. The custodial identity mode includes going to the morgue attendant/medical examiner confirming the accidental death, transporting the victim, and usually a reidentification of the victim. Officer R will have to go the following day to identify the victim in the morgue—standard operating procedure. This role and loss remained unidentified, as the others. Unconscious guilt and annihilation fears were discovered along with nightmares with the repeated motif of death by cauterization as Officer R had been involved in so many identity modes and conflicts hardly resolved.

The importance of using the Socratic method to make the contradictory roles clear cannot be underestimated. The identity modes and the conflicts are brought to awareness with the understanding that they developed in the ecological and ethological influences of what is a tragedy.

I suggest that in working through the insight phase, going through the basic steps, gauging how expansive each antiaffordance is within each identity mode and clarifying the situational demands of command decisions by Officer R within that identity mode is key toward healing. Keep in mind this is not considered a trauma. *Validating the derealization experience of these identity modes is the beginning of working through.* Identification of feelings he is unaware of and has disowned is important.

The officer is an active participant and is likely actively suffering guilt, fear, and revulsion. Keep in mind this event may have been held in silence for years. The beginning of clarifying Officer R's identity modes, conflict, defenses, and emotional upheaval is achieved by placing them in the eco-ethological perspective. In effect, once this process has begun, we have initiated the healing process for Officer R, helping put the trauma in its rightful place in his life.

Case 7: PPS-CPPSD: Det. Q's Altered States of Identity and Dissociation Crystallized

Background

Detective Q is a 41-year-old married Asian American undercover detective. She is a nurturing mom, grandmother, and wife. Her maternal and domestic responsibility is very important in her life. Her husband is also in a service profession. Our work in therapy has been ongoing for a number of years. She is highly perceptive and has a deep spiritual belief that is deistic rather than parochial. Her analytic, practical, and emotional intelligence is sharp and incisive. She recently finished her college degree. Her ecological influences are a combined 19 years of public service in an A House (Extremely Active Command). After three years of patrol, she was put onto a track for detective, and she has excelled in her position. Her command presence is at times aggressive and energetic. She is fully committed to therapy. We work weekly with double and triple sessions. She is warm and likeable. Rage, anxiety, and grief enveloped in multiple trauma have crystallized into what I suggest are different personality identity modes of defensiveness. She is not a Sybil.[1] Maladaptation to chaotic and changing surroundings has framed her separate identity modes through a concrete jungle where guerrilla warfare is a constant and real threat.

Det. Q's Account of Her Most Traumatic Event

I don't use the word trauma, Doc. I feel that is my way of life. Here I don't accept that word. The worst event I can remember is not the shootings, stabbings, and being shot at by perps, but the day during our operation when my man (another undercover she is covering) came to my side helping me during a take down (a planned undercover arrest situation).

The perp said, "I could hurt you, bitch." I told him, "I'll hurt you too. Excuse me, you talking to me? Yeah, okay, you give me something. I give you something." My man (her partner, whose cover is as a dealer) came up to defend me. We had a bad situation. Before I knew it, I took a few slaps. He was talking and I took a few, but maintained. He (her partner) checked out a weapon being taken out to dust me. I didn't see my partner in the hustle. He let off a round to stop the bad guy, and it grazed my head. I mean, I was almost shot. I never thought friendly fire would come down on me by another cop I really respect and would take any hill with him, we are blood (bonding is like brother and sister). It brought my job 180 degrees dealing with the bad guys as the only danger, it made me realize that one of my own could take me out just like that.

I now have 360 degrees of awareness, and constant checking out everyone. A family member of my team could take me out. Always know the person I am with. Dig that, you know, I mean, I always know who on the team I could trust with what, and what not to rely on. That shot really blew my mind, wow! I am happy to talk with you about it! No anger, XX is still my man. We are tight and hang. You know, certain bonding never ends. I forgive him. I know he didn't mean it like that. *It was a deceleration in time for me. Everything slowed down. I have never been the same on the team since then.*

It is the nature of the job for me to deal with perps, but this was new. I didn't think it would happen to me (returning to the event itself). That dude, the bad guy, was a giant that walked over, six-foot plus. The EDP he was with almost cut my face. If I wasn't a certain orientated way knowing I will survive, he would not have held back.

She meant to cut me, and she was the first I totally went face to face with (change in voice is radical, aggressive, and hostile). A minute of total

---

[1] Sybil, who suffered from 16 distinct personality alters which resulted from an extremely dominant mother/father, is distinct from Det. Q's crucible of ongoing immersion in a world of police deep cover trauma and loss (Schreiber, 1973).

aggression, that team is not coming in fast enough. 145 X Avenue. This is one of the buildings I hate going into. I become mean, you hear me, mean! I will go home and my crew as well. It is like the total package when I go inside. You get in that conversation on the street with other hood members, your partner is lost, and you can get taken down. I hate the fact I will get hurt.

I am the only female on my team—that's cool. I got to watch their asses. They had that look, will take her and her man. The only thing that stopped him was my mean ass. I will shoot you if you try to hurt me. My stomach hurts, I come in full force, and that I think stresses me. My gun punches out in the face. They don't play there. Every apartment is dirty. People totaled just like that. I hate that building. The way men perceive me is they know me, my style. I went from bitch mode into my Bette Davis, getting him calm. We did not break cover. I played with him, same man, and night. *I cannot feel sorry for myself. It's my job*; it's a matter of fact, simple as that, you know the deal. (Her voice changes into the voice of one of the hoods) I cased the area to get info. Making the buy and bust. You punk pansy mother f_____ . My team knows: they see me, they give me total respect. I do my share but I kept it from the team.

Eco-Ethological Existential Analytic Intervention with Detective Q: Heuristic Reconstruction of PPS-CPTSD with Detective Q

Detective Q's experience with trauma is not discrete (it is not one incident), it is a continuous experience of quantum psychic moments. Like our prior example of Officer T, trauma is a daily way of life. However, Detective Q's trauma is more complex and elusive. Why? *If we put in perspective her response to what is afforded in her eco-ethological niche, we understand Detective Q must embrace the undercover identities as her own. If she fails to be convincing, the consequence to her is death.*

The layout of antiaffordances Detective Q experiences is a discrete split from her prior adaptations as a patrol officer. The survival value for her is intense. While not traditionally thought of as a trauma, the sacrifice of one's identity to achieve a public service is a severe, indeterminate trauma. Such trauma as Detective Q experiences, while culturally sanctioned, remains largely hidden from others, including one's peers.

A culture of secrecy speaks loudly to the silence of disenfranchised loss in officer-patient Q. That loss is in part effected day in and day out as she attempts to maintain her separate identities in her domestic, civilian identity as a wife, mom, and grandmother. This is in striking opposition to her identity as a deep-cover operative. The expectation of the public-safety department is that Detective Q establish and maintain the same identity, clear in her mind, across her ecological demands as an undercover, as a uniformed police detective, and in her personal life. What we are clear about is that the ecological demands of separate identity modes are in essence so infused with survival value that they warrant being viewed as separate identities. These identity differences we will distinguish as dissociated identity modes, rather than as separate personalities. Detective Q's experience affords radically different meaning for each personality identity mode. Prior to our reconstruction of Detective Q's identity modes, let's examine the context of her eco-ethological niche.

It soon becomes apparent that the rituals, symbols, and the language of the perpetrators she infiltrates imbues her daily interactions. Detective Q accommodates intrapersonal development with the full influence of the eco-ethological meaning of these interactions in human time. Separate and distinct is the fact that not only her survival, but that of each member of her unit relies on a deception being accepted by real criminals. Her status in the unit (her peers and supervisors who really only know the level of her commitment and work) is reinforced from a primal to an existential level. This endowed status is contingent on being able to employ her identity as if she is a member of the gang from which she gathers intelligence. The intelligence gathered in sting operations is critical for making decisions to move in: when, how, and where.

Sting operations can last for days, months, even years. The wartime ego is front line and contingent upon active deception. That deception is expected to be switched on and off at will. It is this impossibility that warrants our attention and our commitment to working on reconstructing the distinct impact on Detective Q's dissociation process as her major presentation of PPS-CPTSD. The identity of being a criminal has its own affordances, behavioral repertoire, cognitions, and mores. This, I hypothesize, becomes imprinted, and like other trauma will remain perhaps lifelong. In this type of trauma, not only are role conflicts, psychophysical stimulation/inhibition extant, but identity itself. Predominantly, Detective Q's mode is intuitive and sensory. Understanding here means appreciating survival as an undercover. It is not playing a role, it is the most serious of business, it is living her multiple identity modes. The impact specifically on Detective Q to live in identity modes and maintain her overall sense of self begs understanding.

As Detective Q initially compartmentalizes her traumatic loss "as a matter of fact," here, I need to find out which identity mode is being presented, when, why, and how. I am keen on finding out what ethological demands and ecological factors have set up what defense, how intense it is, and in my exploration what type of resistance am I likely to encounter. I am respectful, meaning I appreciate the maladaptive sensibility of her behaviors. My empathy and compassion for Detective Q is made explicit as is the hard work we will have to encounter together. My active empathy in handling countertransference feelings of my own disgust over her identity modes that emerge in our work is overcome by my compassion for her ingenuity, courage, and humanity. My stance is that "identity dissociation" is a result of ecological conditioning, shaping through affordances in her unit, and her attempt to maintain meaning in response to cumulative trauma. I avoid using the term "roles," which implies a range of adaptation from acting in a style of which the participant is at least partially aware. The personality style being influenced by eco-ethological motivation cannot be ignored. Judgment of her identity modes is disenfranchising, biased, and furthers blaming the victim.

The value of deception is another critical issue and is contingent upon personal survival, as well as the other members of her niche. The undercover-detective work entails deception of one's own identity. This is a new dimension we will need to understand. Being able to place her identity mode in the perspective of an eco-ethological framework is crucial to reaching her. It also is invaluable in motivating Detective Q to continue in the trauma work all severe dissociation requires. Her relationships with perpetrators is ripe with conflict, for she deals with them, breaks bread, has intimate moments with them, and knows them as individuals. Some losses emerge in this regard. She is sensitive to her necessary double life, which leads to unearned guilt about this often unacknowledged double bind she is left alone to sort through. The beatings she has sustained have no justice, even in prosecution it is not acknowledged but is endured nonetheless. We work on finding existential meaning through suffering. This meaning is not masochism—as in suffering for martyrdom—but, as Detective Q knows better than many, it is necessary to achieve her vocation, as her calling in life.

Suggestions for Approaching PPS-CPTSD with Detective Q

How do we initially intervene with Detective Q's presentation of different modes of identities? Her most significant identity mode is the "Aggressor Perpetrator" but it is critical to realize this is not just a role. Her identity is more than just a relational configuration, it is nested in her (mal)adaptation for survival in earnest. It is evident that drive derivatives of aggression and sexual origin are acted on as compromise formations in the daily adaptation to repetitive trauma. Survival skills can be very sophisticated, and the adaptation requires the lower to higher level coordination of skills that are automatic, reflexive, and sophisticated.

Trust and support is essential in our developing transference, it is key to gaining a hold on countertransference. That we will learn a great deal from Detective Q's adaptive and maladaptive skills is humbling as well as challenging. It enables us to gain skills as a therapist. In a sense, she will partially identify with the aggressor. That identity-mode alter is separate and distinct from her other identity-mode alters. Finding out how much distance and how sharp these boundaries are drawn are important. Her incorporation of the perpetrator's way of thinking has been forged. In her verbatim example, she is likely to express to you the lingo she uses in the street. She has also established a defensive constellation within her ecology; she will not hesitate to act on what she perceives as a threat in that ecology.

It is important to note the differences in cognition, affect, and behavioral responses when she is in that mode of relating to you. Trauma work will support that very ambiance through a vicarious reexperiencing of the full valence of each alter identity. Being respectful and supportive of each alter is important in the work you do. If you think I am accentuating respect of Detective Q's defenses, I am, and I do!

Let us move forward in setting a structure of initial intervention by defining each identity-mode alter Detective Q expresses. In doing so, I will make some specific suggestions about how to approach that alter in general terms of grief work. Remember, her losses include threats and real trauma to her personal integrity. With this in mind, I will not repeat the interventions reviewed in other cases, they can be adapted to working with Detective Q's alter identities. That is especially relevant in role conflicts, situational demands, resistance, and constellations of eco-ethological defenses. Keeping in mind each identity mode develops in the context of multiple permutations evoked in her defensive constellation. When they emerge in therapy, in part they may be a response to the traumatic event we are working on, including transference and countertransference influences. Keep this in mind. An intelligence particular to that alter identity complements a specific type of resistance and defense. Let us put these identity modes in eco-ethological context:

1. Aggressor Perpetrator Identity: This mode may be understood in part through ". . . identification with the aggressor" (Freud, 1936). Detective Q establishes her identity as a perpetrator to develop a deep understanding and to gather evidence for prosecution. However, her intent initially is quite different from what is typically characterized as the Stockholm Syndrome, an identification with the aggressor, although she is not a hostage. However, her relationships with perpetrators must be real, intense, and intimate to be accepted into their cadre. At times, deep-cover officers sustain beatings as has Detective Q. She has received direct threats to her life; invariably and inescapably physical assaults are exacerbated by a culture that often characterizes women as "bitches and holes," the vernacular for prostitutes and objects to be used. Detective Q embraces her alter identity as aggressor perpetrator. If she does not succeed, it is not an issue of losing the case; it is her own and other officers' lives that are endangered with a cruel death. Not to experience overwhelming dissonance by "leaking out a bad vibe," Detective Q protects herself through overidentification with her criminal identity. The value of deception is contingent upon personal survival as well as the survival of other members of her niche. The undercover-detective work entails deception of one's own identity. This is a new dimension we will need to understand. Being able to place her identity modes in the perspective of an eco-ethological framework is crucial to our reaching her. It also is invaluable in motivating Detective Q to continue in the trauma work as all severe dissociation requires.

2. The Elite Police Identity Mode: In the public-service macrocommunity, this mode entails a distinct position of authority and status. It also creates competition among other elite units and patrol officers. Officers in this unit are subject to integrity tests and scrutiny above and beyond most other units. She and her peers are likely to have harsh media and internal investigative probes if something goes wrong. Not that there is a conspiracy on the part of the department or media, but because the elite nature of the unit is akin to celebrity status once exposed. The exposure is unlikely to be for all unit personnel, but publicity destroys confidentiality and confidentiality of officer identity is paramount for safety.

3. The Combat Identity Mode: Protective bonding elicited in unfolding situations is remarkably effective in shielding other officers from assault or assassination attempts. All units in the Uniformed Services support taking responsibility for an officer's partner and his well-being and physical integrity while protecting oneself. However, making a very human mistake can be mercilessly exacting on an officer given the highly skilled training that such elite unit members receive. Detective Q has worked through many difficult courses and has experienced multiple traumas in her cumulative experience. All of which has the added influences of guerrilla warfare in her covert role. She will have to go into full survival combat identity mode if the criminal group she is affiliated with realizes her identity and her cover is blown. If another member is in imminent danger, she will be forced to act, at great risk, on that threat. Detective Q is acutely aware of this risk and calls it standard operating procedure. As with all of these identity alters, we will seek to observe how she deals with these anticipatory schemas bound with survival value.

4. Field Executive Identity Mode: Regardless of any detective's rank, autonomy of decision making at critical moments is demanded when a situation is compromised or contact is lost (e.g., in the apartment of the drug dealer). Command presence is not optimal. It is absolute, for hesitation is death. The mental strain and emotional intelligence required for this position, while unknown, is by necessity high. The officer must keep others convinced and also act as an emotionally stabilizing force in the midst of criminals who live by another set of mores, rules, and taboos at odds with what usually is expected of officers. The constant strain of this identity at the highest levels of responsibility and autonomous decision making is oppositional to the Uniformed Officer Identity Mode.

5. Uniformed Officer Identity-Mode: No matter the assignment, the same responsibility and venue of "use of force" is exacted by internal units and outside agencies, including the U.S. and District Attorney Offices. Some leeway is given, but legal parameters remain intact. This means the accountability of each officer for a high level of integrity is more exacting for deep-cover officers than for their peers on patrol. The stress and strain here is in contradiction to the other identity modes as one must remain constantly vigilant to protect their hidden identity. All aspects of identity are reactionary to situational demands.

6. Peacetime Identity Mode: The homecoming *that veterans of war have experienced is well known in literature. The demands made on the undercover to turn off the hyper-stimulation, hypervigilance, hyperattention of the identities above when in civilian company,* including family and community is largely unknown.

The conflict, opposition, and often-times eco-ethological existential collision of the multiple identity modes with Detective Q's home-front peacetime identity yields a homecoming collision every day with a public-safety combat-related on-and-off switch.

The strain, stress, and existential anguish at the deepest levels of Detective Q's, identity is exemplified by her response to my question about her clarity of her own identity; she responded, "Who am I really? I really just don't know anymore." The question is poignant. I must provide the time and help for Detective Q to find her answer. As we start to intervene in addressing what we do know, we need to define what we don't know about Detective Q. A harsh reality for us is that integration is an ideal worth pursuing, but not necessarily accomplished. What does need to be taken into account is that Detective Q may remain resistant to major changes, no matter how much insight you deliver.

Our good intention that may lead us to persistently confronting Detective Q to leave her unit may backfire if she perceives this as a devaluation of her self. If she believes that she may think we ignore her life work and prized achievements. *This is similar to my own premature, ill placed suggestion to Officer T to change his detail. It could have derailed our alliance. Fortunately it did not.*

Appreciating the difficult truth for the clinician means that small therapeutic changes are keen advantages in improved quality of life. The choice and responsibility for self-actualization and integration may come only from within the patient, not without. That choice and responsibility for self-actualization is incredibly difficult to achieve. At times the patient and clinician need to trade places to be effective. Otherwise, an oak podium may replace the couch, and the navigator the pilot.

Identity dissociation is the least addressed issue of trauma in public service. This may be social denial that filters down to the clinician's denial of the classic psychoanalytic foundation. It may equally be made difficult by sensational account that hardly resemble realistic depictions of identity dissociation. The integration of the identity alters of Detective Q is challenging. This is not a failure of the therapist or patient. Further, our insight is that these dissociative experiences and complex trauma are not part of an insidious plan by uncaring police supervisors, but quite the opposite. Detective Q is immersed on the front lines by living her assignment. Indubitably she is a covert combat veteran behind the lines. Breaking bread, having intimate encounters with gang members, and cultural infiltration works both ways. She is never likely to get acknowledgment for her sacrifice. Her real identity, courage, and value are invisible to others, except her unit members. I have seen no fewer than five different presentations of identity in this complex and wonderfully resilient humane being. This is not in spite of, but because of what she has endured.

It is helpful to pay attention to the different voices (i.e., tone, accent, pitch, semantics, and syntax) presented in the context of trauma. I have also observed different levels of cognitive, emotional, and behavioral intelligence of identity alters. Suggestions that a predisposition for less intelligent officers to choose plainclothes assignment, from anticrime to deep-cover units, is unsubstantiated. I suggest the more successful officers in these assignments have higher intelligence, greater sensitivity, an ability to dissociate, tolerance of frustration, highlighting above-average resilience.

I keep in mind that Detective Q is not a series of alter identity modes, but a whole, unique person. Integration of her identity modes is the long-term goal that requires a clarity on our part as clinicians. To help her heal and move toward a more wholesome lifestyle is an awesome challenge. It is matched by her unusual ability to accommodate to the multiple identity alters without total decompensation. Detective Q's same maladaptation is what can be redirected into our goal of integration. I believe that integration is accomplished through directed insight and supportive therapy. I need her full cooperation as she will be doing the hardest work. Identifying dissociation does not support it, it validates and normalizes a maladaptive process. Rather than perjoration, the need for survival exacts a price. That understanding you make explicit.

Case 8: PPS-CPTSD: Addicted to Trauma through a Social Distance Kaleidoscope

Background

Officer T is a 38-year-old married Irish American, with three children from his first marriage. He is of Roman Catholic faith. Although Officer T is not a fully practicing Catholic, he is faithful to his religious convictions. That conviction as a Catholic includes bearing his suffering well and with humility. Humility is defined by Officer T as having faith in a higher being and bearing unavoidable suffering with human dignity. Officer T intimates his faith has been lost in a whirlwind of police work and in the pits of endless and brutal suffering he has encountered. This spark of faith that is dimmed will be piqued as a center to strike the chord of motivation in the face of what has become distant losses, which have turned a cloud of optimism and ideals into the dark billows of a storm. He has completed one year of college and is seriously considering going back to finish his degree. He let me know his relationship with his wife, a full-time stay-at-home, is stressful. He attributes much of the stress to his public-safety work. His experience of 14 years on patrol has been divided between an A and B House. These houses are characterized as extremely active and very active commands respectively. His cumulative experience on the street is nothing less than that of a combat veteran. What we identified were 48 specific traumatic events out of hundreds estimated. He told me upfront: "I'm fine Doc, nothing is wrong. I feel like vegetating at times, couldn't give a shit attitude. When there is boredom, I need some excitement. My wife asked me to see you. I'll give you a try."

Yet, Officer T kept away from bar hopping, intoxication, alcoholism, and other addictive behaviors, even the topless bars often visited during choir practice. Officer T had no history of bipolar or other disorders. Born into an impoverished area himself, he chose public service to help others, for a secure position, and to pull himself out of that lifestyle. He had a great deal of compassion for the people he observed as victims. He had disdain, hate, and disgust for the inept and indifferent attitude he perceived that afforded an ecology of crime and violence. Officer T's unique skills include being able to construct a cabinet, fix a motor vehicle engine, or open any lock. He is bright, energetic, and acutely aware. He is gifted in practical and creative intelligence.

Officer T's Account of his Most Traumatic Event

In one week I saw the lives of three children ruined. One child was dragged under a car driven by a drunk driver who jumped a curb where this boy was playing hockey in front of his building. The car dragged this kid along a 25-foot entranceway, and all the way up to the stoop of his building. Then we cops and people from the building tipped the car off its wheels and pulled the lifeless kid out. The screams of his family will forever be with me. . . . Later that week, I saw the inhumane and cowardly act of two adults. They left an 11-year-old boy alone to explain to police how his 9-year-old brother was shot to death. It was obvious that the child had been coached by the aunt and uncle he lived with. They had left the boy alone in their apartment with his dead brother and a bad story to take the heat for them. Both kid's lives were destroyed. That was sad.

You know, I have been involved in violent struggles, I had guns pointed at me. I have been shot at. All of it makes me very angry. I have been struck with bottles, thrown off the roof, I had stitches, causing glass to lodge in my eye. I have had bricks thrown from rooftops, smashing the windshield when I was on patrol (from housing projects). I also remember carrying an off-duty cop in my arms who was shot by his girlfriend into Columbia Presbyterian Hospital. I was the first car to pull up behind XX Pct at CPMS as they pulled officer XX out of it and into the hospital where he died.

I have seen several drug dealers meet their end in a bloody mess. I confess it never bothered me. But there was an exception once when one of them was shot as he drove his car and his brains and blood were scattered on his wife and child. I have seen others die as well. One other in a vestibule who was shot several times in the back he was trying to say something to me which I tried to understand, and he held my hand. I just couldn't understand. I'll never know (long pause).

I also was involved in a running gun battle of four armed perps, which began on YY Street and XX Avenue and ended in the Bronx near XX

Avenue. It ended in a fistfight on the XX expressway. I won. He went to jail. I responded with my partner to the sounds of shots near 163rd and XX Avenue. As we drew near, the amount of shots increased dramatically as we turned the corner and joined transit and housing anticrime cops. The perp had wedged his way between the bumpers of 2 parked cars. He was laying on the trunk dying, his gun just out of reach.

I was involved in a chase of armed perp's who robbed a guy in a jewelry store, just a hard working guy on XX Street. He shot the guy. We had to catch this perp. We were in the mode. We got him at an 85 miles per hour clip and he had a collision. I remember watching the perp in the back seat open the door, and for reasons I'll never know, he just stared at me and sat down. I went straight for him to collar him, he pulls out a .38 revolver from his band. I then grabbed his firearm as he pointed at me. Another perp was raising his gun at my head—my partner quickly fired on him. The shot nearly grazed my head, but killed him.

Heuristic Reconstruction of PPS-CPTSD with Officer T

Officer T presents multiple traumas in succession. It seems as if he is in a rush to get it all out, so to speak. His presentation of trauma appears to be offered in a *seemingly haphazard way*. I hypothesize his stream of consciousness is almost manic in his recall of traumatic events. I will later discard the hypothesis. He may have manic-depression. I will affirm that he presents trauma in a manic rush. Some psychodynamic hypotheses emerge (grievance collecting, sadism to share with therapist, condensation of trauma). I keep these emerging working hypotheses in mind to return to later. All hypotheses are tentative predictions. Some will be altered and some dismissed in the process of our approach with Officer T.

We have some immediate groundwork to do. Let's take a view toward reconstructing of Officer T's verbatim narrative of trauma. The sequence of presentation may help us better understand his defenses in response to conflict and multiple trauma. In this perspective, what is likely is that the conflicts in Officer T's mind are repeated in his narrative of the events. That is, the compartmentalization matches the breakdown of each type of trauma into different episodic and discrete memories, which emerge spontaneously in recall. A pattern of overload, and an uninterrupted sequence of different events signals possible categorization. Perhaps a compartmentalization of trauma, an encoded memory, is placed within human time and space as significant. This emotional memory and psychophysiological memory evidenced by Officer T's narrative may become hardwired in police and public-safety officers dealing with cumulative trauma as suggested by the vast literature with combat veterans (Cannon, 1914; Goleman, 1992, 1994; Giller, 1990; Krystal, 1968; Krystal, Kosten, Perry, Southwick, Mason, & Giller, 1989; Southwick, 2005; Thorp, 2005; Van Der Kolk, Greenberg, Boyd, & Krystal, 1985; Yehuda, Resnick, Kahana, & Giller, 1993).

Officer T's recounting of traumatic events assures us that we are reasonably certain of intense loss, anger, and anxiety, all revolving around the loss and existential crisis attendant in how to continue doing his work upstream in a spiral downstream where trauma is without surcease. Why does he continue with his work and not move to a different unit?

In part, we are given clues through Officer T's description of trauma, which is delivered as if he were describing his experiences as a third-party narrator. That social distance is as telling as his mode of disclosure. His social distance is replete with action empathy, while emotional empathy is denied expression.

The affordance of this trauma experience includes experimental traumatic neurosis (conditioned excitation-inhibition), functional dissociation, telescoping, and anticipatory trauma. Yet, Officer T adds an additional distinct dimension: being addicted to trauma. This addiction offers a unique perspective common to those who have remained voluntarily, or involuntarily, in a war zone for many years. The contradiction is, "he did not want to leave this way of life." That choice was his to make as we will see shortly. Why does he choose this war zone, with his considerable gifts of motivation and existential meaning?

We will first seek an answer as to whether there is any pattern to his presentation that is not unseemly or chaotic, but which is sensible within our eco-ethological approach.

The *first trauma cluster is Officer T's involvement in the murder of two children, and, as he put it, the third child's "life is destroyed."* What is important is his estimation that the surviving child's life is full of overwhelming trauma. If he is aware of that for this child, we will have an inroad toward his own interpretation of what he experiences vicariously day in and day out. We are privy to a partial window into the ecology of the trauma Officer T is actively involved in.

Specifically, the first trauma is a child victim killed by a driving-while-intoxicated driver (the family, community, Officer T, and his partner are on the scene). Officer T is actively involved in a rescue-officer role, which is forfeited with the child's death. Officer T's sense of failure is compounded by the community assistance and his simultaneous comforter role also being ineffective as, "the screams of his family will forever be with me." The underlying cause of this tragedy is adult negligence. We are then graduated to another murder caused by adult-negligent homicide, again in which one child is accidentally shot and the brother is left to explain an alibi to Officer T, who is empathically attuned to his young victim's helpless plight.

How are we reasonably assured he is empathically attuned when this is hidden?

Evidence is offered when the surviving child is classified as suffering the conniving and exploitation that does not get past Officer T's awareness. He knows this psychic burden of exploitation and antisocial irresponsibility placed on the dead child's brother as survivor is likely to mar him for life so badly that both the dead brother and the living brother are equated. Officer T articulates his rage toward the uncle and aunt indirectly: "inhumane and cowardly." Officer T achieves a social distance from the perpetrators, placing them in one sphere and himself and the victims in another. Existential despair and rage are summarily treated and closed: "That was sad." I am reasonably certain to probe deeper into what sad means to Officer T, in his own good time, not mine.

The second cluster of ecological trauma continues with an abrupt break from children being killed through adult criminal negligence. Now Officer T presents his own vulnerability as a compromise in which anger replaces loss. *Anger is acceptable when a sacred victim is attacked,* even when that sacred victim is that officer himself. Injuries are alluded to and a rationale for having rage, and perhaps unconscious murderous wishes. We notice he expressed no personal fear or loss, even though Officer T has had bricks thrown at him. The massive denial is a matter-of-fact defense that serves a functional dissociation. But why does this trauma cluster emerge after the context of the first trauma cluster? It may be easier and made sensible in the internal social-distance gauge officers use (see chapter 4). Put in context, an immediate distance is placed in between the helpless children victims, who are uninvolved victims, and the sacred victim where anger toward the offender is not blocked but loss is minimized. This cluster ends with another sacred victim who pays the ultimate price and dies in Officer T's helpless arms. The cluster begins with an assault on Officer T and ends with the murder of a peer (*this most intimate and sacred of violations was descriptive with only anger expressed and devoid of any other emotion). Loss and fear, both taboo, are not mentioned.*

Now we are brought into a third cluster of ecological trauma. We are brought into the bloody mess of drug dealers who pay the price for their malice with death. Note the words "I confess it never bothered me." We are aware this may be a reaction formation, a preemptive declaration felt by the confessor as shameful to express. In other words, Officer T is really saying, "The death of this dealer bothers me, and therefore I need to confess to you." What comes next when heard in this perspective has a new meaning: "But, there was an *exception,* once one of them was shot . . . his brains and blood were scattered on his wife and child. . . ." Officer T finds it impossible to express his direct shock, fear, and loss for a deserving victim. His existential despair is alluded to in his "being bothered," once he qualifies this feeling as exceptional. Why? Because it is taboo to express loss when the person killed is considered a deserving victim within department culture, and within his eco-ethological niche. However, Officer T's loss leaks out through his choice of words, the "bloody mess" that he cannot make sense of within his eco-ethological niche. When such terrorism has been experienced, a compulsion to correct what is unprocessed and emotionally overwhelming may motivate attempts to fix that injustice. Officer T holds the cherished ideal that being a good cop—a good soldier—is to protect and clean up the violence. This goal is furthered by not leaving his brother and sister officers in his niche alone. It may be that motivation, in part, that draws Officer T closer to his solution by staying in the urban war zone while being simultaneously repelled.

He lets us know he witnessed the death of many others. This is followed by the dealer "in a vestibule who was shot several times in the back . . . trying to say something to me . . . I tried to understand . . . he held my hand . . . I just couldn't understand. I'll never know. . . ."

The narration of the dealer being killed in front of his wife is allowed expression in his narrative. This is so because the excuse is presented by declaring innocent uninvolved victims as witnesses to the crime. Now Officer T can express shock, still a far cry from loss. He goes on to describe the dealer (dehumanized) being shot in the back underhanded (unfairly—expectations, even among thieves, being violated) the dealer here is reaching out (grabbing for human relatedness to Officer T), Officer T gives his hand in a symbolic and genuine gesture (evidence his ability for empathy is not dissipated, although on a manifest level he denies it). Now how can he place that interaction in such a cold and callous wanton ecology of violence. It is a departing fare-thee-well. The emotional upheaval is denied, and yet is experienced.

The fourth cluster emerges in this context of dehumanization of the perpetrators. It is back to "us versus them." In Officer T's ecology of trauma, this return to the pursuit-and-chase attack, in which confrontation and social distance escalates, is a line drawn in violence against officers. This motif is different from the second, wherein ambiguity in the situations was evidenced. Emotional is invested with a safe distance from any feelings of loss and attachment for being the sacred victim parallel to the confrontation with the involved victims. The perpetrator here is a competitor who instigates violence, defense, and offensive pursuit. The defense against offense is warranted, sanctioned, and rewarded. Justification of Officer T's role is existentially soothing, because the clarity of the personal assault finishes with justice, custody of the bad guy, "I won." Other traumas continue within the motif of the attempted homicide of sacred victims. This ends with an ironic twist of fate—the perp is killed, wedged between the bumpers of two parked cars, the gun just out of reach, [the bad guy] dying on the trunk. Another victory. Finally, a violent homicide attempt is thwarted after an armed robbery. Here Officer T is almost killed, his partner is reliable, in fact the only reliable person to cover him and save his life. He is letting us know, in his ecological niche of trauma and loss, when reliability and survival value is not abstract, but as tangible as it gets. His self-reliance is contingent upon his partner. The need to give back to his unit buddy is more than a romantic notion of brother and sisterhood, it is an ethological motivation that survival shapes and reinforces. Yet, changing his command is existentially equivalent to abandoning his partner to death and destruction. This bond is perhaps stronger than most bonds one could ever imagine. We have reached, *in part*, another insight about why Officer T has remained in his milieu of death and ongoing threat to his own life.

Officer T's cycle of trauma has exemplified what I described as an internal social distance. The existential vacuum where so many painful events, thoughts, and types of victims moving from one trauma into the other was coherent and sensible in this perspective. Officer T initiated his trauma history with the uninvolved victim, to the sacred victim, to the involved victim. These three clusters laid out disenfranchised fear, anxiety, and existential despair, all in varying levels of loss. Officer T's empathy was connecting all the victims, open to exceptions to rules based upon eco-ethological demands in his niche. Through my empathy and developing trust, disclosure was elicited.

This fourth cluster Officer T presented was that of the sacred and involved victim. This relationship and the type of trauma completes a circle of distance of competition, and one wherein one side wins and the other loses. *It is shaped in the ecological niche of violence and urban warfare.* The emotional expression that began to be expressed when rehumanization moved across all types of victims has come full circle in narrowing degrees of distance, with loss and existential despair dwarfed in the defenses that keep intact the venting of anger, burnout, and righteous rage. *Distance is fulfilled and loss remains buried once again.*

Specifically, the achievement of both participants in therapy is ripe with difficulty and opportunity. The full circle of loss has been exposed and closed. In cluster one, two, and three, our observation of the two murdered children by negligent homicide, the sacred victims are doing their professional duties only to have brick and glass shatter any sense of safety and respect in an intentional assault and bodily threat. We then move to violent dealers of crime who, too, are victimized in such a brutal manner that murder is delivered in the law of the ecological niche, which is purely ethological. Might makes right. This is our thread of loss, when negligence is loss of care and responsibility. The ensuing loss is of security and safety. The next loss is that of human decency and impulse control, the sacred has been made profane. Officer T is left with trauma that has built up where no blood thirst can answer the despair at loss of human life and the victimization or existential questions. Humanizing the inhuman violence to which officer T is subject is given expression (distorted, distanced, and dehumanized at this juncture). That expression offers sensibility under the surface presentation of disparate trauma. I suggest we may have been offered an algorithm of trauma as formed by the evolutionary influences of ecology and ethology in the life of Officer T.

As in the identity mode collision, we are once again given the conflicts and the adaptations necessitated by officers accommodating to an ecology of excessive trauma and loss. Officer T is unconsciously educating us to this severity and letting us know at the same time how to approach our work with him.

Eco-Ethological Existential Analytic Intervention with Officer T

First, why didn't I directly interrupt the flow of Officer T's multiple trauma, and narrow my approach to hone in on his first trauma? In part, my approach was responsive to his presentation of trauma. Officer T barely paused. There was no disruption in his barrage of complex events thrown out at me. The hurried spontaneity of expression in his presentation was directive. His presentation provoked my nascent hypothesis. I first listen to Officer T, I gain an understanding of his style, and how I may be able to disconfirm or confirm what I am tentatively developing as a hypothesis at this point.

What is certain in my mind is Officer T's narrative (verbal and nonverbal presentation) did yield a cumulative presentation of trauma. At first, confusing and fragmented, coherence emerges as I use the heuristic eco-ethological approach.

I keep away from immediate attributions, labeling, and supraordinate interpretation. I take Officer T's narration as an honest accounting, a roll call of his experiences. Clinically, my impression is that his disclosure is genuine. Initially, he is reticent, and said nothing "unusual goes on in his command." That is true. It is not unusual for his experience, it is all too common. Nonetheless, we understand in our approach that events such as he began to describe are as traumatic as an experience can ever be. It is a tragic account of how many multiple traumas emerge within a history of trauma for him. Officer T presents with dissociation in his defenses of denial, addiction, agitation, and anger. To help place his trauma in historical perspective with a goal of achieving insight for himself, I need to be clear about how and why to approach his trauma in relation to his style of presentation. I am not sure how and why his addiction to trauma has become so crystallized. I expect to gain a modicum of insight, but not a definitive grasp.

Approaching Officer T's multiple trauma is made sensible by reviewing sections from other clinical cases I presented in this chapter. What is clear to me is that the affect, cognition, ethological emotions, and the ecological affordances are motivational in shaping an addiction to trauma for Officer T. It appears certain that this level of excitement may develop over time in direct relation to the psychophysiological experience of repetitive trauma that many police, emergency technicians, nurses, physicians, firefighters endure in war zones (Cannon, 1914; Goleman, 1992, 1994; Giller, 1990; Gilmartin, 2002; Krystal et al., 1989; Southwick, 2005; Thorp, 2005; Van Der Kolk et al., 1985; Yehuda et al., 1993).

I realize that Officer T's ecological and ethological affordances are entwined with his identity as an officer, and these expectations emerge in the situational demands and activated roles. It appears Officer T remains in a perpetual existential crisis of meaning versus despair in his addiction to trauma: aggressive, sexualized derivatives, and ethological motivations are extant. His existential problem is framed in psychophysiologic stimulation-inhibition, overinternalized responsibility, survival, and abandonment guilt weighing down freedom and choice. That outlook helps us understand his trauma and place it in perspective with him.

I approached the gestalt of the moment, as Officer T presented it, into clearer and palatable focus. Why? His desire to relate to me how much he had endured in terms of trauma suggested his wish for me to become the "recorder" of his trauma. In police and public safety, usually one partner in a team is the recorder and one the operator. The recorder serves as a navigator and the operator a pilot. I made it explicit with Officer T that he could be the pilot and I the active recorder. In effect, he would narrate the map of his trauma from his pilot's seat. I would record what he had to say and present it to him in terms of navigation and strategy. Clarifying his need by making it explicit and accepting his assuming the pilot's role was not letting him control the therapy, but reinforcing his need for mastery. It helps our alliance and supports his disclosure of trauma.

In our approach as therapists, we initiate our intervention in Officer T's trauma experience by addressing each cluster of trauma, 1-4, by using our heuristic reconstruction as a stratagem. Let us, identify five aspects of social distance and identity modes as follows: Each is related to emotional expression and suppression and making intelligible what appears to be random and non-structured. It is important to go back to the narrative I have highlighted and then look for specific follow-up for each segment of social distance in Officer T's account of his various role conflicts. By doing this, we achieve a tactical initial intervention of each aspect of trauma he experienced.

First, we will try to make sense of why this trauma emerged in the context of multiple traumas. We will use the Socratic method to get to his theme of loss as he expressed in each cluster by first fleshing out each cluster as having a unique social distance and contribution in his overall experience of trauma. Specifically, let's look at cluster one as an example to work on with Officer T. The murder by negligent/alcoholic vehicular homicide is attributed to a negligent/reckless adult. We will also connect this negligence to the "cowardly acts" of adults placing responsibility for murder onto a child. We will explore his investment in his rescue identity mode, which entails saving innocent victims. The expectation of Officer T's wish to rescue the victim's abruptly clashes with the reality of their brutal deaths. Keeping in mind his dominant memory is visual and olfactory for these traumas, our focus is on the most innocent and uninvolved victim—a child who survives and what he imagines happened with him. We note his sadness for the victims and disgust toward the perpetrator. Although he has expressed this, at this point his targeted aggression toward perpetrators is completely absent. We will clarify why this makes sense eco-ethologically with Officer T. We will also clarify his identity modes of arrest and custody with the adults and how and why these roles impact on Officer T, if at all.

Second, we will also look at each cluster to determine what it specifically affords the expression of rage, disgust, anxiety, and guilt. Specifically, let us use cluster 2 as our example. Officer T is attacked, assaulted, and violent struggles ensue. Aggression is expressed as acceptable, grief is not. The assault defines Officer T as a sacred victim. This serves as evidence for his counteraggression, when his pursuit, defense, and confrontation role is acceptable. Ethological aggression becomes a factor within his multiple identity modes. A distance away from grief for the first type of innocent victim is replaced by a focus on an escalated and directed aggression. This is an outlet of justified aggression—justice. What is striking is the absence of expression of grief or loss for self and peers. Although we are aware of why loss is so unacceptable to speak about in terms of sacred victims, we will explore this meaning within the unique vision of Officer-patient T.

Third, we will look at the situational demands of each cluster, identity-mode emergence and conflict, the impact on identity, and dissociation each mode affords Officer T's status in his eco-ethological niche. For example, let's return to cluster 2, where we will explore what, why, and how the sacred identity expands. Fellow officers are murdered off duty, and betrayed. We are given Officer T's intervention in the shooting and death of the off-duty cop he carried. This epitomizes the innocent paragon of an innocent fellow officer being brutally murdered as he dies in his arms. This shift is significant as the aggression is heightened and directed to deserving perpetrators. He expresses no grief, just aggression.

The *fourth* approach will be to work on Officer T's existential despair. The third cluster of trauma provides an excellent example. Existential questions emerge in the depth of the eco-ethological influences. The original innocent victim emerges now as the wife and child of the drug dealer. Questions: Why do the wife and child of the drug dealer get victimized? What was the meaning of the drug dealer's final behavior on a human level, when he reached out to hold Officer T's hand in the final farewell to him? Will Officer T ever know why he is feeling so perplexed about his emotional reaction to the dealers death? Yes. We will eventually work through the overwhelming despair over Officer T's painful loss, his comforter identity mode, and his depth of feeling for another human being in the throes of death.

That existential despair is answered in part by understanding how and why trauma has become addictive within his eco-ethological framework. In part, the spiral of social distance circles around, and the officer has a motivation ethologically to return to his ecology of trauma. The deserving victim receives justice exacted. The drug dealer's threatening the officer's eco-ethological dominance and security by competition for power is a topic for us to clarify. Understanding and relating the officer's perspective is critical. The high level of aggression here is fully confessed to his shrink, a Cop Doc. The drug dealer embodies the deserving victim. I bear witness to the injustice with Officer T. The overwhelming experience of extreme brutality against himself and his peer officers pulled Officer T away from an emerging sense of loss. His addiction to aggression numbs his experiences of existential despair; this numbing of grief blacks out so much of his experience. The social distance with the perp also distances him from the losses of sacred victims, including himself. We are back into a full spiral of pursuit and aggression. Officer T's worthy pursuit role, the final victory, and escape from death, reaches his unconscious epiphany and the perpetrator gets his just death.

The trauma and consequent excitement from aggression acts as an escape from his own overwhelming suffering, pain, and need to distance his own vulnerability. His final account is of his partner saving him from death. That bond is not only understandable on an eco-ethological level, but on the deepest existential level. The one he can trust when he is even blinded is his sacred partner. The reality of his presentation is convincing. This addiction is also occupationally supported in the macro and microculture. But at what price for Officer T and his family? Officer T, as a battle weary patrol and public-safety officer, experiences peace and war event changes multiple times in each of his different roles, to say nothing of home life. Repressed trauma, and its expression, unidentified, usually erupts when officers retire or leave their more violent eco-ethology. Respite from the ecology of excitement of multiple trauma leaves the officer-patient with a labyrinth catacombs of loss and complicated grief.

We can effect a definite difference at this point. Realizing his strengths and redeeming qualities in his identity as an officer-patient, we can help him see his options and clarify choices, which are ultimately Officer T's, and I will respect and support his informed decisions once made. If he leaves his position, it would mean abandoning his partner, his unit, and his whole way of adaptation. Demands of selflessness in his identity as an officer have become overriding in his life. My empathy, challenges, understanding, and encounter will clarify his choices.

Trauma and grief are made meaningful in an adaptive way for Officer T, who remains stuck. His allegiance is not an abstraction of justice, but his ideals provide existential meaning gleaned from excessive and shocking brutality aimed at himself and fellow officers as sacred victims. Is fear of his being labeled for perceived abandonment of his unit experienced as guilt incarnate? The challenge is making sense of this first while acknowledging his resilience.

For example, I started to work on seeing if motivation for Officer T to get out of his war zone existed. My hypothesis was that he would grab onto the offer of a light-duty detail. I was wrong. This was disconfirmed forthright and firmly. When I suggested that I could take action to help him switch to a slower command, he politely refused. He responded directly:

> I would be taking a step backwards, it's the wrong move. That precinct X is a Disneyland of the north. Yeah, a homicide, gun run, serious assault once a month, it's boring. Considering all the changes in faces, switching shifts, buddies, my partner, I don't feel right leaving. I mean, I know my sector like the back of my hand. I know where to get cover, the mugs I could trust, and not. No, it simply will not work, but thanks, Doc.

We built mutual trust and explored understanding why. An REBT assignment I suggested was getting the videotape *Saving Private Ryan* (Rodat, 1998) which he could directly relate to and clarify some of his feelings. I had hypothesized that a strong identification with Private Ryan would help clarify the combat-soldier plight he was in through a safe medium at first. He expressed his feelings as follows:

> It brought on feelings of pride in my country, and much more my admiration for those men who embarked on a mission that was conceived from good intentions. A mission that I know put little value on the battlefield. Just like us grunts in the street who are responsible for the success of getting the violent perpetrators. One aspect of that picture is foreign to me, and that is having a steadfast caring leadership under any circumstance. I always wanted that badly, never had it. With each soldier being murdered, I felt a weird deepening despair that set in. I was touched with James Ryan surviving and leaving his brothers behind.

This helped me in gaining a foothold on how highly Officer T identified with his police unit. His guilt of abandonment was intolerable, even in just contemplating rotation out of the war zone precinct unit. We have achieved an inroad into understanding a different dimension of trauma, to say nothing of the grief work to be done. We are also given an understanding of how to approach Officer T empathically. Good reason exists that evolutionary mechanisms of ethology and ecology influenced Officer T's addiction to trauma. That clarification has moved Officer T from being a victim to survivor at this point.

FINAL COMMENTS AND CONCLUSION: PPS-CPTSD

Taken as a whole the eight cases are a tentative outline for your use in working with Complex PTSD in police and public-safety populations. But our task is not only clinical application. Following our mind's eye, first and foremost we are likely to achieve our therapeutic goals by our clear understanding of PPS-CPTSD. Without a clear foundation, we have only speculation. You have that foundation at this point. It will become apparent that my paradigm may go far beyond that of police and public safety, but the circumference of our work is with the officer-patient at this point in development.

However, another point is necessary before I conclude this advanced guide. I will use a parable to illustrate, that of economics. You may say to yourself, look, a general eco-ethological understanding is a good way to go, but finding out the specifics of each officer-patient is daunting and time-consuming. That point is true! Yet, without understanding the context of the individual officer-patient, your technique and method, which may be right on the money, is likely to be squandered. Why? Because demand can only command a response of supply once that need is established on a fundamental level.

Put another way, the economic laws of supply and demand hold in trauma: what is demanded to be effective is an understanding that reaches the reality of what is experienced in the field of meaning for your officer-patient. Until you can relate that field of meaning in the individual officer-patient's way of looking at his construction of loss in trauma, you are making a pitch in a sea of unanchored chance.

Ethology and ecology are disciplines with great potential for our population of police and public safety. It speaks to the experience of officer's traumas and losses in the field of their historical evolution. That evolution is relevant to cultural competence and individual development. Doing our work requires challenges to our own intellect, and more so to our passion and the existential meaningfulness we invest in our own work and those with whom we work.

Yet, that is not an impossible task, but one where patience and curiosity engenders an attitude that is likely to facilitate a probable humane and scientific understanding that is effective. *To achieve your task, learning the language goes beyond the macroculture and the official line of the public-safety department.* It entails your understanding and knowledge of the experience of demands in the officer-patient's ecological niche. Personal expectations, intensity of those expectations, investment, and gains as well as losses are experienced in terms of survival value, suffering, resilience, and optimism. That understanding is the currency we need to invest and trade in the market economy of trauma and loss with the officer-patient.

A demoralized participant may opt out of the journey of life. Their investments may be largely in destructive stock. Our challenge to that option is possible if we are clear on what currency the participant is using, what options for reinvestment may be considered, and if we have a meaningful investment available to redirect the officer-patient investor. Once that is known, then all your training and experience is put to the best selective advantage in a competitive market economy. While you and I may not prefer to speak of trauma and loss in terms of trade and market economies, it may be the most economical metaphor available. That is markedly salient in a market economy anchored in limiting therapy to briefer as better. However, when you meet the needs of a goldfish you can use a bowl, when you need to meet the needs of a blue whale you had better be thinking expansion. That blue whale is trauma being hidden in our bathtub, and something's gotta give.

Understanding the economy and the specific investments the officer-patient has made may help us suggest a reinvestment of static into dynamic redirection and growth. I suggest that grasping this reality deepens insight, boosts realistic assessment, and sharpens strategic treatment in working through Complex PTSD with the five police personality styles we are likely to encounter in our expanded domain of trauma work.

CONCLUSION

The vast majority of public-safety officers will be referred by agencies, and some will be walk-ins without any prodding and seeking out a mental health practitioner for the first time. Many will come forward with the dysfunctional myths we discussed. Some will be green with idealism, some tarnished with the gray of pessimism, and many soaked in the red shock of war wounds—so many tattered rags on the domestic warfronts—in the intrapsychic conflicts of their psyches. At our departure, I have offered you effective interventions that are evident in each chapter throughout this book.

However, many, but not all, of my mistakes in my interventions have been omitted. Hopefully, your own techniques will be inspired by my interventions. I would suggest taking nothing for granted and using your own skill as a therapist. Existential meaning is invariably personal and relates back to being invested in the patient's way of looking at the universe without losing yours. If you conceptualize this approach as a multicultural venture with a specific goal of understanding culture of the ecological and ethological influences, you can connect with an increased chance of encounter.

A potential caveat is a misinterpretation of the stance I advocate throughout this book. That is working on an antireductionistic approach to eco-ethological etiology with the gestalt in mind.

If as clinicians we reduce our approach to a formula, we are in danger of prepackaging the human being, invariably winding up caught in the lining from which we construct our web-like designs. That snare has always been alluring to me. I suggest that sharing the real person behind the therapist's approach is the way to bring out the real patient one is evolving with. Each real interaction is a step in one's own choice to grow, regress, or stagnate. That intangible encounter is irreducible and is the apogee of the intervention's crest to take away as a crosswind from this book on your own rewarding voyage with public servants of red, white, or blue hues. To infuse the wisdom of Talmudic sages, "to save one life is to save a world," if you prevent an officer's suicide, you have saved a world, not only their own but the world at large!

REFERENCES

Balter, R. (2004). Personal correspondence re: *Uni-dimensional protocols in treating losses. American Psychological Association, Chair Division of Media and Attorney, Psychologist and Professor in Criminology & Psychology.*

Barnes, R. (2005). Personal correspondence re: *Trauma and police issues from a logotherapy and forensic perspective retired Veteran and Psychologist President Viktor Frankl Institute, Harding Simmons Professor and Chair of Psychology and Counseling.*

Benner, A. (1999). Personal correspondence re: *Cop Doc and the forging of a new role for the uniformed psychologist by founder of Cop Doc's National Association and Co-founder of West Coast Post Trauma Retreat, United States Marine Corp Pilot and Captain San Francisco Police Department.*

Benner, A. (2004). Personal correspondence re: *Cop Doc guide and emotional exhaustion fatigue in peer support officers and Uniformed Psychologist Cop Docs.*

Brenner, C. (1974). *An elementary textbook of psychoanalysis.* New York: Anchor Books.

Brenner, C. (1976). *Psychoanalytic technique and intra-psychic conflict.* New Haven, CT: International University Press.

Brenner, C. (1982). *The mind in conflict.* New Haven, CT: International University Press.

Brenner, C. (2004). Personal correspondence re: *The iatrogenic casting of trauma without accounting for the deeper layers of personality—why an individualized approach optimal.*

Cannon, W. B. (1914). The emergency function of the adrenal medulla in pain and the major emotions. *American Journal of Physiology, 3,* 356-372.

Einstein, A. (1954). *Ideas and opinions.* United States: Crown Publishers Incorporated.

Frankl, V. (1978). *The unheard cry for meaning.* New York: Simon & Schuster.

Frankl, V. (2000). *Man's search for ultimate meaning.* Cambridge, MA: Perseus Publishing.

Freud, S., Ferenczi, S., Abraham, K., Simmel, E., & Jones, E. (1921). *Psychoanalysis and the war neuroses.* London & New York: International Psycho-Analytic Press.

Freud, A. (1936). *Ego and the mechanism of defense.* New York: International University Press.

Gibson, J. J. (1966). *The senses considered as perceptual systems.* Boston: Houghton Mifflin.

Gibson J. J. (1986). *The ecological approach to visual perception.* New Jersey: Lawrence Erlbaum Associates.

Gibson, J. J., & Gibson, E. (1955). Perceptual learning: Differentiation or enrichment? *Psychological Review, 62,* 32-41.

Giller, E. L. (Ed.). (1990). *Biological assessment and treatment of post traumatic stress disorder.* Washington, DC: American Psychiatric Press.

Gilmartin, K. (2002). *Emotional survival for law enforcement: A guide for officers and their families.* Tucson, AZ: ES Press, Inc.

Goleman, D. (1992, January). Wounds that never heal. How trauma changes your brain. *Psychology Today,* pp. 62-68.

Goleman, D. (1994, October). Emotional memory of trauma: Cahill's study. *New York Times, Science Time Tuesday.*

Heller, J. (1961). *Catch 22.* New York: Dell Publishing Company.

Howell, M., & Ford, P. (1981). *The true history of the elephant man.* Middlesex, England: Penguin Books Publishing Company.

Kalayjian, A. (2003). Impact of 9/11 terrorism on mental health practitioners in the New York Tri State Area. *Eye on Psi Chi Magazine.* Vol. 2.

Ker Muir, W. (1977). *Police: Street corner politicians.* Chicago & London: University of Chicago Press.

Krystal, H. (1968). *Massive psychic trauma.* New York: International Universities Press.

Krystal, J., Kosten, T., Perry, B., Southwick, S., Mason, J., & Giller, E. (1989). Neurobiological aspects of PTSD: Review of clinical and pre-clinical studies. *Journal of Behavior Therapy, 20,* 177-198.

Mansfield, V. (2004a). Personal correspondence re: *A chief's viewpoint of three decades of executive police leadership and Rudofossi's construct of PPS-CPTSD.*

Mansfield, V. (2004b). Personal correspondence re: *Chief of police issues and trauma issues from a police department and United States military veteran.*

Myers, C. (1940). *Shell shock in France 1914-1918.* Cambridge: Cambridge University Press.

Pavlov, I. (1941). *Conditioned reflexes and psychiatry.* New York: International Publishers.

Rado, S. (1939). Developments in the psychoanalytic conception and treatment of the neuroses. *Psychoanalytic Quarterly, 8,* 427.

Rado, S. (1956). *Psychoanalysis of behavior.* New York & London: Grune and Stratton, Inc.

Reese, J. (1991). *Critical incidents in policing.* Washington, DC: Department of Justice, Federal Bureau of Investigation.

Reese, J. (1996). Personal correspondence re: *Federal Bureau of Investigation Agent Cop Doc advice in setting up a program for trauma and support in conducting research on PTSD and services.*

Richards, A., & Willick, M. (1986). *Psychoanalysis: The science of mental conflict.* Ersdale, NJ: The Analytic Press.

Rodat, R. (1998). *Saving Private Ryan.* Produced by Steven Spielberg. Amblin Entertainment Productions.

Rudofossi, D., & Ellis, R. R. (1999, August). *Differential police personality styles use of coping strategies, ego mechanisms of defense in adaptation to trauma and loss.* Symposium conducted at American Psychological Association, Boston, Massachusetts.

Rudofossi, D. M. (2007). *Working with traumatized police officer patients: A clinicians guide to complex PTSD.* Amityville, NY: Baywood.

Scharf, R. (2004). Personal correspondence re: *Trauma and organizational character traits and issues from a psychoanalytic perspective,* New York Psychoanalytic Institute and Society.

Schiff, W. (1979). *Perception: A text book.* New York: New York University Press.

Schiff, W. (1994). Personal correspondence re: *Trauma and risk taking experiment with police officers at New York University Laboratory,* New York University.

Schreiber, F. R. (1973). *Sybil.* Chicago, IL: Henry Regnery Company.

Solomon, H., & Yakovlev, P. (1945). *Manual of military neuropsychiatry.* Philadelphia & London: W. B. Saunders Company.

Southwick, S. (2005). Personal correspondence re: *Trauma and police issues from a logotherapy and forensic perspective retired veteran and police officer physician,* Yale University Professor, Chief National Division of Clinical Neuroscience Veterans Administration, United States.

Thorp, J. (2005). Personal correspondence re: *Trauma and Police Issues from a logotherapy and forensic perspective retired medical professional and Police Officer.*

Van Der Kolk, B., Greenberg, M., Boyd, H., & Krystal, J. (1985). Inescapable shock, neurotransmitters and addition to trauma: Toward a psychobiology of post traumatic stress disorder. *Journal of Biological Psychiatry, 20,* 314-325.

Wambaugh, J. (1972). *The blue knight.* Boston, MA: Little Brown.

Worden, J. (2001). *Grief counseling & grief therapy.* New York: Springer.

Yehuda, R., Resnick, H., Kahana, B., & Giller, E. (1993). Long lasting hormonal alterations in extreme stress in humans: Normative or maladaptive? *Journal of Psychosomatic Medicine, 55,* 287-297.

Toward an Antidote to Terrorism:
An Eco-Ethological Existential Analysis

This epilogue is not an epiphany it is an attempt to find a beginning: A limited aperture rightfully owned by me as a Cop Doc, that is, as a Cop and Doc. I make no claim that my suggested antidote has efficacy greater than any human being's attempt to acknowledge the fallibility, vulnerability, and susceptibility of being put in situations that are without doubt very difficult to imagine much less experience on a personal level. My eco-ethological existential analysis of Police Complex Trauma offers another dimension toward understanding an ancient phenomenon hiding under the umbrella of a new name that attempts to horrify its recipients. That ancient phenomenon is despotism, tyranny and what is now called terrorism. It is interesting to note from the onset that there is no such thing as enlightened terrorism.

The first step is to not glorify or romanticize what is on one hand human illness, and on the other human depravity and evil. If we pause and think about it, any behavior used to control another against his own volition outside of persuasion, vehement polemics and short of forceful violence—is unacceptable. To a degree, we all experience this painfully in life at one time or another—usually in small and palatable doses.

However, at a large and intense dosage, most of us are not ready to assimilate the experience of forceful control. Once control **becomes** forceful, random, and intense violence it becomes psychopathological by definition, while victimization results are perniciously psycho-physiological. Most psychopathology is not intentional but fueled by extreme passion and cognitive and existential distortions. Some aspects of insidious control are effective and yet more subtle.

For example, intellectual elitism in movements that popularizes a motto of eliminating differences and equating the ability to persuade others as equal with terror tactics stigmatizes those who disagree with public hysteria and fads to correct the "evils" of society. However popularized and under the guise of whatever title currently used we call it political correctness, or in the past national democratic socialism and regardless of how nice such titles sound where differences of opinion are squelched in mass hysteria a subtle form of fascism may be the new wave to inundate the defiant power of the human spirit.

Terrorist tactics rely on counter tactics that are nested in the other side of our strength for democratic equality which is our greatest weakness, and our blind spot. That blind spot is politically correct uniformity in conformity with a need to impose sweeping reactionary agendas. That blind spot cannot elude the existential realm and is clearly the domain of psychology and psychiatry. Any response to terrorism must clearly identify terrorism and its components inherent in our own democracy which may unwittingly and at times explicitly aid terrorist's tactical advantage. We would not be the first democracy to succumb to national terrorism or fascism, to ignore that possibility is to ignore the facts of history and terror-ism tactic's. Professor Santayana (1906) in his inimitable style said it straight from the desk of experience,

> Progress far from consisting in change, depends on retentiveness. When change is absolute there remains no being to improve and no direction is set for possible improvement: and when experience is not retained as among savages, infancy is perpetual. **Those who cannot remember the past are condemned to repeat it** . . . this is the condition of barbarians in which instinct has learned nothing from experience.

The experience of terror-ism like all of fascism is that *Terrorists are violent and use violence to achieve their means*—conversely persuasion that relies on one party convincing another party that one option is better then another and is not violence nor terror. This remains true no matter how distasteful the attempt to persuade without violence as long as the other party has the ability to move on and tune out and off. To actually move on is a consequence of free will and personal responsibility, to assert different is not only infantilizing another party— but stigmatizing him/her as being shorn of free-will. It is clear that as a scientist the ability to discriminate is an asset, as a humane being it is a virtue one cannot exist without. Without the moral compass to discriminate between human good and evil we have no compass to select what is worthwhile to fight for and how and when to do so. Without this ability we could not defend ones civil and religious rights to practice without harm or violence. By fighting for what is crucial all things are not equal, and in achieving equality as opportunity to chose freely one needs to realize no human being is the same as another—similarities not withstanding. However, all human beings have a right to be fully human and fully unique in choice and that choice brings anxiety. The ability to tolerate anxiety is crucial to maintaining a free society.

It is important to identify in this context that in the face of anxiety a positive outgrowth is if we are recipients of terror tactics each of us always have one choice if we are to survive the physical onslaught, that choice is what to do in our attitude toward the attempt terrorists use individually and collectively to terrorize. The attitude one chooses to believe in and to confront the physical terror is layered in the psychological realm, specifically the existential.

Terrorists target the existential realm of human behavior, thought, and belief while denying their very existence. Terrorists and their faith in terrorism is without any genuine ideal, exerting change by infusing terror into the life-source of those targeted and affected by their willful and premeditated attack. As in most narcissistic offenses terrorists *attack our personal sensibility* we all use (consciously and unconsciously) in our daily living as anchored in our existential differences as individuals. Terrorists also *lay waste* to our *common sensibilities* by the attack on our (ecology) in which is nested in our culture with its attendant mores, and philosophical stances on life within our specific sphere of living and being. Terrorists attempt to displace our transcendental essence as human beings which is unique and beyond the grip of the rational and ego-interest based functions in society (eco-ethological).

A lesson that is helpful is in order to flesh out the antidote for dealing with terrorism, is understanding what poison that has been ingested. The corollary to that understanding is to know the persons individual response to that type of poison and why. To ignore confrontation is to ignore the aspect of passivity inherent in being silent to extreme aggression. This passivity which as human a tendency in most of us displaces what is sacred in not only being human, but our responsibility to other human beings outside of ourselves. Meaning it is not only I who am egocentric; it is my group of affiliation and my eco-ethological niche and even my larger choices of likes and dislikes.

In speaking frankly being a Cop Doc is not only a major affiliation for me, it is a calling. As a street cop in New York City pounding the beat green to blue as well as in becoming a psychologist, as an imperfect, fallible, and innately stubborn learner I opened up to a learning process of higher tolerance for peoples foibles in the context of common sensibility. I also learned the invaluable lesson of responsibility as a clinician is being a journeyman: I am better able to receive, analyze, and Socratically, help the officer-patient "internally-witness" (Rudofossi, 2007) their hidden resilience through the re-narration of their own experiences of trauma including vicarious and actual terrorism. The process of what I have called "internal witnessing" distills the crushed flour of disenfranchised losses through a kneading process of reflecting back with the officer-patient—his own *hidden compassion and courage*—into the sweetness of Sourdough which leavens gain—rein-franchised for living. It is in a personal odyssey that an antidote from an eco- ethological existential analysis provides a solution. That solution is in identifying terrorism as one form of potentially pernicious complex traumatic events. It is by you and I as healers, who cannot alter the event but can alter the understanding of the ecological, ethological-experiential, and existential-spiritual personal and common sensibilities that are conscious, uncon- scious and conscience in not only damage control but in potential sources of energy that the individual may use in healing.

As clinician you and I become a journeyman facilitator in educating ourselves through the humility of the Socratic method and dialectical approach in filling the narrow gaps in the bridge of meaning lost in trauma but also in regaining tragic optimism (coined by Frankl) and soul revival from soul sickness (Solevetchik) with the officer-patient, not exclusive from the process (Frankl, 1955; Solevetchik/Peli, 1980). The counter-transference is on a transcendental dimension that compliments a dynamic one (Brenner, 1976), it is not in denial of our drive derivatives that we rise to the essence of who we are, it is in the crux of the temptation to escape from our inner need for meaning that we come back with the full transformation of despair into meaning in-deed!

Our journey values the human being as a whole not partial person by means of what is paradoxical and even possibly counter-intuitive through the breakdown of each dimension from the ground up, from the deeper layers to the wholesome higher processes of spiritual development and its response toward healing and compassion.

With this context in mind it is our time to move toward our first task of begging to define the complexities we encounter in terrorism. Definitions lead to an ability to communicate with a reference point and are not ever written in stone; however, when held to dogmatically they at times can lead to borders etched in blood.

Terrorism is a concept that rightfully earns its place as the crowning definition of the heel in a book written about complex trauma and in the context of those sworn to fight it—without forgetting they too experience it. The front line soldiers and officer-patients are not "them," but, without apology, are "we," as well.

The dissolution of terrorism is not an ideological challenge of debate, terrorism is never justified! To open conversations with terrorists is to condone and add legitimacy to victimization and trauma of the most complex sort with its recurrent nightmare effects: It is truly Kafkaesque to label the victim guilty for being victim; it is even more nonsensical to stigmatize the officer-patient for being the rescuer, than it is to label the healer as socially and morally guilty. Terrorism is murder as much as it is genocide. Yet genocide does not cover the term well, it is too broad and loses meaning in the masses and swarming numbers that numb its potent impact.

One lesson learned is *creating a highly individual language that is specific and sensitive to the suffering of the individual officer-patient which suffices!* The word murder is an elegant term with a distinct meaning which does not minimize human value and the dignity afforded a victim.

Murder holds ownership to those individuals who commit human atrocity, whether against citizens of Israel, Rwanda, Sudan, Pennsylvania, Japan, India, or New York City. It is a trait of terrorists to label all peoples of a religion or an ethnic group as dehumanized targets. Examining this way of thinking let us pause, and think of the premise in reverse here and how distorted this labeling is. We would not ever think it sensible to highlight collective genius for example to Einstein's family and friends, rather then to Albert Einstein himself as the creative mind behind the theory of relativity—in the same way—we may not descend to insensibility to judge all peoples of a specific religion for those radicals who abide by a code of violence and evil to their fellows by the bonfire of terror. It is never all people of one geographic region that are all evil, and certainly not human to allow the leaders of such human atrocity to go unnoticed and merge in the crowd of anonymity they seek to find refuge in. Again individual responsibility and choice is key to dismantling terrorisms attempt to dehumanize a people and notwithstanding their own group affiliation.

Another lesson learned is *personal responsibility is strategic in the eco-ethological existential analysis of understanding the perpetrators of terrorism, as well as healing the survivors.*

It is in giving enormous credit and power to a delusion that we make terrorism all encompassing—disenfranchising the survivors, invalidating the victims—while empowering the wielders of terror. It is here with an antidote to terrorism, we as clinicians, as well as public service officers, may dismantle the terrorist networks not only physically but by understanding the act of terror as an eco-ethological moment that is quantum in existential magnitude (see Rudofossi, 2007). The existential magnitude is a highly personal experience no matter how much commonality exists—it is how and why one officer-patient is effected that is crucial in helping her re-gain her losses into meaningful gain and motivation to make a stand. It is the eco-ethological existential analysis that gives coordinates to the senses that have been lost in the bitter necrosis through the light of vitality, one officer-patient at a time.

A third lesson learned is the *ecological and ethological dimensions of an act of terrorism colludes in the hidden variability of how and why an individual officer-patient experiences a specific freezing of meaning* connected to her senses lost in time and space in the first place. It is always nested in the eco-ethological dimension which is impacted and colored by the existential frame. To ignore the complexity of this reality is to disenfranchise the cost and the impact on each person effected. *The solution is in part the hidden aspect of meaning that is nested in the choice of what is lost in that experience of the officer-patients ecological niche and ethological motivation that brings the contour of what and how to address existentially. It is from the ecological niche and its ethological impact that we draw out the unique and individualized existential need and place it in a context of meaning and re-enfranchised motivation to live and move in with the fluidity of life.*

Arguably even the perpetrators are victims of their own human illness and human depravity we have become afraid to characterize for what it genuinely is, "evil"! It is not to their plight that I address this small attempt to add to the understanding and hopeful fruit of what has been characterized as the "sociological–imagination" (Goffman, 1967; Mills, 1959) which nowadays may be viewed as the existential imagination. With a foundation of what we are all grappling with—we will define "terrorism."

Terror-ism: It is in-deed an ism. Ism's that are linear tend to be rigid and closed to choice and options but condemn and use the force of self-righteous indignation to imagined violations to do what is antithetical to creativity, analytic process of an open mind, and a practical compromise. Terrorism holds the promise of death, destruction, and an end to creativity by violent control or at times by calling the victim the offender. Note when a minister of terror can deny the Holocaust and we as humane and civilized humane beings can aid and abet this philosophy— we narrow creativity to darkness overshadowing light and damming the door of any foundation sealed shut including life and love.

A fourth lesson gleaned is Terrorism is a bridesmaid of her dark prince, Fascism. Terrorism seeks its *legitimacy by the motto of right* by might, fascism by controlling all into one corner too far left, without a center, which falls on itself and like an abyss sucks all in with it. It is one who leans to far to the right or to far to the left where the twain is crushed by the sheer force of its controlled chaos. It is the echo of narcissus without the reflection of hearing ones voice of conscience. This is not unusual to the anti-social personality that uses force simply because she/he can and then proclaims her victory in the name of a god with a small g.

Fascism incorporates an all encompassing goal of violence, notice it is a corollary to malevolence. . . . I was a cop, as I have written before I became a doc. In that capacity as a cop I learned well that crimes are in two categories. The first category is that of commission which is easily recognizable by an action done with intent. The other is a crime that is done by omission. That is one chooses with intent to ignore the consequences of being complacent when action is warranted, the absence of a stand is a definite perspective of action in inaction.

Keep this in mind when we move on in our discussion of expanding the meaning of terror-ism and then how we may be able to learn in some small way how my emerging therapy as a Cop Doc may help officers and others they live with, work with and experience life with.

Terrorism and the struggle for human survival is sadly complicated by commercializing and marketing it with a supply that is endless and dehumanizing. In this book as well as its predecessor in this series I highlight what has been disenfranchised as loss, and left in its complex melee of interpersonal to intrapersonal collateral damage. Damage may better be understood in regard to an economic motive in terrorism as a situational demand in an ecology that has evolved its territorial markings with evolutionary motivation that is in its production and demand supplied in its destructive potential. The physical destruction is answered in terms of dollars and no-sense.

In regards to psychological and mental damage we can assess the damage as the terror it spawns in the victim, the culture around the victim and the potential targets and their responses. The existential response is the meaning lost in one strike which assumes a concentric circle with the effect of psychological aftershocks. Terrorism is nested in being sudden and shocking as all trauma events are.

It may be rated on an *F* scale as severe weather patterns and like a tornado is always intense and targets coordinates to maximize the after shock effects. It is in reality never as large as we process it, and it is never controllable just as a tornado. Unlike a tornado it is manmade and is deliberate with full intent to cause maximal destruction, yet it follows a similar path of destruction in human cost. Like a tornado it terrorizes because it is so sudden and with little warning it causes shockwaves of after effects.

Still our efforts to control terrorists and devastate its targets is logistics; to act against terrorism by politics is tactics; all important components. It is in the strategy that a war against terrorism is made an oxymoron as a war cannot be fought on a guerilla basis entirely. It is tactical genius to hit targets manned by terrorists and halt activities in military fashion, it is necessary, highly effective, but it is not a strategy.

A strategy implies a strong and meaningful perspective that is resistant and one envisioned by creativity as a counter point to what is destructiveness inherent in all fascist cults. Cults are not manipulated by stupid people nor by the uneducated: To the contrary, the fact is most cults are started and maintained by men and women of religion, politics and money that are highly educated and highly intelligent including on how to manipulate others at times where they are in search of meaning which is cached as meaning but is self importance offering the gilded panacea for G-d, in the figure of a woman/man who is here today and gone tomorrow.

All fascists are cult bound and form around rituals that create a unique adherence to rules as sacred, the non-sacred meaning is projected onto those who expose the cult leader as a dictator. The cost is that when humane opposition to tyranny is initiated the label of profane, dispensable, and inhuman is likely to emerge, while in reality the leader of opposition is unusually humane, and courageous.

A fifth lesson learned is that dehumanization and de-sacredizing life as a core component for a purpose of conquest by terrorists is almost always nested in the quest for perfectionism and control of others. It is a method that denies compassion and ultimately hubris at its height—attempting to be selfless to an ideal, leading to the arrogance of forcing others to worship what is alien to all humans a relinquishing of self which is what makes us personally viable and sensibly intelligent toward a common goal.

It is relevant to include one of the sources of pointing out the hypocrisy in any society and that is the intuitive, the science fiction writers are uncommonly sensible in this regard: Fiction in scientific forecasting may permeate with alacrity the veil of hypocrisy and expose through science-fiction the solution to what is equivalent to Mind Snatching that occurs in all terrorists' strategy: It is no accident that Jack Finney's, *Invasion of the Body Snatchers* (1954) and John Wyndham's *The Day of the Triffids* (1951), and his follow up with *The Chrysalids* (1954) all coalesce the theme of cells that mimic what is human in us all—with the myth of purity as a cleansed race in totality—excluding anyone outside of the fundamental utopian community as evil, superfluous, and worthy of immediate persecution and sudden annihilation.

Both writers of moderate acclaim in the fifties have ascended the forests of tomes laid to recycling rest as revived best sellers in our time when intellectual fascism has terrorized the market economy of ideas freely exchanged into a time when ideas are policed into the parody of ordered chaos.

The buoyancy of these writers is captured in what terrorists seek to do, not a military takeover, but one that seeks to present an omnipresence of their potency while snatching our aptitude as humans which is nested in our ability of choice, responsibility, direction, and attitude.

A **sixth lesson to be embraced** is Terrorist's feign being as-if they are gods but in their finite spectrum of conscience and transcendental cruelty with a small g, they would hardly be noticeable. They infiltrate by hoping we will miss the obvious which is the fact that we will not see that the antidote lies in our own existential attitude and never relinquishing being fully human and fully alive: It is in our stand as human beings, that glimpsing our own courage to transcend the tactics to terrorize us that yield the internal witnessing of Ultimate Meaning which shines its source beyond the illusions of our own castles made in the darkness of our own backyards.

A **seventh lesson** is in a society that is racked by the death of creativity via the hysteria of over-reactivity and fueled by fear of being politically-incorrect, or hitting a bottom line that has bottomed out in health care—the collapse of freedom paradoxically may be ensured: An anxiety free world aids the terrorist's agenda with alacrity. The converse is true that for the healer to effect thera-peutic gain—he/she needs to listen and reflect the officer-patients healthy anxiety to unearth his/her *own hidden dimensions of courage, compassion, mercy, and the unique ability to care for others by transcending his own sphere of self preservation.*

It is critical to cull out and help re-assess the humane responses heard by the clinician's third ear to create optimism out of tragedy that is otherwise dismissed as "routine" or "part of the job."

The examples given in this book and in my first book offer how to use the Eco-Ethological Existential Analysis to shine light on what is anything but routine in public safety (Rudofossi, 2007).

An **eighth lesson** is derived from the seventh lesson above: When the hidden dimensions of human transcendence are submerged under the sea of anonymity that excludes the personal journey of each officer-participant—guilt, self blame, and withdrawal emerge with a fury that enables the terror in terrorists agenda to win inter-personally and even more critically intra-personally with not only victims, but rescuers as officer-patients, and the healers that try to effect change.

Hippocrates admonition in treatment to us as healers offers a solution. It is not the disease we attempt to cure but knowing the person who has the disease. The strategy informs us that the layers of personality commingle with each persons strategy of dealing with losses, and losses are at the core of terror-ism and the economics that fuel the process of those very losses.

The **ninth lesson** learned follows the eighth lesson and that is in doing an eco-ethological existential analysis we make tangible to the officer the how and why he/she is invaluable as a humane being and their experiences of complex losses may be reinfranchising by the very means of their own attitude and motivation to transcend those very losses by achieving the gains that link attitude with courage and faith. A faith that cannot be diminished in the face of human fallibility and judgment, but in the optimism within tragedy of the **Infinite Hope and Ultimate meaning.** Infinite hope and ultimate meaning in the face of random terror tactics act as an antidote in a clinically personal approach incorporating officer-patients personality and individuality which opposes all fascists and cult practices. It is the inoculation against burnout and extreme cynicism that emerges when fighting the aggressors tactics by existentially infusing meaning in the face of dehumanizing strikes of terror by not losing sight of ones own human responses to loss.

The **tenth lesson** is the strategic effort of dismantling terrorism by taking away the motive novelty and the express goals of terror-ism by looking at it as a branch of fascism. That is simply being real and not apologizing for murder—but painting it as evil in its destructive vortex. It is in-deed small and desperate individuals that use hate, and destruction to motivate the experience of chaos in the common sensibilities and private sensitivities of the effected.

We as healers are one of the effected folks and can individualize the intra-personal recovery by inoculation into an inter-personal recovery ourselves. It is in healing that we heal as well, to accept this is to accept an aspect of being human ourselves and to use our transference with patients as an "internal witnessing" for ourselves with each officer-patient we work through complex trauma events with.

Terrorism is one deed that keeps on paying until it is countered by inter-vention. It is a strategic strike that is psychological and it is a counterstrike that must counter from a superior vantage point to be an effective antidote. That antidote as a psychological existential one serves as inoculation borne in resilience, and derived in the existential analysis of the here and now for maximum effect.

A case example will follow that I have used with officer-patients time and again that significantly impacted on their ability to deal with some of the most difficult losses in complex trauma including acts of terrorism. Being no less immune to the impact of trauma and losses in terror-ism myself shape my own method of intervention titled, the eco-ethological existential analytic approach. The terrorism of the worst sort was Nazism and the hero (mine as well) *is none other then Viktor Frankl.*

WHY VIKTOR FRANKL?

Because his humanity lives on and his connection to all of us is through his integrity and his moral compass as a decent humane being was unshaken. This voice of freedom and responsibleness [owned responsibility as a choice and direction chosen] is an aspect of his indefatigable soulfulness and the Ultimate Source it ascended from—in fact his remarkable genius is dwarfed by his irreducible humanity. That humanity is shared by members of all denominations that are of the decent race, the one divide between indecent and decent, the humane and inhumane and the fulcrum in any antidote that is the Viktor in a war on terror.

Professor Dr. Frankl probably is one of the most quoted and read authors with some hidden aspects of his unique contributions missed in the crucible of his suffering and his stands toward that suffering. Frankl underscored his achievement of survival of trauma in very average terms in comparison to his incredible task of remaining humane and compassionate balanced with a sense of justice that was indefatigable. His sense of justice drove him to being a witness for all human beings and transcending his own fear of death in maintaining his faith as a Jew who was targeted for murder for being born to a people who have traversed the world of trauma and loss. Frankl's message spreads a message of decency and responsibility in an increasing narrowing cusp of politics achieved in blood and violence. His message was his life and the way he lived it in the face of terror-ism and the hell it produced called Auschwitz. He had an incredible will to live and to share that will to meaning with all of us directly—refusing to compromise his faith in a message of unity and strength to strength—in the face of attacks that would appear absurd if it not so tragic. If this seems past history or not as relevant it is too modern and to much of an agenda of hatred and narrowness Terrorists employ. Further even the most gifted of science fiction writers failed to imagine the genuine horror of one of the finest democratic societies such as the Weimer Republic that descended into a Fascism where human beings were collected and murdered systematically in what terrorist mathematicians called a final solution where humans were exchanged for the product of the accumulated ashes they produced. It is to Frankl then as an exquisite human being that transcended his own time and space in courage to stand up to terror as a healer that honesty beckons tribute that is timeless. It is to Frankl's genius that is realized in his books peroration with the optimism we can hold unto in the face of the tragic,

> We can know who man really is. After all, man is that being who invented the gas chambers of Auschwitz; however, he is also that being who has entered those gas chambers upright, with the Lord's prayer or Shema Yisrael on his lips. (Frankl, 1963, pp. 213-214)

The Viktor Frankl Institute via Dr. Bob Barnes, President, Dr. Graber, Professor Thorpe and Dr. Steve Southwick have helped that dream live on in and through the ground gained in ensuring Logotherapy. In a privilege of receiving an international award for public service by the Viktor Frankl Institute and an invitation where I wrote about the resilience of the Elephant Man, Sir John Merrick (Rudofossi, 2008) whose unique ability to transcend the most complex trauma and loss that the idea to yield evidence in the value of the eco-ethological existential attitude and the fruits of its produce to learn from—must include Frankl himself. The lesson that resounds in the inner sanctum of ones intuitive ears is the reverberations of the highest levels of courage are borne as the air that flows under ones wings in a storm when one has not even recognized they are in flight. It is not in yet another iteration of Dr. Frankl's genius or even history that I am culling the antidote in part to terrorism, but in his own personal courage and indefatigable soulfulness he called us to heed. It is in the lessons learned in-deed from a small corner of Dr. Frankl's rich life that seven more invaluable lessons emerge. I try to use them in my life as well...the lessons presented here are my own not Frankl's but are taken from his life example as inspiration for living terror-free.

STRATEGIC BALANCE:
SEVEN MORE LESSONS LEARNED

Disabusing Ourselves of Terror Tactics!

Lesson One: *That no matter what one experiences in loss there is a power to regain the will to live, the will to live is inherent in the experience of meaning. No one person, group, or natural disaster has or ever will be able to wipe out our lives and ability to transcend tragedy. As the great sage says, "If you believe that it's possible to ruin, then believe that it's possible to rectify . . . there's no despair in the world at all!"* (Besancon & Breslov, 2007)

It is always an individual journey to affirm the humane in being. For example, Dr. Frankl watched his wife and children sent to the crematorium and yet chose to witness his own future by knowing there is a G-d and ones humanity can never be stolen. He knew that no one could take away meaning and he held onto that infinite truth in the bowels of hell and lived to make it tangible in your life and mine.

Lesson Two: *Meaning transcends the darkest moment with the light within that can never know darkness. Even in death: There is no darkness where light cannot illuminate a way out!*

It is in ones ecological niches that one is tested with what is meant to be a meaningful choice and consequent responsibility. It is within the very context of ones ecological niches and the affordances that limit ones language from a cultural and evolutionary perspective that choices are forged. It is in the layers of evolution that we are tested to transcend the primal drives and their derivatives by the creative focus on life, living, and love.

It is relevant to the particular means of destruction that we find the very key to resistance of strength to that force of evil in its most physical manifestation. For example it is in giving ones life that the martyred priest Father M. Kolbe, wearing the star of David chose to take the place of a man who in his twenties was sentenced to die. After multiple heroic acts of extreme courage and his indefatigable will to transcend he did in a final act of eternal courage to respond to the fascist's final act of human perfidy. Father Kolbe died physically, but his essence lives on in his humanity which could not be terrorized as he wore his Star of David in his own way and faith in his choice for ultimate meaning he was faced with. His record is one of eternity as heroes truly never die. His light inspires us today even in darkness his fulgent pith emerges in the moment of choice.

Lesson Three: *In relinquishing ones own eco-ethological motivation for survival at any cost and choosing with responsibility to inspire faith in a higher being and uncommon private sensibility one paradoxically wills oneself to transcend the terror-isms of common insensibility.*

For example, a key factor in Frankl surviving the holocaust was in a choice—visiting his ancestor's desecrated tombstones that Frankl sought meaning and derived meaning from terrorists [Nazi's] in their attempt to make him inhuman. His choice to be humane and to stay with his parents by realizing the tombstone epitaph was to respect his father and mother transcending his own psycho-physiological conscious survival instinct, inspired his own existential transcendental unconscious one. Resilience is not a happy attitude or a positive one but one that is an attitude of meaning made from the very element that attempts to destroy that spark of hope. It is in his desire to suffer with his family that he choose to be profoundly faithful to his G-d and personally humane. He transcended his own ethological motivation to survive and be secure in his ecological niche and by doing so paradoxically survived the horror and multiple traumas of terrorism.

Lesson Four: *If we have one person to love and care for we transcend our self and are able to find our self and the other which makes one all too human and so wonderfully humane.*

A fourth lesson as Frankl put it is if we have one person to love and to care about more then ourselves we are alas able to be human and in being human we add color to the palette of decency. In decency we can never be defeated for it is in our fallibility and humanity that we become what and whom we are meant to be. It is never accidental but always with intent we must act in the world. It is in our will to live and to be alive that we affirm the eternal in the finite.

Frankl lived this lesson by holding on to life in war torn and crumpled Post War Germany/Austria and marrying his best friend and lover his wife (Tilly Frankl) who helped him regain his hope in love and commitment after the shock of what may be overwhelming losses (Frankl, 1977). He refused to leave his hometown for he realized the enemy was not a people, but a spiritual malice in people. He refused to believe an entire people were responsible for atrocities but rather he believed in accounting them as individuals who committed these atrocities. In overcoming his fear to love another and lose her, he regained love, commitment and a life of love and loving by risking his love to only have it regained and renewed in its splendor.

A modern novelist of note Nicholas Sparks based his novel *The Notebook* on a similar premise, the love he witnessed his grandparents live, speaks for itself,

> I am nothing special of this I am sure. I am a common man with common thoughts and I've led a common life. There are no monuments dedicated to me and my name will soon be forgotten, but I've loved another with all my heart and soul, and to me, this has always been enough.

Lesson Five: *We are the only animal that knows we will die, we are the only one that can even make death a meaningful process to experience now while we all know we know nothing and control nothing, it is in human bravery and faith we all can learn to relinquish that drive to control . It is what makes us human and decent to care for another beyond our selves. In our decency we become humble and in our humility we glimpse eternity in the ineffable ether of eternal light which is an illusion we can never fully know but embrace with grace which is what makes us human and decent no matter what the challenge. It is not measured by material success but by the stand we make.*

For example, it is no secret Frankl as others of genius before and likely after him will confront their own losses and trauma to transcend the terror-ism they have experienced. It is in his choice to let go, let G-d; that he forged his therapy of logo-therapy and existential analysis. It is clear that he held his need to heal infused in the science of his calling that transcended his history of trauma that distinguished why Frankl became the leader of the third school of Viennese Psychology and Psychiatry and not an obsequious co-conspirator of a Mengle. Dr Frankl lived his tragic optimism by not discarding the suffering he experienced—he brought meaning to line his suffering journey with its creases and crevices within the texture of direction to transcend his own pain to suffice in uplifting others.

For example Dr. Professor Frankl with his M.D., Ph.D. chose to dig ditches rather then plumb the depths of mans inhumanity in genetic engineering that would have given him a few more days of life as some of his cohorts chose. It is in his indefatigable humility and his faith in a higher being that he emerged from the ashes with a tome of which from his memory he was able to regain what appeared lost forever the **original** copy lost in the flames of Auschwitz's terrorism.

Frankl's reactive depression and near Suicidality to the thousands of shocks he endured only made him more human and esteemed as one who transcended the abyss to make the pyrrhic a flame to inspire in the days we need to heed our third ear and hear our intuitive senses. It is this book that has emerged as *Man's Search for Meaning. . . .* This scrap of papers Frankl "internally witnessed" for himself and almost lost for prosperity in the ashes of his soul-fellows was recounted by finding within himself the hidden ability to rebound the pages lost and make it his life work to give it to us.

Lesson Six: *There is never any decree made by any group or person, no matter how so called 'powerful' in which one cannot emerge unscathed in their soul no matter how dire and challenging the situation.*

Frankl's ancestor was the Maharal of Prague whose cry for meaning preceded Frankl's by a few hundred years. He lived through his own series of trauma and losses. In his work no doubt inspired by longstanding suffering without losing the balance of meaning he writes that one suffers a decree by others as long as the person perceives himself to be under the control of human physical forces. When a person sees that ones faith in the Higher being can life one even out of the gates of hell, one is elevated to see tomorrow and to be sheltered from any storm (Feuer, 1964).

For example the terror seekers of the world including the Nazi's swore to a thousand year Reign of terror, and yet their Reich lasted for six years and the seventh they were put to eternal arrest. Ones faith in ones ability to transcend the evils of the world and the attempts to control ones personal choice and responsibility is more then just a challenge, it is a call to make a stand! The stand we make during a storm leaves behind seeds that are gathered on the wind of turbulence and nestle in the soil of fertile dreams that nurture healing and restoration. The challenge for us as healers that work with public safety officer-patients is to create a haven where mutual respect, validation and the full array of what makes us human and beyond our limited vista is not embellished with an esoteric tower but one made of dust that whirls its way around our mind and into the infinite reach of our souls and the timeless essence of its source. . . .

Terrorists and fascists cannot reach it and neither could the insults they wage on man and his essence—in their choice to ignore the human in themselves he/she create the choices unique to the destructive cells we must transcend and disarm— our bridge is a choice of the heart and soul as much as the psyche and the body. It is our deepest source within that is infinite and that has no end point to this challenge which is why I believe we need to know each officer one at a time and in so doing unravel the terror-ism in rich ways using my method of Eco-Ethological Existential Analysis and supplanting it with the inestimable value each officer-patient yields in the labor of meaning hidden in his/her suffering stories re-deemed.

Lesson Seven: *We all have a transcendent Unconscious which derives from a source which transcends our own time and space and culture: It is a voice that is universal and embraces all cultures and adheres to none in particular. It* *is fully human and fully alive and transcends all trauma and losses. Frankl's introspection led him to realize in life one must confront death and that meaning is not taught it is experienced and must be found one individual at a time.*

Their can be no prescription for meaning—that experience I do not have the wisdom to offer you, I suggest it cannot be culled from a mass consensus but only derived by an inner journey leaving the officer-patient and doctor with adaptive intuition. Adaptive intuition can only be a guide to expand ones voice and ear to listen and perceive his/her own voice of conscience. Adaptive intuition which includes the courage to have faith in ultimate meaning transcends all attempts to control or to force by terror—the antidote to terrorism as well is its greatest threat relies on our ability to chose responsibly.

In realizing our unique strengths we acknowledge our limitations and our experience of unseen infinite power, the contracted power behind the word we call—awesome. That unseen infinite power of creativity lies not in relinquishing our own choice and responsibility to other humans—but in our ability to transcend our nature and grasp for the infinite while being human. The source of the infinite can never come from the finite. The awesome experience of the source of all transcendence which defies explanation and definition cannot be diminished by mans attempt to control or terrorize man—it can only be derived from the humility of transcending our own by disabusing ourselves that any force can take away the power of love and compassion for life—which in the service of protecting the public from those who seek to destroy freedom can never succeed in doing so. That is the motive force of faith and transcendence it is the cornerstone of my approach to healing the force of terror and traumatic losses via each eco-ethological existential analysis—it is as healing to doctor as patient if one allows him/herself the ability to listen, learn and transcend—it is in our service that the common power rises above the denominator. Freedom has no better advocate then a man who lives by example of his life. Frankl lived his philosophy through a lifetime of service. Spreading mankind's search for meaning in the face of terror has never been more important then in our time—the message is Optimistic Responsibility on The West Winded Coast standing without a monument—it remains quite naked.

A poem is a symbolic reminder that binds the East Winds Tragic Assault On Freedom in NY Harbor as a 911 call for all the Public Servants and Citizens from Coast to Coast with responsible freedom: Let us remember or we are bound to lose what is so hard fought for—without Freedom that has limits who will cry out to stop trampling on others rights while Tyrants Sing Freedom Songs, as nations worst despots decried there woes in the name of being Social and Democratic. . . . As the ancient sage Hillel, cried, "If not us, whom?"; "If not now? When?" Lest we forget tyrants must not rest, we will never sleep in the peaceful tranquility that freedom is secure in—responsibility. . . . Dr. Frankl's life was a living example of how the human pledge for responsibility is the timeless surety of our liberty from the East Coast to the West Coast as he desired to Have a Statute of Responsibility (Frankl, 1977). A Higher being assures us of a higher calling and that calling is made higher then the fright of might makes right tyrants may come and go with their terrorism in the bough of their hull—the ballast of weight lies in liberty with the responsibility of our message that we do care and we do rather then just talk—that led to the United States where we choose faith in G-d We Trust, to that dream, to officer-patients and to you the reader my poem is written in my pen to inspire "our calling" to service of justice tempered in compassion: where inner-sight enlightens darkness in Ultimate Meaning that blossoms in the swells of the narrow straits of tragedy unfurled . . .

Lay down your steel armor—tyrants around the world,
Invincibility in Ultimate Meaning—through the face of the Supreme Being,
Being without limit or beginning—peace to strangers in needful grace,
Eternal Light through the darkest tunnels of despot's illusions—unfurl,
Rumbling thunder hush goes the lull of the poor cast aside upon un-free shores,
Triumphant Liberty—we heed your plea for freedom for all marked for deaths glee,
Yank open our harbor ports and rest in the sanctuary of Americas open haven.

Pour in your orphans and refugees from terror and oppressions slate,
Lay down your weary heart in your hope for love agape,
Untoward toward those who hate American liberty and responsibility,
Soar in rapture human decency and fair play—cherish living forever and a day . . .

Resolved are our huddled masses in white, black, red and yellow hues resplendent,
Equal as the rainbows prisms—un-repentant,
Special in prayer as gems cast forth along our coasts as shining pendants,
Prosperous in justice, our ideals radiant as glowing pearls,
Offerings to G-d's mercy—never will we relinquish freedoms call,
Never will the clasping hands of a purposeful prayer be unheard,
Silent in bowed head for our heroes—ultimate sacrifice when each has been—roll   called,
In unison with our palms upward we beseech the Creator—our Maker forever and   a day,
Begging wisdom: We know that, we know—not at all,
In all we aspire to dreams untold—what we Americans have left—is yet to unfold,
Lighting our souls afire—terrorists fail to squelch what we have—sacred and bold,
If we only pause and listen to our own neighbors call for peace unrequited,
Tilling our conscience—set in the hearth—of our very hearts rhythms and unique birth,
Yell do we from every street corner and district, we challenge defeat, our call to meet . . .

Endless in how many have entered our shores and achieved responsibility anew,
Question: Why?—Oh where else has this hard earned right alien to so many still un-free,
Ubiquitous Justice resound on our harbors shore—raise the jets where Eagles soar,
A desire to create a haven for a world threatening our ports of responsibility,
Lay down twin towers articulate heights to the soul's effigy in the Eternal's sight.

Oh how blessed in freedoms martial tune which is willing to fight for liberties bellow,
Underpinning our sacrifice—which is never free,
Republic—suffering tears and losses—regains meaning each time we say tis of thee . . .

Fire will not burn out our spirit and water will not drown our plight,
Relinquish our freedom—sooner die—and give up our sight,
Equal to our own responsive call: Mercy temper your chalice with justices pearls,
Ever present to guard our hard won dreams and ideals,
Dare to say yes with bowed head to the Ultimate meaning and stance,
Offer our heart and soul in clasped hands to our real founder invisible and eternal,
May G-d balance the scales we choose to embrace, justice and liberty **to eternities grace!**

REFERENCES

Besancon, I. I., & Breslov, R. N. (2007). *Courage.* Los Angeles, CA: Breslov Center.

Brenner, C. (1976). *Psychic conflict and psychoanalytic technique.* New York: International University Press.

Feuer, A. C. (1964). *The Ramban's ethical letter with an anthology of contemporary rabbinic expositions* (p. 64). Brooklyn, NY: Mesorah Publications.

Finney, J. (1954). *Invasion of the body snatchers.* New York: Dell Publishing Company.

Frankl, V. (1955). *The doctor and the soul.* New York: Alfred A. Knopf.

Frankl, V. (1963). *Man's search for meaning. An introduction to logotherapy* (pp. 213-214). New York: Washington Square Press.

Frankl, V. (1977). *Recollections: An autobiography.* New York: Plenum Press.

Goffman, I. (1967). *Interaction ritual.* Garden City, NY: Doubleday & Company, Inc.

Mills, C. W. (1959). *The sociological imagination.* London: Oxford University Press.

Peli, P. (1980). *The oral discourses of Rabbi Solevetchik.* New York: K TAV Press.

Rudofossi, D. (2007). *Working with traumatized police officer-patients: A clinician's guide to complex PTSD syndromes in public safety professionals.* Amityville, NY: Baywood.

Rudofossi, D. M. (2008). An eco-ethological existential analysis via a psychological autopsy of Sir John Merrick: How an anomalous case example challenges the paradigm of the human regression hypothesis paradigm. *The International Forum for Logotherapy, 31*(1), 19.

Santayana, G. (1906). *The life of reason: The phases of human progress.* New York: Scribners.

Sparks, N. (1996). *The notebook.* New York: Time Warner Books.

Wyndham, J. (1951). *The day of the triffids.* New York: Doubleday & Company.

Wyndham, J. (1954). *The chrysalids.* London: Michael Joseph Ltd.

GLOSSARY

In understanding PPS-CPTSD as a clinical and developmental psychological syndrome that interacts dynamically with officer-patient's personality, an expansion of my taxonomy of operational definitions in an earlier work is necessary (2007). The following operational definitions will orient you in establishing coordinates for approaching loss in trauma from a perspective of individual differences.

PPSS-CPTSD: Operational Definitions— Coordinates for Balance

Anger refers to a primary incited aggression toward a specific attacker in immediate protection of self, a fellow officer, or victim's life. A secondary frustrated anger is unrealized wishes of hostility toward those identifiable as offenders. This hostility is diffuse, free-floating, and can be explosive. An example is a disorder-control event, with injuries to both police and protestors. Injury to a sacred victim may increase a diffuse expression of rage, psychophysically heightened to an apex, becoming potentially and ethologically contagious.

Depressive Affect is an original contribution to the science of conflict as conceptualized by Brenner (Brenner, 1974, 1976, 1982; Freud, 1926). Depressive affect provokes conflict as a defense against unpleasure, and over a believed calamity that has already happened. Early experience of such trauma influences and affects the ever-present and evolving conflicts that are grounded in both realistic and defensive behavior. In terms of catastrophe that emerges in early life and throughout adult life, object loss, loss of love, fear of being mutilated, guilt, and other losses in general, while not exclusive to depressive affect, is an important component. Brenner suggests,

> Mourning is not the same for everyone, nor is there a uniform norm by which to judge it. What is important is . . . to understand as thoroughly as possible what are the psychic conflicts that determine the particular features of the reaction of the particular patient in question to the loss of the object. (Brenner, 1976, p. 24)

Using and implementing Brenner's original assertion that "unpleasure is responsible for defense and conflict"; and that unpleasure is of two kinds: anxiety (toward a calamity) and depressive affect (that calamity has happened) (Brenner, 1982, pp. 7, 62, 94). While Brenner identified unpleasure as infantile instinctual wishes, that in no way detracts from our focus on the direct intervention, in terms of trauma as loss (mourning) that in part emerges in the here and now of therapy. Listening to the individual officer-patient's experience of loss as intrapsychic conflict moves a one cast one dimensional approach to trauma into a complex multidimensional approach to trauma. A critical incident may be made more sensible when the therapist can move beyond his own standard conceptualizations and approach to trauma therapy. This may be achieved by the therapist learning what is critical in terms of what is selected as traumatic.

The therapist's approach toward understanding how depressive affect has developed, and the pursuit of why a certain episodic experience is experienced as an unpleasurable calamity in the individual officer-patient's experience of cumulative losses in trauma becomes critical. Anxiety may occur side by side with depressive affect. That anxiety may be approached as conflict and anticipation of how the unfolding of more loss may emerge in the individualized impact of his depressive affect. The compromise formations that become patterns of behavior and cognition and affect the officer-patient's present are focused in this book through the more recent trauma and loss experienced as an officer. As I illustrate, the present may telescope back to early experiences in each officer-patient's life history (chapters 3 and 4). While my focus in this book is on the more recent developmental presentations of loss in trauma largely disenfranchised, it is by no means an endpoint of what is already superbly covered in the enormous body of experience of dealing with early and childhood loss in trauma. Understanding the emergence of personality styles (see chapters 2 and 3) in terms of more current loss in trauma as police and public-safety officer-patients may be appreciated in large part by the therapist considering this developmental context.

I suggest *trauma is a core component of conflict; it is non-sense to speak of trauma without loss. Loss always occurs in a context (ecology) and motivation (ethology and its drive derivatives). Without context and motivation, no conflict would ever emerge. Fundamental to life is struggle, movement, and change; without these components of conflict, life as we know it would cease.*

By thinking of trauma as the disruption of what has been afforded and invariant in an existential way, and related to ethological survival value, we can understand why time is so important and why it becomes fixed to the loss. The motivation is to find how, what, and why trauma has disrupted and is experienced as loss. Our task as therapists is to help the officer-patient identify loss in part as to what was afforded and invariant in their ecological niche and is disrupted through the antiaffordance he experiences as an ethological insult.

Clinically, this is presented by an officer's functional ability, while developmental change is stagnant. I call this adaptive functional dissociation. The practical consequence is that officers may be assessed fit for duty and yet be experiencing complicated trauma through loss. These trauma events shape attempts to assimilate, accommodate or (mal)adapt through attempts to overcompensate for what is breached in affordances to the participant. In this context, antiaffordances make sense of a core aspect of searching tendencies to compensate for loss on an eco-ethological level. I suggest what has been lost in meaningful human time by destruction of ethological invariants is compensated for by meaning shaped by the overcompensation through antiaffordances in traumatic events. In other words, the traumatic events serve as perpetual influences maladaptation to loss and are evident in stereotype and fixed responses to different situations of trauma by an officer-patient.

Practically therapeutic interventions are guided by a refocusing on finding out what that meaningful something is. This loss emerges in focused free association. Lost invariants are found through verbal markers. Examples of such markers are descriptions of some place being surreal. The therapist initially followed up on the patient expressing a surreal situation by asking, "What is surreal—what comes to mind right here and now?" What follows first is what has been keenly noticed as disrupted in the patient's experience of important markers. Practical direction leads to deeper associations regarding the loss of invariants, while clarifying existential meaning attached to the more intimate losses (see chapter 3).

Indestructible Officer is a schema of an officer-patient's perceived invulnerability to injury. When the officer-patient is faced with sudden, violent, and unpredictable injury, including natural and unnatural accidents (guerrilla type warfare, terrorism, etc.), a strong sense of loss and confusion may be experienced. In this schema, it is the abrupt intensity of change between the previous investment in one's identity as indestructible, in comparison with the reality of loss experienced through the reality of vulnerability and injury. This superhuman image may engender self-recrimination in many police officers actively identifying with the public portrayal of their professional identity when vilified.

Professional identity may become submerged in this motif, which supports anticipatory schemas of guilt, shame, and legal recriminations. This invulnerable presentation of the officer-patient supports denial, rather than trust. The exposure of his vulnerability is necessary in gaining social support, so critical during times of trauma. Keen awareness and avoidance of labels of vulnerability are made sensible in its evolutionary value as I describe above (see ethological affordances). This invulnerability supports a schema of emotional alexythymia. The personality style of officers most impacted by this tendency is the Addictive Hyperexcited (see chapter 3).

Public-Safety Personality Styles are defined in the context of survival, adaptation, maladaptation, and intra/interpsychic defenses from an evolutionary perspective. Existential meaning in larger part not only illuminates the understanding of personality styles, it makes it comprehensible as a unique human phenomenon (see chapter 3).

The clinical goal is adaptation and repositioning of trauma and grief without a focus on psychopathology. The definition of maladaptation may be considered in the context of developmental tendencies of each active participant. The therapy method derived from this paradigm is one that seeks the unique why and how the maladaptation has emerged within that officer-patient's individual manifestation of his personality style. Having the patient understand how and why these tendencies emerge in a nonpejorative manner is part of the assessment and therapy stance (Horowitz, 1974, 2003; Millon, 1996; Sperry, 1995).

Original Quantum Psychic Moments emerge in the context of an officer's adaptation, framed by the ethological invariants afforded within the ecological context of his unit. I choose that descriptive term not as literal but as metaphoric. Specifically, the intensity of disruption by a quantum psychic moment is set by a prior level of adaptation. This former level of adaptation is laid out by an existential sense of normalcy and reality through ethological invariants that afford behavior, cognitions, and emotional expressiveness. Real life and death decisions out on the street happen in a split second. That choice may impact on ongoing or disrupted meaning in that officer's lifelong development (see chapters 1, 3, and 4 for detailed examples).

A quantum psychic moment can be perceived as a disruption of an expected outcome as an anticipatory schema (Gilmartin, 2002; Horowitz, 2003; Rudofossi, 1997; Silverstein, 1992). In public safety, the quantum psychic moment shatters the officer-patient's sense of survival value invested thus far in what is afforded in their eco-ethological niche. Extreme disruption between explicit and normative reality by a quantum psychic moment may alter the officer's prior adaptation level to the present maladaptation. This may result in what I call functional ambivalence. This active numbing is apparent in the officer's professional performance, which may well be up to par functionally, but cognitively, emotionally, and existentially his development may be marked by confusion and being overwhelmed. An example arises when the officer-patient retreats into frenetic involvement in his work, which serves as a mask to cover his loss in trauma.

A quantum psychic moment is not gradual, but an immediate punctuation in human equilibrium. They are split-second decisions—a simultaneous barrage of conflicting choices. What are the legal consequences of actions as one is defending one's own life? How do I survive while saving others, to name a few? Quantum moments impact on a whole universe of expectations and stability shattered by traumatic events that are unpredictable. This is more than just a single loss; critical incident does not capture the complexity of the experience. I suggest it is a new perceptual experience hitherto unprocessed emotionally.

REFERENCES

Brenner, C. (1974). *An elementary textbook of psychoanalysis.* New York: Doubleday Dell Publishing.

Brenner, C. (1976). *Psychoanalytic technique and psychic conflict.* New Haven, CT: International Universities Press.

Brenner C. (1982). *The mind in conflict.* New Haven, CT: International University Press.

Freud, S. (1926). *Inhibition, symptoms and anxiety.* London: Hogarth Press, Vol. 2.

Gilmartin, K (2002). *Emotional survival for law enforcement: A guide for officers and their families.* Tucson, AZ: ES Press, Inc.

Horowitz, M. (1974). Stress response syndromes. Character style and dynamic psychotherapy. *Archives of General Psychiatry, 31,* 177-198.

Horowitz, M. (2003). *Treatment of stress response syndrome.* Washington, DC: American Psychiatric Press.

Millon, T. (1996). *Disorders of personality: DSMIV and beyond.* New York: John Wiley.

Rudofossi, D. (1997). *The impact of trauma and loss on affective profiles of police officers.* Ann Arbor, MI: Bell & Howell Company.

Rudofossi, D. (2007). *Working with traumatized police officer patients. A clinicians guide to Complex PTSD.* Amityville, NY: Baywood.

Silverstein, R. (1992). *The correlation between combat related trauma processing and ego development.* Ann Arbor, MI: Bell & Howell Company.

Sperry, L. (1995). *Handbook of diagnosis treatment of the DSMIV personality disorders.* New York: Brunner/Mazel.

Index

In Praise

Once again, in this sequel to his earlier book on traumatized police officers, Dr. Rudofossi has blended theoretical and practical applications of psychology and law enforcement. His approach of identifying the five varieties of public safety personality styles provides critical information for both mental health practitioners working with law enforcement personnel and law enforcement managers. This is an excellent book that should be read by all who work with, or are interested in, law enforcement officers.

Thomas Creelman, M.A., CEAP
Employee Assistance Program Coordinator
New York State Office of the Attorney General

Dr. Rudofossi has been successful in defining the private and public faces of law enforcement officers, encapsulating them within the five police personality styles that he presents. His work provides the insight required when dealing with men and women engaged in enforcing our laws. This is a valuable resource for clinicians providing mental health service to that population.

Stanley D. Smoote, Ph.D., ABPP
Diplomate in Forensic Psychology
American Board of Professional Psychology
Ret. Police Officer-Licensed Psychologist
COP DOC, DEA, and Border Patrol, OHS

A gifted scientist, Dr. Rudofossi expertly integrates the disciplines of psychology and law enforcement in this critical volume. *A Cop Doc's Guide to Public Safety Complex Trauma Syndrome* fills a gap in the literature by providing a method to guide assessment and interventions with the five varieties of public safety personalities. As a clinician providing services to law enforcement staff and their families, I find Dr. Rudofossi's work enables me to better guide officer patients to use insight into the meaning of loss and its impact. Layered deeply and convincingly in Dr. Rudofossi's work is his adherence to the humanness, wholeness, and resilience of these officer patients, by regarding their unique strengths.

Stephanie Kutzen, Ph.D., L.C.S.W.
Director, Employee Consultation Services
Professor of Social Work

Dr. Rudofossi's "Epilogue: Toward an Antidote to Terrorism" is worthy to stand alone as an article or booklet that would help us grasp the nature of our battle against those who would wield terror as a weapon. He shows us that terrorism ranks with despotism and tyranny as "psychopathological" behavior, with "victimization results [that] are perniciously psycho-physiological." This is a powerful insight, which he uses to illuminate a path toward defeating terrorism while protecting our own national and individual psyches. As he so well states, we must "not glorify or romanticize what is on one hand human illness, and on the other human depravity and evil. . . . In order to flesh out the antidote for dealing with terrorism, we must understand the poison that has been ingested. . . . Arguably even the perpetrators are victims of their own human illness and human depravity we have become afraid to characterize for what it genuinely is, 'evil'!" And "It is in healing [this evil, psychopathological behavior] that we heal as well."

Dr. Dan has served as both a cop and a therapist. From this unique perspective he can well and truly say: "To serve is a profile in courage! Therapists serve, too. The deeper the excavation the more resplendent the shine of darkness into the fulgent light of hope." Well done, Dr. Dan. And many thanks for the bright light of hope that you have shone on our brave men and women who go in harm's way, on those who would wield terrorism against us, and on ourselves. I take up the prayer with which Dr. Rudofossi concludes his book: "May G-d balance the scales we choose to embrace, justice and liberty to eternities grace!"

Lt. Col. Dave Grossman, US Army (Ret.)
Author, On Killing and On Combat

Dr. Rudofossi has provided for clinicians working with law enforcement and public safety personnel a unique clinical tool. The psychometrically based personality styles he presents offer an insightful structure with which to understand how traumatized officers cope with the violence and loss that is all too commonly a part of their duties. However, he emphasizes that we treat individuals, not faceless categories. To this end, Dr. Rudofossi embodies each personality style with a wealth of personal detail gathered from extensive clinical interviews and therapeutic encounters. The goal of treatment is to help traumatized personnel cope with the sadness and suffering they experience. However, even within such tragedy there are opportunities for the officer to grow and find meaning. Dr. Rudofossi offers therapeutic strategies and clinical insight to assist providers in enhancing the process of treatment, while continually emphasizing the fundamental importance of empathic listening and relationship-building. This book will benefit even experienced law enforcement clinicians.

John A. Dooley, Ph.D.
Clinical Assistant Professor, Department of Psychiatry & Behavioral Neuroscience Wayne State University School of Medicine
Area Clinician, Drug Enforcement Administration

Dr. Rudofossi presents here a timely and valuable resource for our generation, filled with wisdom that is, most importantly, based on the beginning of wisdom, which is faith in the Lord, and recognition of the underlying spiritual element in all things. May the Almighty bless him and his work.

Rabbi Joseph Kolakowski
Congregation Kol Emes/Young Israel of Richmond Virginia

Daniel Rudofossi not only offers a wealth of psychological insight but brings to the literature on the mental health of law enforcement and public safety personnel a special personal and spiritual sensitivity.

Rabbi Kalman Packouz,
Aish HaTorah Shabbat Shalom Weekly

Dr. Daniel Rudofossi's most recent work, *A Cop Doc's Guide to Public Safety Complex Trauma Syndrome: Using Five Police Personality Styles,* is a valuable contribution for the clinician who seeks insight into the complex and often misunderstood issues affecting the psychological well-being of the men and women of law enforcement. Dr. Rudofossi is a unique and rare individual who can combine his decades of experience in the multiple worlds of police officer, clinician, and academician to provide us with a much-needed understanding of the dynamics taking place. This is a must read for the mental health clinician who wants to assist the men and women who work in law enforcement.

Kevin Gilmartin, Ph.D.
Clinical Psychologist (retired Law Enforcement)
Author, *Emotional Survival for Law Enforcement:
A Guide for Officers and Their Families*

In *A Cop Doc's Guide to Public Safety Complex Trauma Syndrome*, Daniel Rudofossi manages to connect complex psychological theories of personality to the common sense of a police officer. He has a unique ability to see the world from the point of view of both a well-educated psychologist and a street cop trained under fire on the streets of New York City. Dr. Rudofossi promotes his *eco-ethological analytic* approach to looking at traumas in an officer's life, which takes into account the defenses, drives, and motivations of an officer and the ecosystems that sustain the resulting behavior. From there, he describes five police personality styles modifying Millon's personological approach of personality and psychopathology. The book is philosophical and insightful, and will advance the thinking in psychological science applied to public safety professionals. This book should be required reading for anyone wanting to do therapy with police officers.

Gary S. Aumiller, Ph.D.
Executive Director, Society for Police and Criminal Psychology
Author, *Keeping It Simple: Sorting Out What Really Matters in Your Life*
Red Flags! How to Know You're Dating a Loser
Walk Like a Chameleon: Animal Instincts that Control Your Relationships and Your Life